THE LIBRARY
ST. MARY'S COLLEGE OF MARYLAND
ST. MARY'S CITY, MARYLAND 20686

D1804219

CLASSICS IN PSYCHOLOGY

CLASSICS IN PSYCHOLOGY

Advisory Editors
HOWARD GARDNER
AND
JUDITH KRIEGER GARDNER

Editorial Board
Wayne Dennis
Paul A. Kolers
Sheldon H. White

A NOTE ABOUT THE AUTHOR

CHARLES S. SHERRINGTON was the major investigator of the lower functions of the nervous systems for close to a half century. Born in England in 1857, he studied physiology at Cambridge, received medical training in London, and then visited Goltz' and Ewald's laboratories in Strasbourg. There Sherrington saw the reactions of a dog who had a high spinal cord transection; the effect of such lesions on the reflexes of the nervous system. More generally, the nature of neural connections remained Sherrington's scientfic preoccupation until he retired as Waynefelete Professor of Physiology at Oxford in 1935.

In addition to his pioneering work in the physiology of the nervous system, Sherrington also published philosophical writings, *Man on his Nature* (1940) and poetry, *The Assaying of Brabantius and Other Verse* (1925). He embraced a dualistic view of mental phenomena, yet the thrust of his work served to encourage the emergence of a psychology based on stimulus and response. Recipient of the Nobel Prize for Medicine in 1932, Sherrington died, much honored, in 1952 at the age of 95.

THE INTEGRATIVE ACTION
OF THE
NERVOUS SYSTEM

by

SIR CHARLES SHERRINGTON

ARNO PRESS
A New York Times Company
New York ★ 1973

Reprint Edition 1973 by Arno Press Inc.

Classics in Psychology
ISBN for complete set: 0-405-05130-1
See last pages of this volume for titles.

Manufactured in the United States of America

Library of Congress Cataloging in Publication Data

Sherrington, Sir Charles Scott, 1857-1952.
    The integrative action of the nervous system.

    (Classics in psychology)
    Reprint of the 1948 ed. published by the University
Press, Cambridge, England.
      Includes bibliographical references.
    1. Psychology, Physiological. 2. Nervous system.
I. Title. II. Series. [DNLM: 1. Psychophysiology.
WL102 S553 1947F]
QP355.2.S53   1973   612'.8   73-2989
ISBN 0-405-05162-X

THE INTEGRATIVE ACTION
OF THE
NERVOUS SYSTEM

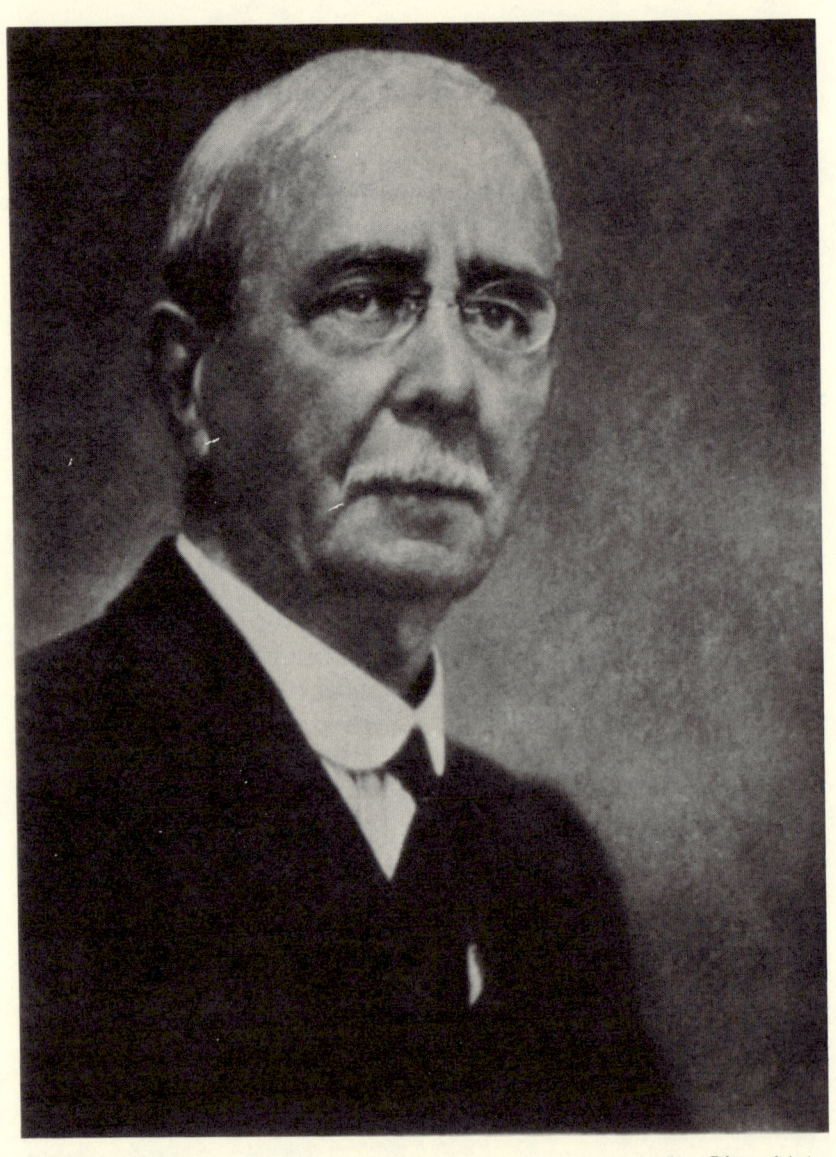

A. H. Bodle, photographer   Emery Walker Ltd. ph. sc.

Ch. S. Sherrington

THE INTEGRATIVE ACTION
OF THE
NERVOUS SYSTEM

by

SIR CHARLES SHERRINGTON

O.M.

WITH A NEW FOREWORD
BY THE AUTHOR
&
A BIBLIOGRAPHY OF
HIS WRITINGS

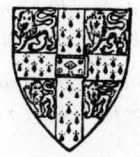

CAMBRIDGE
AT THE UNIVERSITY PRESS
1948

This book, which has as its basis a course of lectures given at Yale University under the Hepsa Ely Silliman Memorial endowment, was first published by Charles Scribner's Sons in 1906, and reprinted in 1911, 1914, 1916, 1918, 1920. The present edition has been entirely reset, 1947. Reprinted June, 1948.

*Printed in the United States of America by Yale University Press
and published by the Cambridge University Press
(Cambridge, and Bentley House, London)*

*Agents for Canada and India: Macmillan
Agents for U.S.A: Yale University Press*

CONTENTS

Portrait of the Author	Frontispiece
Editorial Note	vii
Curriculum Vitae	xi
Foreword to 1947 Edition. By Sir Charles Sherrington	xiii

THE INTEGRATIVE ACTION OF THE NERVOUS SYSTEM

LECTURE I. Introductory—Co-ordination in the simple reflex	1
II. Co-ordination in the simple reflex (*continued*)	36
III. Co-ordination in the simple reflex (*concluded*)	70
IV. Interaction between reflexes	116
V. Compound reflexes: simultaneous combination	152
VI. Compound reflexes: successive combination	182
VII. Reflexes as adapted reactions	236
VIII. Some aspects of the reactions of the motor cortex	270
IX. The physiological position and dominance of the brain	308
X. Sensual fusion	353
BIBLIOGRAPHICAL REFERENCES	391
Bibliography of the Writings	401
Index	421

EDITORIAL NOTE

The Integrative Action of the Nervous System was first published in 1906. It was immediately acclaimed as a work of outstanding importance which had refashioned neurophysiology by reason of the wealth of the original experimental observations that it contained, its wide generalizations, its philosophic insight and the stimulus that it gave to subsequent research. It determined in large measure the lines of development of the subject. The book has, however, been out of print for a generation, and it is no longer available—as it should be—to be read by all students of physiology and to be re-read by their teachers and by mature investigators in this field. The Physiological Society felt that it must remedy this unsatisfactory state of affairs, and that it owed a duty to Physiology to bring out a new edition of this work for the benefit of the many who would be inspired by it. Such an action also seemed to be a fitting tribute to the author, who had served not only Physiology, but the Society itself for so long and in so outstanding a manner. Sherrington was for fifty years (1885–1935) an 'ordinary' member of the Society; he became a member nine years after the formation of the Society; he served the Society as its Secretary, member of the Committee, and Editor of its *Journal*. The Society which had notably honoured itself by electing Sherrington to its honorary membership hoped that it might give him pleasure by making one of the works, by which his name will go down to posterity, live once more in the minds of grateful readers. Sherrington readily and generously agreed to the Society's suggestion; I was asked to take charge of the venture. He wrote to me of the proposal that "it is a most generous compliment and I value it accordingly; all that it proposes is very welcome to me". He continued with characteristic modesty: "I have long looked on the book as dead and buried and the suggestion that it has still got a fraction of life is a pleasing thought to me—but whether it has enough to make some resuscitation worth while I must leave to others." The 'others' think

Editorial Note

the resuscitation very worth-while. The Yale University Press, the owners of the copyright of *The Integrative Action*, with equal generosity transferred their rights in the book to the Physiological Society without cost, on the sole condition that in the new edition the entire text was reprinted—a condition which exactly expressed the Society's wishes.

The new edition contains the entire text completely reset with the skill and good taste found in all the work of the Cambridge University Press. The text has been carefully read, misprints have been corrected and minor doubtful points cleared up; throughout I have had the benefit of Sir Charles Sherrington's guidance and advice. As the original blocks were worn out all the figures have been redrawn by Mr Edwards and new blocks prepared. The tracings have been most faithfully reproduced but where necessary the 'apparatus of interpretation' has been modified to bring out the significance of the records more clearly and, where necessary, the legends have been appropriately altered. Sir Charles Sherrington has written a new Foreword for which we are most grateful; in addition we have provided an attractive signed photograph (taken by Mr Bodle), a curriculum vitae and a complete bibliography of all the published writings. This last is based on the bibliography prepared by Professor J. F. Fulton which appeared in Denny-Brown's *Selected Writings of Sir Charles Sherrington* published by Messrs Hamish Hamilton. We are indebted to Professor Fulton, Professor D. Denny-Brown and Messrs Hamish Hamilton for permission to use the bibliography in this way.

The Physiological Society has decided to present a copy of this new edition to every member of the XVII International Congress of Physiology, meeting at Oxford in July 1947. It was thought that members of the Congress, both for sentimental and practical reasons, would be glad to possess a copy of this work. And in addition there is something specially apt in the Congress gift-book being a work written by a man who has done so much to promote and consolidate the international brotherhood of Physiologists. Sherrington served the International Congress as Secretary at Liége (1892), Berne (1895), Cambridge (1898), Turin (1901), Brussels

Editorial Note

(1904), and Heidelberg (1907), and some of his outstanding discoveries were demonstrated at these Congresses. Interesting details about Sherrington's demonstrations at the International Congresses are given in K. J. Franklin's "Short History of the Congresses" (*Annals of Science*, 1938, III, 241). I give a few brief extracts. 1892 (Liége): C.S.S. "with faultless operative technique" (Fredericq) demonstrated in a monkey the cortical control of the anus and vagina. 1898 (Cambridge): "ebenso eleganter Versuch" (quotation from Magnus's diary) on reciprocal innervation of antagonists. 1901 (Turin): cerebral localization in anthropoids including a gorilla; "in questa esperienza fatta sopra un animale di forza erculea, non sappiamo se debbasi di piu ammirare l' abilita o il coraggio dello sperimentatore". 1904 (Brussells): scratch reflex in the spinal dog. In 1907 at Heidelberg the Congress President (Kossel) "informed the meeting of Sherrington's resignation of the office of general secretary for the English language. He expressed the general regret that his decision must evoke and the gratitude that all must feel to Sherrington for the distinguished way in which he had for so many years fulfilled his arduous duties."

I wish to thank the Cambridge University Press for the trouble they have taken in these difficult times to bring out this attractive new edition at short notice in time for the International Congress. Sir Charles Sherrington has helped me at every stage of my editorial work. The Physiological Society trusts that he will accept this new edition with the affectionate homage of his friends, colleagues, pupils, admirers and well-wishers the world over.

SAMSON WRIGHT

June 1947

SIR CHARLES SHERRINGTON: CURRICULUM VITAE

1871. Ipswich School.
1880. Matriculated Gonville and Caius College, Cambridge.
1881. Part I. Natural Sciences Tripos. First Class.
1883. Part II. Natural Sciences Tripos. First Class.
Student-Demonstrator in Anatomy to Professor Sir George Humphry.
Shuttleworth Scholarship for Physiology, Gonville and Caius College.
1884. Student at St Thomas's Hospital, London.
George Henry Lewes Student for Physiological Research.
Worked in Physiological Institute, Strassburg (Profs. Goltz and Ewald).
1885. M.R.C.S.
Member of the Physiological Society.
Investigated cholera epidemic in Spain.
1885–86. M.B. Cambridge. Physiological Laboratory.
1886. Commission on Asiatic cholera. Investigated cholera in Italy, examining anatomical material in Prof. Virchow's laboratory at Berlin.
1887. L.R.C.P.
Thruston Triennial Prize, Gonville and Caius College, for research in physiology.
Experimental physiology in Prof. Zuntz's laboratory, Berlin.
Fellow of Gonville and Caius College, to 1893.
Research in Bacteriology under Prof. Koch.
Lecturer in Systematic Physiology, St Thomas's Hospital.
1889–1905. Secretary, Physiological Society.
1891. Professor-Superintendent of the Brown Institute.
1892. M.D.
Anglo-American Secretary, International Congress of Physiology, Liége, 1892; also Berne, 1895; Cambridge, 1898; Turin, 1901; Brussels, 1904; Heidelberg, 1907.
1893. Fellow of the Royal Society.
1895. Holt Professor of Physiology, Liverpool.
1897. Croonian Lecturer, Royal Society.
1904. Physiological Secretary, British Association, Cambridge.
Silliman Memorial Lecturer, Yale.

Curriculum Vitae

1906. *The Integrative Action of the Nervous System.* Charles Scribner's Sons, New York.
1910. Page May Memorial Lecture, London University.
Member of Board of Trade Sight-Tests Committee.
1913. Croonian Lecture, Royal College of Physicians.
Member of Home Office Committee on Lighting of Factories and Workshops.
Waynflete Professor of Physiology, Oxford, to 1935.
1914–17. Fullerian Professor of Physiology, Royal Institution.
1916–17. War Office Committee on Tetanus.
Alcohol Committee, Central Board of Control.
1918. Chairman, Industrial Fatigue Research Board.
1919. *Mammalian Physiology. A course of practical exercises.* Clarendon Press.
1920–25. President of the Royal Society.
1922. President, British Association, Hull.
1925. *The Assaying of Brabantius and other verse.* Oxford University Press.
1925–34. Member of Medical Research Council.
1926–34. Editor, *Journal of Physiology.*
1927. Dunham Lecturer, Harvard.
Lister Oration, Canadian Medical Association, Toronto.
1929. Ferrier Lecture, Royal Society.
1932. *Reflex Activity of the Spinal Cord,* with Creed, Denny-Brown, Eccles and Liddell. Clarendon Press.
Nobel Laureate, Medicine, with E. D. Adrian.
1934. Rede Lecture, Cambridge.
1937–38. Gifford Lecturer, Edinburgh.
1940. *Man on his Nature.* Cambridge University Press.
1946. *The Endeavour of Jean Fernel.* Cambridge University Press.

FOREWORD TO 1947 EDITION

Let me here tender thanks to the Physiological Society, its Officers and all its Members and quite particularly to Professor Samson Wright, for the present generous compliment paid to my rather elderly book. I comply with pleasure to their request for a foreword to it. Owing to various circumstances, the text of the book has remained exactly as when first published. This seems a suitable opportunity to deal with some ambiguities which have in course of time arisen.

(*a*)

To describe the action of nerve as integrative is, although true, hardly sufficient for a definition. If the nature of an animal be accepted as being that of a whole presupposed by all its parts, then each and every part of the animal is integrative. This is illustrated strikingly by cancer, the growth of which being outside the integrative plan of the body is destructive both to the normal body and to itself. Our search for a more satisfying definition of nerve has then to ask what is the specific contribution which nerve makes to animal integration. Finger-pointings toward an answer are that nerve in any strict sense of the term is not an element of the plant-world. Nor is it found in unicellular animals, although it is practically universal in the multicellular. In these latter, similarly universal, is an organ of mechanical work, muscle, executant of movements and attitudes, the animal's motor behaviour. This behaviour falls into two divisions. One digestive, excretory, in short visceral; the other inclusive of all which is not merely visceral. This latter behaviour is that of external relation, so called. In it, motor behaviour reaches its highest speeds and precision, nerve attains its greatest and supreme developments.

The volume here reprinted concerns itself predominantly with the type of motor behaviour which is called 'reflex'; it might give the impression that in reflex behaviour it saw the most important and far-reaching of all types of 'nerve' behaviour. That is in fact

Foreword to 1947 Edition

not so. But reflex action presents certain advantages for physiological description. It can be studied free from complication with the psyche: also free from complication by that type of 'nerve' activity which is called autochthonous (or 'spontaneous') and generates intrinsically arising rhythmic movements, e.g. breathing, etc. But taken in comparison with the great field of behaviour in general, pure reflex action of itself cannot be seen to cover such extensive ground as do the instincts actuated by 'urges' and 'drives'. But the mechanism of these has hardly yet been analysed sufficiently for laboratory treatment. The pure apsychical reflex has a smaller role. Studied in that self-contained animal group, the Vertebrates, behaviour seems to become less and less reflex as the animal individual becomes more and more complexly individuated. The 'spinal' man is more crippled than is the 'spinal' frog.

(b)

A 'reflex' can be diagrammatized as an animal reacting to a cosmical 'field' containing it. Animal and 'field' are of one category, both being comprised within the physicist's term 'energy'. They are machines which interact—a point taken by Descartes. His wheelwork animals geared into the turning universe. Cat, dog, horse, etc. in his view had no thoughts, no ideas; they were trigger-puppets which events in the circumambient universe touched-off into doing what they do. It was a view less strange than might seem from this condensed epitome. But it lets us feel Descartes can never have kept an animal pet. Experiment to-day does, however, put within reach of the observer a puppet-animal which conforms largely with Descartes' assumptions. In the more organized animals of the vertebrate type the shape of the central nerve-organ allows a simple operation to reduce the animal to the Descartes condition. An overlying outgrowth of the central nerve-organ in the head can be removed under anaesthesia, and on the narcosis passing off the animal is found to be a Cartesian puppet: it can execute certain acts but is devoid of mind. That it is devoid of mind may seem a dogmatic statement. Exhaustive tests, however, bear the assertion out. Thoughts, feeling, memory, percepts, conations, etc.; of these

Foreword to 1947 Edition

no evidence is forthcoming or to be elicited. Yet the animal remains a motor mechanism which can be touched into action in certain ways so as to exhibit pieces of its behaviour.

An outline of the spatial arrangement of nerve illustrates how this comes about. From points within and on the surface of the animal, nerve-threads run to its muscles, but in their course thither are engaged by the central organ and are there relayed; the central organ becoming a sort of switchboard where muscles can be switched on or off. The starting-point of the nerve-thread is not equally responsive to all the various types of the field forces. Each starting-point is armed with a structure, the receptor, which reacts to one specific class of field agency, e.g. one to light, not heat, another to heat, not light. The reaction of the nerve-thread itself is, in all nerve-threads, to generate a repetitive series of brief and minute electric currents which run away from the starting-point and, by relays through the central organ, reach this or that set of muscles determined by the topography of the starting-point concerned. As the play of the 'field' shifts over the animal, different sets of receptors come into and go out of action. The receptors thus analyse the successive situations occurring between animal and field in terms of the selective receptors, and ultimately in terms of the muscles of the limbs, etc. Change in the external situation brings corresponding change in the muscles brought into and released from contraction. A train of motor acts results therefore from a train of successive external situations.

The movements are not meaningless; they carry each of them an obvious meaning. The scope commonly agrees with some act which the normal animal under like circumstances would do. Thus, the cat set upright (Graham Brown) on a 'floor' moving backward under its feet walks, runs or gallops according to the speed given to the floorway. Again, in the dog a feeble electric current ('electric flea') applied by a minute entomological pin set lightly in the hair-bulb layer of the skin of the shoulder brings the hind paw of that side to the place, and with unsheathed claws the foot performs a rhythmic grooming of the hairy coat there. If the point lie forward at the ear, the foot is directed thither, if far back in the loin the foot goes

Foreword to 1947 Edition

thither, and similarly at any intermediate spot. The list of such purposive movements is impressive. If a foot tread on a thorn that foot is held up from the ground while the other legs limp away. Milk placed in the mouth is swallowed; acid solution is rejected. Let fall, inverted, the reflex cat alights on its feet. The dog shakes its coat dry after immersion in water. A fly settling on the ear is instantly flung off by the ear. Water entering the ear is thrown out by violent shaking of the head. An exhaustive list would be much larger than that given here. The experiments of Graham Brown and of R. Magnus give excellent examples. But when all is said, if we compare such a list with the range of situations to which the normal cat or dog reacts appropriately, the list is extremely poverty stricken as a conspectus of behaviour. It contains no social reactions. It evidences hunger by restlessness and brisker knee-jerks; but it fails to recognize food as food: it shows no memory, it cannot be trained or learn: it cannot be taught its name. The mindless body reacts with the fatality of a multiple penny-in-the-slot machine to certain stimuli, all of them, as in the case of the penny-in-the-slot machine, physical, and not psychical.

A point is that these mindless acts yet treat the animal's motor machinery as a united whole. Thus the mindless machine can walk, and run, and gallop; it can also spring. These acts include 'balance' and adjustments of poise as well as phasic movements duly co-ordinated. There is integration although purely motor integration. What is noteworthy is that such acts should be carried out in absence of mind, that is to say of mind in any ordinary acceptation of the term. Of course we do not forget that here what we observe is an artefact; but it is an analytic artefact. And that an artefact of such effectiveness should obtain in animals so highly mentalized as cat and dog, suggests that in creatures less mentalized than they a residuum of behaviour still larger relatively to the total behaviour will be 'reflex'. The behaviour of the spider is reported to be entirely reflex; but reflex action, judging by what we can sample of it, would go little way toward meeting the life of external relation of a horse or cat or dog, still less of ourselves. As life develops it would seem that in the field of external relation 'conscious' behaviour tends to replace reflex, and

Foreword to 1947 Edition

conscious acts to bulk larger and larger. Along with this change, and indeed as part of it, would seem an increased role for 'habit'. Habit arises always in conscious action; reflex behaviour never arises in conscious action. Habit is always acquired behaviour, reflex behaviour is always inherent and innately given. Habit is not to be confounded with reflex action.

The examples of reflex action taken for study here have been for the most part isolated artificially by extracting them so to say from animal lives of relatively highly* developed external relation, e.g. cat and dog. Examples of reflex behaviour could have been taken under much less artificial conditions by resort to animals of less complex external relations (of lower animal type), e.g. the frog. But then the reactions, though more naturally obtainable, would have been more open to equivocal interpretation as to purpose and less rich in executive complexity.

(c)

We turn to behaviour of a different kind, some say even of a different category of act. The field of the psyche is entered. An old adage has it that to the trodden worm its own trodden self is the world's greater half. That anthropomorphic worm may typify ourselves to us; the 'self' of each of us goes far to epitomize the integration we are now to look at. We can retain the scheme of spatial nervous arrangement we used before, this time, however, not mutilating the central organ, but keeping the animal—the human animal if you will—intact. The receptors at the starting-points of the nerve-thread we find now to be, by conspiracy with a psyche in the central organ, sense-organs. The full panel of the 'five-senses' is in session, and by further collaboration with the psyche, a world of subject and object for the individual is in being. The individual has attained a psychical

---

* The terms 'higher' and 'lower' as applied to animals in this book regard range of life of external relation. Mr K. W. Monsarrat expresses this: "by a higher animal is meant here one that displays a greater range and variety in its dealing with its surrounding than some other with which it is being compared." *Myself, My Thinking and My Thoughts* (1942), p. 117. Some biologists use the terms more broadly.

Foreword to 1947 Edition

existence. Phases and moods of mental life accrue. Each waking day is a stage dominated for good or ill, in comedy, farce or tragedy, by a *dramatis persona*, the 'self'. And so it will be until the curtain drops. This self is a unity. The continuity of its presence in time, sometimes hardly broken by sleep, its inalienable 'interiority' in (sensual) space, its consistency of view-point, the privacy of its experience, combine to give it status as a unique existence. Although multiple aspects characterize it it has self-cohesion. It regards itself as one, others treat it as one. It is addressed as one, by a name to which it answers. The Law and the State schedule it as one. It and they identify it with a body which is considered by it and them to belong to it integrally. In short, unchallenged and unargued conviction assumes it to be one. The logic of grammar endorses this by a pronoun in the singular. All its diversity is merged in oneness.

How habitually and unwittingly the self regards itself as one is instanced by binocular vision. Our binocular visual field is shown by analysis, to presuppose outlook from the body by a single eye centred at a point in the midvertical of the forehead at the level of the root of the nose. It, unconsciously, takes for granted that its seeing is done by a cyclopean eye having a centre of rotation at the point of intersection just mentioned. In this visual field it obtains visual depth by unknowingly combining besides the actually identical fixation points, the host of homonymously—and heteronymously—crossed images of not too great lateral disparation. The combining of these last rests on a cancelling out—an algebraical submental summation—of the two disparations of right and left eye images respectively. Oneness is obtained by compromise between differences, if not *too* great, offered to the perceiving 'self'. There are other perceptual instances. The brightness of a binocular field differs hardly sensibly from that of either of two equally illuminated uniocular fields composing it. But the quantity of stimulus received by the eyes is roughly double in the binocular observation that which it is in the uniocular. If, with relatively simple fields, the brightness of one uniocular field is less, but not too greatly less, than that of the twin field offered to the other eye, the binocular brightness

Foreword to 1947 Edition

is intermediate between that of the two uniocular fields. If the difference of brightness between the two uniocular fields is too great there is alternating oscillation, rivalry instead of binocular fusion. Again, with colours, binocular fusion results in an intermediate tint: thus the red and green postage stamps give a sheeny bronze when binocularly united. The well-known outline-figures, often called equivocal-figures, with which while we gaze at what depicts for instance an overhanging eave the interpretation suddenly changes to a set of ascending steps, have the character of giving always wholly either the one thing or wholly the other. The meaning is never at the same time partly this and partly that. Doubtless because to be so would be to have no meaning. Psychical integration is immensely influenced by meaning. An early trouble for the squinter is the 'doubling' of things. He has to school himself to accept that doubleness not as of the things but of himself, the visual self. Each of the two-of-a-thing which the squint gives enters at first convincingly enough as a separate item into the visual picture of the moment. The squint prevails at first despite the self's reasoned criticism that there are truly not two of the thing. But the self learns to suppress one of them. Conjunction in time *without* necessarily cerebral conjunction in space is thus an element in the unification of the mind. Simultaneity will of itself make a mental unity. It is somewhat as if two persons of similar make-up could pool their separate psychical experiences to one.

(*d*)

There remains yet another type of integration which claims consideration, although to saddle it upon nerve may perhaps encounter protest. Integration has been traced at work in two great, and in some respects counterpart, systems of the organism. The physico-chemical (or for short physical) produced a unified machine from what without it would be merely a collocation of commensal organs. The psychical, creates from psychical data a percipient, thinking and endeavouring mental individual. Though our exposition kept these two systems and their integrations apart, they are largely complemental and life brings them co-operatively together at

Foreword to 1947 Edition

innumerable points. Not that the physical is ever anything but physical, or the psychical anything but psychical. The formal dichotomy of the individual, however, which our description practised for the sake of analysis, results in artefacts such as are not in Nature. Each such is a quasi-organism which does not resemble ourselves, nor does it, *pace* Descartes, resemble dog or cat. For our purpose the two schematic members of the puppet pair which our method segregated require to be integrated together. Not until that is done can we have before us an approximately complete creature of the type we are considering. This integration can be thought of as the last and final integration.

But theoretically it has to overcome a difficulty of no ordinary kind. It has to combine two incommensurables; it has to unite two disparate entities. To take an example: I see the sun; the eyes trained in a certain direction entrap a tiny packet of solar radiation covering certain wave-lengths emitted from the sun rather less than 10 minutes earlier. This radiation is condensed to a circular patch on the retina and generates a photo-chemical reaction, which in turn excites nerve-threads which relay their excitation to certain parts of the brain, eventually to areas in the brain-cortex. From the retina onward to the brain the medium of propagation is wholly nervous; that is to say, the reaction can be subsumed as electrical. Some of this electrical reaction generated in the eye does not reach the brain-cortex but diverges by a side-path into nerve-threads which relay it to a small muscle, which by contracting prevents excess of light attaining the retina. The electric current propagated to the muscle activates the muscle. The chain of events stretching from the sun's radiation entering the eye to, on the one hand, the contraction of the pupillary muscle, and on the other to the electrical disturbances in the brain-cortex are all straightforward steps in a sequence of physical 'causation', such as, thanks to science, are intelligible. But in the second serial chain there follows on, or attends, the stage of brain-cortex reaction an event or set of events quite inexplicable to us, which both as to themselves and as to the causal tie between them and what preceded them science does not help us; a set of events seemingly incommensurable with any of the events leading

Foreword to 1947 Edition

up to it. The self '*sees*' the sun; it senses a two-dimensional disk of brightness, located in the 'sky', this last a field of lesser brightness, and overhead shaped as a rather flattened dome, coping the self, and a hundred other visual things as well. Of hint that this scene is within the head there is none. Vision is saturated with this strange property called 'projection', the unargued inference that what it sees is at a 'distance' from the seeing 'self'. Enough has been said to stress that in the sequence of events a step is reached where a physical situation in the brain leads to a psychical, which however contains no hint of the brain or any other bodily part. We cannot of course suppose that in the instance taken, the 'seeing the sun' breaks into a visual vacuum; in the waking day 'seeing' of some sort is always going on: on the physical side similarly electrical waves in the brain from one source or another must be practically unremitting during the waking day. The supposition has to be, it would seem, two continuous series of events, one physico-chemical, the other psychical, and at times interaction between them.

This is the body-mind relation;* its difficulty lies in its 'how'. As to the utility of the liaison that appears patent enough, namely that the psychical may influence the physical act. In illustration—a simple everyday illustration—a morsel of food in the mouth is subject to the movements of the lips, tongue, cheeks, etc. The conscious self is aware of it, perhaps, acutely—if it is savoury or distasteful. In the former case the self can swallow it, in the latter reject it. If the former, the tongue and fauces push it from the mouth into the grasp of the gullet. That done, our conscious self is aware of the morsel no more, although the morsel is still within the grasp of muscle and nerve and they skilfully deal with it further. The conscious self has, however, lost it and control of it. Even if the morsel be poison the self can no longer directly intervene. That is, the morsel vanishes from an experience at the moment when our choice in regard to it becomes inoperative. The psyche does not persist into conditions which would render it ineffective.

Further it is claimed that the psychical can increase the reactivity

* For luminous treatment of this point see W. Russell Brain, *Philosophy* (1946), vol. XXI, p. 134.

Foreword to 1947 Edition

of the body's physical system. Thus, it is shown that under favourable circumstances the reaction of the retina to as few as six photons can be perceived; and a visual reaction can release motor behaviour of the whole body. But without the visual perception there would be no general reaction. The process by which a reaction of merely 'quantum' order is biologically raised to molar dimensions is called by some biologists 'amplification'. A means to 'amplification' is emotion. As physical stimulus a ghost may be of barely threshold power; but given emotion, and it can convulse the whole individual. Intensification of behaviour by emotion accompanies animal life very widely. I once had opportunity to watch under the microscope a flea 'biting'. The act, whether reflex or not, seemed charged with the most violent emotion. Its Lilliput scale aside, the scene compared with that of the prowling lion in 'Salâmbo'. It was a glimpse suggesting a vast ocean of 'affect' pervading the insect world. An inference is, that part at least of the *raison d'être* for our psychical experience is to exert influence on the body's physical acts. The service of the psychical to the individual life seems to lie in influencing the body's acts, in the interest of self-conservation, an aim innate in the individual from a primordial outset. The psychical therefore implements more fully a principle already implicit in life.

When this situation is viewed broadly to-day it reveals a circumstance at first sight strange. We perceive that the immemorial principle of self-conservation is being challenged by a 'new deal'; a novel order of things antagonizes a preceding; a new moral value is appearing over the horizon. The principle of altruism has arisen. A great antinomy is shaping. A behaviour actuated by 'charity' even to the extent of sacrificing one's own self for the sake of another's self. The soldier gives his own life for that of others. This new spirit seems to be largely correlated with the development of man on our planet. Lord Acton had in purpose a History of Liberty. A history of Altruism might be not less worth while. This may be thought to be digressing from physiology, but in fact I do not think it is. St Augustine's *De Civitate Dei* contains not a little physiology. In so far as physiology involves man as a physio-

Foreword to 1947 Edition

logical factor on our planet this great antinomy of which he is the protagonist is not alien to the scope of physiology.

Agreeing that the biological function of the physico-psychical liaison is to enhance the organism's power of disposing of its acts, a further question asks of what service is the physical organism to the psychical? This question is only in part a reciprocal of the other, because only some organisms possess the psychical component. In such as do, however, it is clear that the body-mind liaison provides in a largely physical world the physical means of giving expression to the psychical.

In all those types of organism in which the physical and the psychical coexist, each of the two achieves its aim only by reason of a *contact utile* between them. And this liaison can rank as the final and supreme integration completing its individual. But the problem of *how* that liaison is effected remains unsolved; it remains where Aristotle left it more than 2000 years ago. "There is, however, one peculiar inconsistency which we may note as marking this and many other psychological theories. They place the soul in the body and attach it to the body without trying in addition to determine the reason why, or the condition of the body under which such attachment is produced. This, however, would seem to be a real question."*
Instead of, as is usual in physiology, leaving that impasse unmentioned, it seemed better to draw attention to it by the experimental observations in this book's final chapter.

The demand for discussion of this liaison between two incommensurable factors can be avoided, but at a cost, by adopting either of two other courses. If for instance we start out from the notion of the psychical self and proceed thence to its apprehended world including its apprehended body, the whole scheme is a mental one, and the body-mind incompatibility falls. The self and its world are then one in their nature. Or again, remembering that common sense and physics and chemistry, from their analysis of our body and its cosmical surround reduce these ultimately to a single factor, 'energy', we can suppose that our thinking is likewise an outcome of 'energy'. Then again the body-mind disparation

* *De Anima*, I. 3, §§ 22-3 (Wallace's translation, p. 35).

Foreword to 1947 Edition

disappears, because both have become forms of 'energy'—though in this case by means of an assumption which seems to many an unjustified one.

Of these two views Cajal tells how he was for a time a zealous disciple of the former, and noticed that to his practical life adherence neither to the one nor other seemed to make any difference whatever. I should myself have supposed that the Berkeleian view would impair the 'zest' of the waking day, nor can I imagine the achievements of ancient Rome emerging from such a doctrine.

That our being should consist of *two* fundamental elements offers I suppose no greater inherent improbability than that it should rest on one only.

C. S. SHERRINGTON

June 1947

THE

INTEGRATIVE ACTION

OF THE

NERVOUS SYSTEM

BY

CHARLES S. SHERRINGTON
D.Sc., M.D., Hon. LL.D. Tor., F.R.S.
*Holt Professor of Physiology in the University of Liverpool,
Honorary Member of the American Physiological Society,
&c.*

WITH ILLUSTRATIONS

NEW YORK
CHARLES SCRIBNER'S SONS
1906

[*Facsimile title-page
of the first edition*]

To
DAVID FERRIER
In token of recognition of his many services
to the experimental physiology of
THE CENTRAL NERVOUS SYSTEM

Lecture I

INTRODUCTORY—CO-ORDINATION OF THE SIMPLE REFLEX

ARGUMENT: The nervous system and the integration of bodily reactions. Characteristics of integration by nervous agency. The unit mechanism in integration by the nervous system is the reflex. Co-ordination of reflexes one with another. Co-ordination in the *simple reflex*. Conduction in the reflex-arc. Function of the receptor to lower for its reflex-arc the threshold value of one kind of stimulus and to heighten the threshold value of all other kinds of stimuli for that arc: it thus confers selective excitability on the arc. Differences between conduction in nerve-trunks and in reflex-arcs respectively. These probably largely referable to the intercalation of synaptic membranes in the conductive mechanism of the arc. Latent time of reflexes. Reflex latency inversely proportional to intensity of stimulation. Latency of initial and incremental reflexes. None of the latent interval consumed in establishing connexion between the elements of a resting arc. *After-discharge* a characteristic of reflex reactions. Increase of after-discharge by intensification of the stimulus, or by prolongation of short stimuli. 'Inertia' and 'momentum' of reflex-arc reactions.

NOWHERE in physiology does the cell-theory reveal its presence more frequently in the very framework of the argument than at the present time in the study of nervous reactions. The cell-theory at its inception depended for exemplification largely on merely morphological observations; just as these formed originally the almost exclusive texts for the Darwinian doctrine of evolution. But with the progress of natural knowledge, biology has passed beyond the confines of the study of merely visible form, and is turning more and more to the subtler and deeper sciences that are branches of energetics. The cell-theory and the doctrine of evolution find their scope more and more, therefore, in the problems of function, and have become more and more identified with the aims and incorporated among the methods of physiology.

The physiology of nervous reactions can be studied from three main points of view.

In the first place, nerve-cells, like all other cells, lead individual lives—they breathe, they assimilate, they dispense their own stores of

Introductory

energy, they repair their own substantial waste; each is, in short, a living unit, with its nutrition more or less centred in itself. Here, then, problems of nutrition, regarding each nerve-cell and regarding the nervous system as a whole, arise comparable with those presented by all other living cells. Although no doubt partly special to this specially differentiated form of cell-life, these problems are in general accessible to the same methods as apply to the study of nutrition in other cells and tissues and in the body as a whole. We owe recently to Verworn and his co-workers advances specially valuable in this field.

Secondly, nervous cells present a feature so characteristically developed in them as to be specially theirs. They have in exceptional measure the power to spatially transmit (conduct) states of excitement (nerve-impulses) generated within them. Since this seems the eminent functional feature of nerve-cells wherever they exist, its intimate nature is a problem co-extensive with the existence of nerve-cells, and enters into every question regarding the specific reactions of the nervous system. This field of study may be termed that of *nerve-cell conduction*.

But a third aspect which nervous reactions offer to the physiologist is the *integrative*. In the multicellular animal, especially for those higher reactions which constitute its behaviour as a social unit in the natural economy, it is nervous reaction which *par excellence* integrates it, welds it together from its components, and constitutes it from a mere collection of organs an animal individual. This integrative action in virtue of which the nervous system unifies from separate organs an animal possessing solidarity, an individual, is the problem before us in these lectures. Though much in need of data derived from the two previously mentioned lines of study, it must in the meantime be carried forward of itself and for its own sake.

The integration of the animal organism is obviously not the result solely of any single agency at work within it, but of several. Thus, there is the *mechanical* combination of the unit cells of the individual into a single mass. This is effected by fibrous stromata, capsules of organs, connective tissue in general, e.g. of the liver, and indeed the fibrous layer of the skin encapsulating the whole body. In muscles

Integration by Nervous Agency

this mechanical integration of the organ may arrive at providing a single cord tendon by which the tensile stress of a myriad contractile cells can be additively concentrated upon a single place of application.

Integration also results from *chemical* agency. Thus, reproductive organs, remote one from another, are given solidarity as a system by communication that is of chemical quality; lactation supervenes *post partum* in all the mammary glands of a bitch subsequent to thoracic transection of the spinal cord severing all nervous communication between the pectoral and the inguinal mammae (Goltz). In digestive organs we find chemical agency co-ordinating the action of separate glands, and thus contributing to the solidarity of function of the digestive glands as a whole. The products of salivary digestion on reaching the pyloric region of the stomach, and the gastric secretion on reaching the mucosa of the duodenum, make there substances which absorbed duly excite heightened secretion of gastric and of pancreatic juice respectively suited to continue the digestion of the substances initiating the reaction (Bayliss & Starling,188[*] Edkins311). Again, there is the integrating action effected by the circulation of the blood. The gaseous exchanges at one limited surface of the body are made serviceable for the life of every living unit in the body. By the blood the excess of heat produced in one set of organs is brought to redress the loss of heat in others; and so on.

But the integrative action of the nervous system is different from these, in that its agent is not mere intercellular material, as in connective tissue, nor the transference of material in mass, as by the circulation; it works through living lines of stationary cells along which it dispatches waves of physico-chemical disturbance, and these act as releasing forces in distant organs where they finally impinge. Hence it is not surprising that nervous integration has the feature of relatively high *speed*, a feature peculiarly distinctive of integrative correlation in animals as contrasted with that of plants, the latter having no nervous system in the ordinary sense of the word.

The nervous system is in a certain sense the highest expression of

[*] The reference numbers in the text refer to the bibliographical list at the end of the volume.

Introductory

that which French physiologists term the *milieu interne*. With the transition from the unicellular organism to the multicellular a new element enters general physiology. The phenomena of general physiology in the unicellular organism can be divided into two great groups; namely, those occurring within the cell, intracellular, and those occurring at the surface of the cell, in which forces that are associated with surfaces of separation have opportunity for play at the boundary between the organism and its environment. But in the multicellular organism a third great group of phenomena exists in addition; namely, those which are *inter*cellular, occurring in that complex material which the organism deposits in quantity in the intercellular interstices of its mass as a connecting medium between its individual living units.

When the intercellular substance is solid, e.g. in many connective tissues, the physiological agencies for which it affords a field of operation are mechanical rather than chemical. The organism obtains from it scaffolding for supporting its weight, levers for application of its forces, etc., and in this degree the intercellular material performs an integrative function. Where the intercellular material is fluid, as in blood, lymph, and tissue juice, it constitutes a field of operation for agencies chemical rather than mechanical. The intricacy of the chemistry of this *milieu interne* is shown by nothing better than by the specificity of the precipitins, etc., the intercellular media for each separate animal species yielding its own particular kinds. The cells of a multicellular organism have therefore in addition to an environmental medium in which the organism as a whole is bathed, and to which they react either directly or through the medium of surface cells, an *internal medium* created by their organism itself, and in many respects specific to itself.

But the internal interconnexion of the multicellular organism is not restricted to intercellular material. Intercellular material is, after all, no living channel of communication, delicately responsive to living changes though it may be. An actually living internal bond is developed. When the animal body reaches some degree of multicellular complexity, special cells assume the express office of connecting together other cells. Such cells, since their function is to

Reception, Conduction, and End-Effect

stretch from one cell to another, are usually elongated; they form protoplasmic threads and they interconnect by conducting nervous impulses. And we find this living bond the one employed where, as said above, speed and nicety of time adjustment are required, as in animal movements, and also where nicety of spatial adjustment is essential, as also in animal movements. It is in view of this interconnecting function of the nervous system that that field of study of nervous reactions which was called at the outset the third or integrative, assumes its due importance. The due activity of the interconnexion resolves itself into the co-ordination of the parts of the animal mechanism by reflex action.

It is necessary to be clear as to what we understand by the expression 'reflex' action.

In plants and animals occur a number of actions the initiation of which is traceable to events in their environment. The event in the environment is some change which acts on the organism as an exciting *stimulus*. The energy which is imparted to the organism by the stimulus is often far less in quantity than the energy which the organism itself sets free in the movement or other effect which it exhibits in consequence of the application of the stimulus. This excess of energy must be referred to energy potential in the organism itself. The change in the environment evidently acts as a releasing force upon the living machinery of the organism. The source of energy set free is traced to chemical compounds in the organism. These are of high potential value, and in immediate or mediate consequence of the stimulus decompose partly, and so liberate external from internal energy. It is perfectly conceivable, and in many undifferentiated organisms, especially in unicellular, e.g. amoeba, is actually the case, that one and the same living structure not only undergoes this physico-chemical change at the point at which an external agent is applied, but is subject to spread of that change from particle to particle along it, so that there then ensue in it changes of form, movement. In such a case the initial reaction or *reception* of the stimulus, the spatial transmission or *conduction* of the reaction, and the motor or other *end-effect*, are all processes that occur in one and the same living structure. But in many organisms these

Introductory

separable parts of the reaction are exhibited by separate and specific structures. Suppose an animal turn its head in response to a sudden light. Large fields of its body take part in the reaction, but also large fields of it do not. Some of its musculature contracts, particularly certain pieces of its skeletal musculature. The external stimulus is, so to say, led to them by certain nerves in the altered form of a nervous impulse. If the neck nerves are severed the end-effect is cut out of part of the field; and the nerves themselves cannot exhibit *movement* on application of the stimulus. The optic nerve itself is unable to enter into a heightened phase of its own specific activity on the application of light. Initiation of nervous activity by light is the exclusive (in this instance) function of cells in the retina, i.e. retinal receptors. In such cases there exist three separable structures for the three processes—*initiation, conduction* and *end-effect*.

These reactions, in which there follows on an initiating reaction an end-effect reached through the mediation of a conductor, itself incapable either of the end-effect or, under natural conditions, of the inception of the reaction, are 'reflexes'. The conductors are nerve. Usually the spaces and times bridged across by the conductors are quite large, and easily capable of measurement. Now there occur cases, especially within the unicellular organism and the unicellular organ, where the spaces and times bridged are minute. In them spread of response may involve 'conduction' (*Poteriodendron, Vorticella*) in some degree specific. Yet to cases where neither histologically nor physiologically a specific conductor can be detected, it seems better not to apply the term 'reflex'. It seems better to reserve that expression for reactions employing specifically recognizable nerve-processes and morphologically differentiated nerve-cells; the more so because the process of conduction in nerve is probably a specialized one, in which the qualities of speed and freedom from inertia of reaction have been attained to a degree not reached elsewhere since not elsewhere demanded.

The conception of a reflex therefore embraces that of at least three separable structures—an *effector* organ, e.g. gland cells or muscle cells; a conducting nervous path or *conductor* leading to that organ; and an initiating organ or *receptor* whence the reaction starts. The

The Simple Reflex

conductor consists, in the reactions which we have to study, of at least two nerve-cells—one connected with the receptor, the other with the effector. For our purpose the receptor is best included as a part of the nervous system, and so it is convenient to speak of the whole chain of structures—receptor, conductor, and effector—as a *reflex-arc*. All that part of the chain which leads up to but does not include the effector and the nerve-cell attached to this latter, is conveniently distinguished as the *afferent-arc*.

The reflex-arc is the unit mechanism of the nervous system when that system is regarded in its integrative function. *The unit reaction in nervous integration is the reflex*, because every reflex is an integrative reaction and no nervous action short of a reflex is a complete act of integration. The nervous synthesis of an individual from what without it were a mere aggregation of commensal organs resolves itself into co-ordination by reflex action. But though the unit reaction in the integration is a reflex, not every reflex is a unit reaction, since some reflexes are compounded of simpler reflexes. Co-ordination, therefore, is in part the compounding of reflexes. In this co-ordination there are therefore obviously two grades.

THE SIMPLE REFLEX

There is the co-ordination which a reflex action introduces when it makes an effector organ responsive to excitement of a receptor, all other parts of the organism being supposed indifferent to and indifferent for that reaction. In this grade of co-ordination the reflex is taken apart, as if separable from all other reflex actions. This is the *simple reflex*. A simple reflex is probably a purely abstract conception, because all parts of the nervous system are connected together and no part of it is probably ever capable of reaction without affecting and being affected by various other parts, and it is a system certainly never absolutely at rest. But the simple reflex is a convenient, if not a probable, fiction. Reflexes are of various degrees of complexity, and it is helpful in analysing complex reflexes to separate from them reflex components which we may consider apart and therefore treat as though they were simple reflexes.

The Simple Reflex

In the simple reflex there is exhibited the first grade of co-ordination. But it is obvious that if the integration of the animal mechanism is due to co-ordination by reflex action, reflex actions must themselves be co-ordinated one with another; for co-ordination by reflex action there must be co-ordination of reflex actions. This latter is the second grade of co-ordination. The outcome of the normal reflex action of the organism is an orderly coadjustment and sequence of reactions. This is very patently expressed by the skeletal musculature. The co-ordination involves orderly coadjustment of a number of simple reflexes occurring *simultaneously*, i.e. a reflex pattern, figure, or 'complication', if one may warp a psychological term for this use; orderly *succession* involves due supersession of one reflex by another, or of one group of reflexes by another group, i.e. orderly change from one reflex pattern or figure to another. For this succession to occur in an orderly manner no component of the previous reflex may remain which would be out of harmony with the new reflex that sets in. When the change from one reflex to another occurs it is therefore usually a far-reaching change spread over a wide range of nervous arcs.

This compounding of reflexes with orderliness of coadjustment and of sequence constitutes co-ordination, and want of it incoordination. We may therefore in regard to co-ordination distinguish co-ordination of reflexes simultaneously proceeding, and co-ordination of reflexes successively proceeding. The main secret of nervous co-ordination lies evidently in the compounding of reflexes.

CO-ORDINATION IN THE SIMPLE REFLEX

It is best to clear the way toward the more complex problems of co-ordination by considering as an earlier step that which was termed above, the first grade of co-ordination, or that of the simple reflex. From the point of view of its office as integrator of the animal mechanism, the whole function of the nervous system can be summed up in the one word, *conduction*. In the simple reflex the evidence of co-ordination is that the outcome of the reflex as expressed by the activity induced in the effector organ is a response

The Receptor

appropriate to the stimulus imparted to the receptor. This due propriety of end-effect is largely traceable to the action of the conductor mediating between receptor and affector. Knowledge of the features of this 'conduction' is therefore a prime object of study in this connexion.

But we have first to remember that in dealing with reflexes even experimentally we very usually deal with them as reactions for which the reflex-arc as a whole and without any separation into constituent parts is laid under contribution. The reflex-arc thus taken includes the receptor. It is assuredly as truly a functional part of the arc as any other. But, for analysis of the arc's conduction, it is obvious that by including the receptor we are including a structure which, as its name implies, adaptation has specialized for excitation of a kind different from that obtaining for all the rest of the arc. It is therefore advantageous, as we have to include the receptor in the reflex-arc, to consider what characters its inclusion probably grafts upon the functioning of the arc.

Marshall Hall[23] drew attention to the greater ease with which reflexes can be elicited from receptive surfaces than from afferent nerve-trunks themselves; and this has often been confirmed (Eckhard, Biedermann). Steinach[190] has measured the lowering of the threshold value of stimulation when in the frog a reflex is elicited by a mechanical stimulus applied to skin instead of to cutaneous afferent nerve. The lowering is considerable. There are numerous instances in which particular reflexes can be elicited from the receptive surface by particular stimuli only. Goltz[45] endeavoured in vain to evoke the reflex croak of the female frog by applying to the skin electrical stimuli. Mechanical stimuli of non-nocuous kind were the only stimuli that proved effective. By direct stimulation of the afferent nerve itself the reflex could but rarely be elicited at all. Later Goltz's pupil Gergens[68] succeeded in provoking the reflex by applying to the skin a mild discharge from an influence machine.

A remarkable reflex[304] is obtainable from the *planta* of the hind-foot in the 'spinal' dog. The movement provoked is a brief strong extension at knee, hip, and ankle. This is the 'extensor-thrust'. It

The Simple Reflex

seems obtainable only by a particular kind of mechanical stimulation. I have never succeeded in eliciting it by any form of electrical stimulation, nor by any stimulation applied directly to an afferent nerve-trunk.

Again, a very characteristic reflex in the cat is the pinna-reflex.[304] If the tip of the pinna be squeezed, or tickled, or in some cases even touched, the pinna itself is crumpled so that its free end is turned backward, as in Darwin's[550] picture of a cat prepared to attack. The afferent nerve of this reflex appears to be in part at least not the cranial fifth nerve, but the foremost cervical. The reflex emerges very early from the shock of decerebration and is submerged very late in chloroform narcosis. This reflex, easily elicitable as it is by various mechanical stimuli to the skin, I have never succeeded in provoking by any form of electrical stimulation.

The same sort of difference, though less marked in degree, is exhibited by the scratch-reflex.[87,126,251,252,300] This reflex is one in which various forms of innocuous mechanical stimulation (rubbing, tickling, tapping) applied to the skin of the back behind the shoulder evoke a rhythmic flexion (scratching movement) of the hind-limb, the foot being brought toward the seat of stimulation. This reflex in the spinal dog, although usually elicitable, varies much under various circumstances in its degree of elicitability. When easily elicitable it can be evoked by various forms of electrical stimulation as well as by mechanical; but when not easily elicitable electrical stimuli altogether fail, while rubbing and other suitable mechanical stimuli still evoke it, though not so readily or vigorously as usual.

A question germane to this is the oft-debated sensitivity of various internal organs. Direct stimulation of various afferent nerves of the visceral system is itself well known to yield reflexes on blood-pressure, etc. But in regard to the sensitivity of the organs themselves we have, on the one hand, the passage of bile-stones, renal calculi, etc., accompanied by intense sensations, and on the other hand the insensitivity of these ducts and various allied visceral parts as noted by Haller[6] and observed by surgeons working under circumstances favourable for examining the question. The stimula-

Adequate Stimulus

tion which excites pain in these internal organs is usually of mechanical kind, e.g. calculus, and the surgeon's knife and needle provide mechanical stimuli, and Haller and his co-workers in their research employed multiform stimuli, many of them mechanical in quality. But though mechanical, the latter are remote in quality from the former; the former are distensile. The action of a calculus can be imitated by injecting fluid of itself innocuous. Marked reflex effects can then be excited[194] from the very organs (Fig. 1), the cutting and

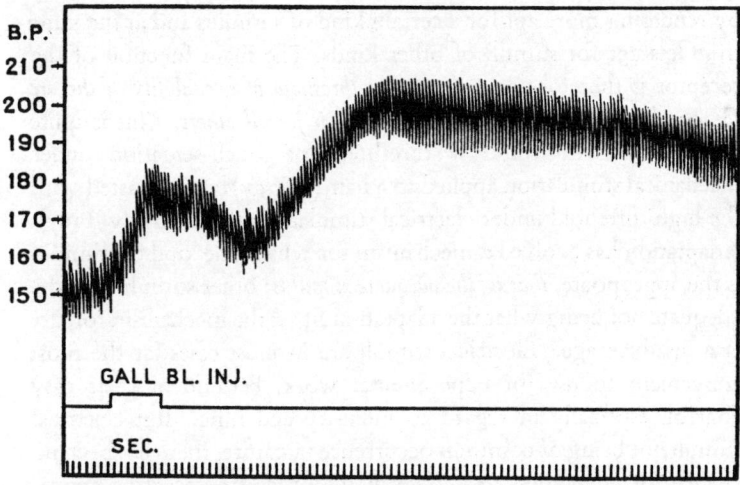

Fig. 1. Effect of distension of common bile duct on arterial blood-pressure
Cat under $CHCl_3$ and curare; double vagotomy.
Records from above downwards:
    Arterial blood-pressure: scale in mm. Hg.
    Signal line: rise of signal indicates rapid injection of 2·5 c.c. of saline solution into the common bile duct.
    Time in sec.
Distension of the duct produces a rise of arterial pressure. (Cf. Bibliography, no. 194.)

wounding of which remain without effect. For Haller's and the surgical experience to be harmonized with the medical evidence from calculi, etc., all that is necessary is that the mechanical stimulation be *adequate*, and to be adequate it must be of a certain kind. Thus we see that when the mechanical stimulation employed resembles

The Simple Reflex

that occurring in the natural accidents that concern medicine, the experimental results fall into line with those observed at the bedside.

Therefore we may infer provisionally—for the facts justify only a guarded judgement—that the part played by the receptor in the reflex-arc is in the main what from other evidence it is inferred to be in the case of the receptors as *sense*-organs; namely, a mechanism more or less attuned to respond specially to a certain one or several of the agencies that act as stimuli to the body. We may suppose this special attuning acts as does specialization in so many cases, namely by rendering more apt for a certain kind of stimulus and at the same time less apt for stimuli of other kinds. The main function of the receptor is therefore[205] *to lower the threshold of excitability of the arc for one kind of stimulus, and to heighten it for all others*. This is quite comparable with the low threshold for touch-sensation under mechanical stimulation applied to a hair (v. Frey)[172] contrasted with the high threshold under electrical stimulation of the skin (v. Frey). Adaptation has evolved a mechanism for which one kind of stimulus is the appropriate, *that is, the adequate stimulus*: other stimuli than the adequate not being what the adaptation fitted the mechanism for, are at a disadvantage. Electrical stimuli are in most cases far the most convenient to use for experimental work, because of their easy control, especially in regard to intensity and time. But electrical stimuli not being of common occurrence in nature, there has been no chance for adaptation to evolve in the organism receptors appropriate for such stimuli. Therefore we may say that electricity never constitutes the adequate stimulus for any receptor, since it is always an artificial form of stimulus, and every adequate stimulus must obviously be a natural form of stimulation. It is therefore rather a matter for surprise that electrical stimuli applied to receptor organs are as efficient excitors of reflexes as they in fact prove to be. It is particularly in regard to a class of reflexes whose receptive cells seem attuned specially to react to nocuous agents, agents that threaten to do local damage, that electrical stimuli are found to be excellently effective. But the conditions of adaptation to stimuli appear here peculiar; and there will be better opportunity of considering them later.

We infer, therefore, that the main contribution made to the

Conduction in Reflex-Arc

mechanism of the reflex-arc by that part of it which constitutes the receptor is *selective excitability*. It thus contributes to co-ordination, for it renders its arc prone to reply to certain stimuli, while other arcs not having that kind of receptor do not reply, and it renders its arc unlikely to reply to certain other stimuli to which other arcs are likely to respond. It will thus, while providing increase of responsiveness on the part of the organism to the environment, tend to prevent confusion of reactions (inco-ordination) by limiting to particular stimuli a particular reaction.

On the whole, we may regard the receptor as being concerned with the *mode of excitation* rather than with the features of conduction of the reflex-arc, and may now return to that conduction, which itself has important co-ordinative characters.

Nervous conduction has been studied chiefly in nerve-trunks. Conduction in reflexes is of course for its spatially greater part conduction along nerve-trunks, yet reflex conduction *in toto* differs widely from nerve-trunk conduction.

Salient among the characteristic differences between conduction in nerve-trunks and in reflex-arcs respectively are the following:

Conduction in reflex-arcs exhibits: (1) slower speed as measured by the latent period between application of stimulus and appearance of end-effect, this difference being greater for weak stimuli than for strong; (2) less close correspondence between the moment of cessation of stimulus and the moment of cessation of end-effect, i.e. there is a marked 'after-discharge'; (3) less close correspondence between rhythm of stimulus and rhythm of end-effect; (4) less close correspondence between the grading of intensity of the stimulus and the grading of intensity of the end-effect; (5) considerable resistance to passage of a single nerve-impulse, but a resistance easily forced by a succession of impulses (temporal summation); (6) irreversibility of direction instead of reversibility as in nerve-trunks; (7) fatigability in contrast with the comparative unfatigability of nerve-trunks; (8) much greater variability of the threshold value of stimulus than in nerve-trunks; (9) refractory period, 'bahnung', inhibition, and shock, in degrees unknown for nerve-trunks; (10) much greater dependence on blood-circulation, oxygen (Verworn, Winterstein,

The Simple Reflex

v. Baeyer, etc.); (11) much greater susceptibility to various drugs—anaesthetics.

These differences between conduction in reflex-arcs and nerve-trunks respectively appear referable to that part of the arc which lies in grey matter. The constituents of grey matter over and above those which exist also in nerve-trunks are the nerve-cell bodies (perikarya),[170] the fine nerve-cell branches (dendritic and axonic nerve-fibres), and neuroglia.

Neuroglia exists in white matter as well as in grey, and there is no good ground for attributing the above characteristics of conduction in reflex-arcs to that part of the arcs which consists of white matter. It is improbable, therefore, on that ground that the features of the conduction are due to neuroglia. Indeed, there is no good evidence that neuroglia is concerned directly in nervous conduction at all. As to perikarya (nerve-cell bodies) the experiment of Bethe[178] on the motor perikarya of the ganglion of the second antenna of *Carcinus*, and the experiments of Steinach[190] on the perikarya of the spinal-root ganglion, also the observation by Langley[220] that nicotine has little effect when applied to the spinal-root ganglion, though breaking conduction in sympathetic ganglia, all indicate more or less directly that it is not to the perikarya that the characteristic features of reflex-arc conduction are referable. Similarly, the experiments of Exner,[71] and of Moore & Reynolds,[193] detecting no delay in transmission through the spinal-root ganglion—though observations by Wundt[69] and by Gad & Joseph[121] had a different result—withdraw from the perikaryon the responsibility for another feature characteristic of reflex-arc conduction. Again, histological observations by Cajal, van Gehuchten, and others, indicate that in various cases the line of conduction may run not through the perikaryon at all, but direct from dendrite stem to axone.

As to the nerve-cell branches (dendrites, axones, and axone-collaterals) which are so prominent as histological characters of grey matter, they are in many cases perfectly continuous with nerve-fibres outside, whose conductive features are known by the study of nerve-trunks; they are also themselves nerve-fibres, though smaller in calibre than those outside. It seems therefore scarcely justifiable to

Conduction in Reflex-Arc

suppose that conduction along nerve-fibres assumes in the grey matter characters so widely different from those it possesses elsewhere as to account for the dissimilarity between reflex-arc conduction and nerve-trunk conduction respectively.

In this difficulty there rises forcibly to mind that not the least fruitful of the facts which the cell-theory rests upon and brings together is the existence at the confines of the cells composing the organism of 'surfaces of separation' between the adjacent cells. In certain syncytial cases such surfaces are not apparent, but with most of the cells in the organism their existence is undisputed, and they play an important role in a great number of physiological processes. Now in addition to the structural elements of grey matter specified above, there is one other which certainly in many cases exists. The grey matter is the field of nexus between neurone and neurone. Except in sympathetic* ganglia, the place of nexus between neurone and neurone lies nowhere else than in grey matter. We know of no reflex-arc composed of one single neurone only. In other words, every reflex-arc must contain a nexus between one neurone and another. The reflex-arc must, therefore, on the cell-theory, be expected to include not only *intracellular* conduction, but *intercellular* conduction. But on the current view of the structure of the nerve-fibres of nerve-trunks the conduction observed in nerve-trunks is entirely and only *intra*cellular conduction. Perhaps, therefore, the difference between reflex-arc conduction and nerve-trunk conduction is related to an additional element in the former, namely, *inter*cellular conduction. If there exist any surface or separation at the nexus between neurone and neurone, much of what is characteristic of the conduction exhibited by the reflex-arc might be more easily explicable. At the nexus between cells if there be not actual confluence, there must be a surface of separation. At the nexus between efferent neurone and the muscle-cell, electrical organ, etc., which it innervates, it is generally admitted that there is not actual confluence of the two cells together, but that a surface separates them; and a surface of separation is physically a membrane. As regards a number of the features enumerated above as distinguishing reflex-arc

* = Autonomic.

The Simple Reflex

conduction from nerve-trunk conduction, there is evidence that *similar features, though not usually in such marked extent, characterize conduction from efferent nerve-fibre to efferent organ*, e.g., in nerve-muscle preparation, in nerve-electric-organ preparation, etc. Here change in character of conduction is not due to perikarya (nerve-cell bodies), for such are not present. The change may well be referable to the surface of separation admittedly existent between efferent neurone and effector cell.

If the conductive element of the neurone be fluid, and if at the nexus between neurone and neurone there does not exist actual confluence of the conductive part of one cell with the conductive part of the other, e.g. if there is not actual continuity of physical phase between them, there must be a surface of separation. Even should a membrane visible to the microscope not appear, the mere fact of non-confluence of the one with the other implies the existence of a surface of separation. Such a surface might restrain diffusion, bank up osmotic pressure, restrict the movement of ions, accumulate electric changes, support a double electric layer, alter in shape and surface-tension with changes in difference of potential, alter in difference of potential with changes in surface-tension or in shape, or intervene as a membrane between dilute solutions of electrolytes of different concentration or colloidal suspensions with different sign of charge. It would be a mechanism where nervous conduction, especially if predominantly physical in nature, might have grafted upon it characters just such as those differentiating reflex-arc conduction from nerve-trunk conduction. For instance, change from reversibility of direction of conduction to irreversibility might be referable to the membrane possessing irreciprocal permeability. It would be natural to find in the arc, each time it passed through grey matter, the additive introduction of features of reaction such as characterize a neurone-threshold (Goldscheider[187]). The conception of the nervous impulse as a physical process (du Bois Reymond) rather than a chemical, gains rather than loses plausibility from physical chemistry. The injury-current of nerve seems comparable in mode of production (J. S. Macdonald[234]) with the current of a 'concentration cell', a mode of energy akin to the expansion of a

The Synapse

gas and physical, rather than chemical, 'volume-energy'. Against the likelihood of nervous conduction being pre-eminently a chemical rather than a physical process must be reckoned, as Macdonald well urges, its speed of propagation, its brevity of time-relations, its freedom from perceptible temperature change, its facile excitation by mechanical means, its facilitation by cold, etc. If it is a physical process the intercalation of a transverse surface of separation or membrane into the conductor must modify the conduction, and it would do so with results just such as we find differentiating reflex-arc conduction from nerve-trunk conduction.

As to the existence or the non-existence of a surface of separation or membrane between neurone and neurone, that is a structural question on which histology might be competent to give valuable information. In certain cases, especially in Invertebrata, observation (Apathy, Bethe, etc.) indicates that many nerve-cells are actually continuous one with another. It is noteworthy that in several of these cases the irreversibility of direction of conduction which is characteristic of spinal reflex-arcs is not demonstrable; thus the nerve-net in some cases, e.g. Medusa, exhibits reversible conduction (Romanes, Nagel, Bethe, and others). But in the neurone-chains of the grey-centred system of vertebrates, histology on the whole furnishes evidence that a surface of separation does exist between neurone and neurone. And the evidence of Wallerian secondary degeneration is clear in showing that that process observes strictly a boundary between neurone and neurone and does not transgress it. It seems therefore likely that the nexus between neurone and neurone in the reflex-arc, at least in the spinal arc of the vertebrate, involves a surface of separation between neurone and neurone; and this as a transverse membrane across the conductor must be an important element in intercellular conduction. The characters distinguishing reflex-arc conduction from nerve-trunk conduction may therefore be largely due to intercellular barriers, delicate transverse membranes, in the former.

In view, therefore, of the probable importance physiologically of this mode of nexus between neurone and neurone it is convenient to have a term for it. The term introduced has been *synapse*.[170]

The Simple Reflex

The differences between nerve-trunk conduction and reflex-arc conduction are so great as to require for their exhibition no very minute determination of the characters of either; but we may with advantage follow these differences somewhat further. In doing so we may take the reflexes of the hind-limb of the spinal dog as a field of exemplification.

REFLEX LATENCY

A dissimilarity between nerve-trunk conduction and reflex-arc conduction which has often been stressed is the slowness of the latter as measured by the latent interval between application of stimulus and appearance of end-effect. In nerve-trunks the interval between the moment of stimulation and the appearance of response (electrical) at any distant point is strictly proportional to the distance of that point from the seat of stimulation. There is in the nerve-trunk no measurable delay or latent interval for the response at the seat of excitation. The latent time for nerve-trunk response is therefore entirely a propagation time. The speed of propagation in frog's nerve at 15° C. is about 3 cm. per sigma ($\sigma = 0.001$ sec.). We may compare with this the latent period of the flexion-reflex of the 'spinal' dog's hind-leg. The movement of this reflex is a flexion at knee, hip, and ankle. It is easily and regularly evoked by nocuous or electrical stimuli applied to the skin of the limb or to any afferent nerve of the limb. For measurements of the reflex latency I have stimulated with break or make shocks of regular but varied frequency. Assuming that in warm-blooded nerves the conduction is the same (Helmholtz found it faster) as in the frog, and that the length of the reflex-arc of the dog's knee is two-thirds of a metre, and assuming that we may add 5σ for mechanical latency of the flexor contraction of the limb, we should have about 27σ as the latent time for the flexion-reflex, supposing its conduction proceeded as does nerve-trunk conduction. But, as a fact, a period double that is common enough for the latency of this reflex under ordinary moderate intensities of stimulation.

But with intenser stimuli the latent period of this reflex is much less. A period of 30σ from commencement of stimulus to commencement of mechanical response is not then uncommon. I have

Reflex Latency

met, at shortest, with 220σ. There is little difference here between speed of reflex conduction and speed of nerve-trunk conduction. Similarly François Franck[111] has recorded latent periods for reflex action differing little from those of simple nerve-trunk conduction. Thus, 17σ were obtained for a reflex contraction of the crossed gastrocnemius evoked by stimulation of the afferent root of the first lumbar nerve. These short latencies Franck obtained with strong stimuli.

It would seem, therefore, that the more intense the stimulation the more the conduction along the reflex-arc comes to resemble in speed the conduction along simple nerve-trunks.

It is with mild stimuli that the difference in speed between reflex conduction and nerve-trunk conduction becomes most obvious. The latent period for the flexion-reflex, then, lies usually between 600σ and 1200σ. I have met with it as long as 2000σ. There is no good evidence that the speed of propagation in nerve-trunk conduction is in response to weak stimuli appreciably slower than to strong. This slackening of propagation speed under weak stimuli (Fig. 2) is, I would urge, a more significant difference between reflex-conduction and nerve-trunk conduction than is the mere greater slowness of the former than of the latter. Another difference between the two in regard to conduction-speed is that in the various cerebrospinal nerve-trunks of the same animal species the conduction-speed appears to be practically the same. But reflex conduction-speed as measured by the latent period differs greatly in the various type-reflexes of even one and the same limb. The latent time of the scratch-reflex is, on the average, much longer than that of the flexion-reflex or extensor-thrust, although the spatial distance of the nerve-fibre conduction is not greater. The latency of the former usually in my experience lies between 1400σ for intenser stimulation and 5000σ for weaker, and I have seen it extend to 24400σ and even to 35400σ. So that although a weakly provoked flexion-reflex may have a lengthier latency than a strongly provoked scratch-reflex, the latency of the scratch-reflex is nevertheless on the average very characteristically longer than that of the flexion-reflex. Now there is no evidence that this is referable to a difference in the conduction rate along the nerve-trunks of the

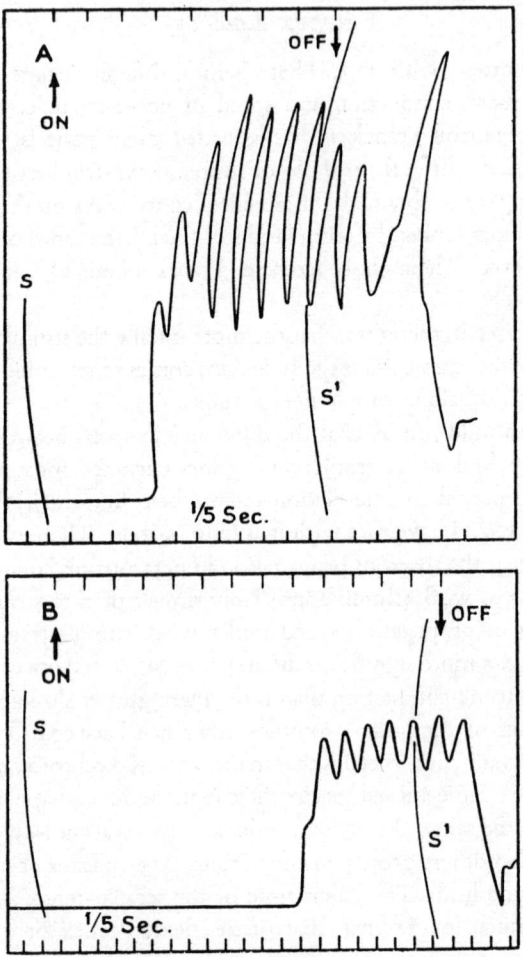

Fig. 2. Scratch-reflex. Lengthening of latency on reducing the intensity of stimulation

Records (in A, B) from above downwards:

Signal line showing frequency of repetition of the double induction shocks used as stimuli (from ON to OFF). The *frequency* is the same in A and B (the tracings are unequally reduced), but the *intensity* is weaker in B than in A.

Myograph curve of scratch-reflex: the vertical arc S indicates onset and S^1 cessation of stimulation.

Time in $\frac{1}{5}$ sec.

The reflex movement began after delivery of three stimuli in A and after delivery of nine stimuli in B. The greater intensity of the stimuli in A is also evidenced by the greater amplitude of the reflex movement and by the longer 'after-discharge'.

Long Latency of Weak Reflexes

two reflexes; indeed, the efferent nerve-trunks for the two reflexes are the same.

The speed of travel of nervous impulses along nerve-trunks is fairly known. On the not improbable assumption that their velocity along the myelinate fibres of the white tracts of the central nervous system is about the same as along the myelinate fibres of nerve-trunks, the latent period of reflex-actions of moderate intensity is obviously greater than can be accounted for by travel along such conductors of the same length as the reflex-arc itself. The delay in speed occurs whenever the impulses pass through grey matter. This has been especially clearly shown by Exner.[149] The delay in the grey matter may conceivably be due to slower conduction in the minute, branched, and more diffuse conducting elements—perikarya, dendrites, arborizations, etc.—found there; or it may be referable to a fresh kind of transmission coming in there, a process of transmission different in nature from conduction along nerve-fibres. The neurone itself is visibly a continuum from end to end, but continuity, as said above, fails to be demonstrable where neurone meets neurone—at the synapse. There a different kind of transmission may occur. The delay in the grey matter may be referable, therefore, to the transmission at the synapse.

And if the delay occur at the synapse, the possibility suggests itself that the time consumed in the latent period may be spent mainly in establishing active connexion along the nervous-arc, which connexion once established, the conduction in the arc then proceeds perhaps as speedily as does conduction in a simple nerve-trunk. The latent time would then be comparable with time spent in closing a key to complete an electric circuit or in setting points at a railway junction. The key once closed, the points once set, the transmission is as expeditious there as elsewhere. Measurements of reflex times deal customarily, so far as I am aware, with the latent time of reflexes initiated in arcs *not in action at the moment* when the exciting stimulus is applied to their afferent end. How the latent time is spent can receive some light from observation on the latent time of an increase of action in an arc already active in the same direction as the incremental action.

The Simple Reflex

To examine this the flexion-reflex was excited by a sub-maximal stimulus, and after its appearance the intensity of the exciting stimulus was abruptly increased by short-circuiting a definite resistance from the primary circuit. The stimulus was a series of break shocks of regular interval given by a key rotating at constant speed in the primary circuit of the inductorium. An electromagnet marked the interruptions of the primary current; the electromagnet was arranged to show by more ample excursion of its armature the point of time from which onward the primary current was increased. The shocks were applied by a needle-point (kathode) to the skin of a digit: the other electrode, large and diffuse, was wrapped round a fore-foot, i.e. headward of the spinal transection. In these experiments the earlier reflex elicited may be termed the *initial reflex*. Its sudden increase on sudden intensification of the stimulus may be termed the *incremental reflex*. The latent times of the initial reflex and incremental reflex, when compared, showed almost always that the latency of the latter was rather the shorter. But the difference often was not great (Figs. 3 and 4). The average for thirty of the initial reflexes was 48σ, and for the thirty corresponding incremental reflexes was 38σ. This difference seems too small to support the supposition that the latent time of the initial reflex is chiefly consumed by 'setting' the synapse, which, once set, conducts in much the same way as regards speed of transmission as does the rest of the arc. It might be that the incremental reaction involved the 'setting' of other additional synapses. But such an explanation demands that none of the augmentation occurs through the synapses already in action, for the latent time is measured to the first beginning of the steplike incremental ascent of the curve.

In the incremental stage of the reaction the reflex is usually a relatively intense one. Now the length of reflex latency is *ceteris paribus* inversely as the intensity of the reflex. If the reflex as produced in two stages be compared with the reflex produced by delivery of the stimulus in its full strength at the outset, the latent time of this latter is found shorter than that of either the initial or incremental reaction of the other reflex (Fig. 4). The latent time under the same external stimulus is thus less in circumstances that

Latent Time of Incremental Reflex

ex hypothesi involve building a bridge and then sending impulses across it, than when the bridge already having been built the impulses have merely to pass. This argues against an amoeboid movement of the protoplasm of the cell being the step which determines

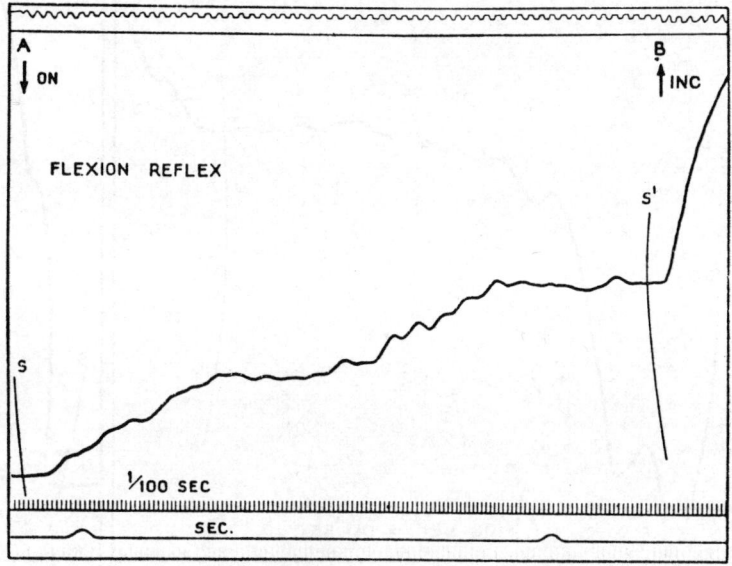

Fig. 3. Flexion-reflex. Spinal dog. Latent period of incremental reflex compared with that of initial reflex

Records from above downwards:
 Signal line: unipolar faradization by break shocks. Electromagnet recording the shocks. Kathode at needle point in plantar skin at outermost digit. A weak stimulus is delivered at A (ON) and maintained and then when the resulting reflex movement has become steady the stimulus is increased in intensity by short-circuiting 5 Ω from the primary circuit at B (INC).
 Myograph curve of flexion-reflex: the vertical arc S indicates the onset of the 'initial' stimulus and S^1 the onset of the 'incremental' stimulus.
 Time in $\frac{1}{100}$ sec. and 1 sec.
The latent time of the incremental reflex (after S^1) is distinctly shorter than that of the initial reflex (after S).

its conductive communication with the next (Demoor, Cajal, Renaut, Monti, Duval, Lugaro). It also seems conclusive against any major portion of the latent period being consumed at the synapse in a

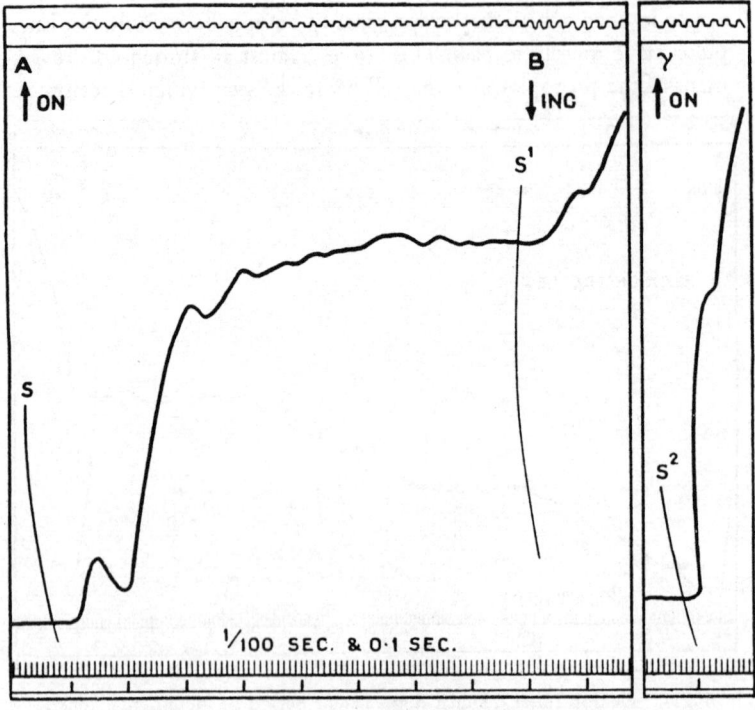

Fig. 4. Flexion-reflex. Spinal dog. Latent period of incremental reflex compared with initial reflex

Same as Fig. 3, but with somewhat stronger initial stimulus and reflex. Records from above downwards:

Signal line: electromagnet records stimulating break shocks, unipolar faradization. Kathode at needle point in plantar skin of outermost digit.

A (ON): a weak stimulus is delivered and maintained and then when the resulting reflex movement has become steady the stimulus is increased in intensity at B (INC) by short circuiting 5 Ω from the primary circuit.

At the extreme right of the figure, at γ (ON) the intensity of the stimulus used incrementally at B (INC) is thrown in at the outset.

Myograph curve of flexion-reflex: the vertical arc S indicates onset of *initial* stimulus, S^1 of *incremental* stimulus and S^2 of the *total* stimulus.

Time in $\frac{1}{100}$ and 0·1 sec.

There is little difference between the latent times of the 'initial' and the 'incremental' reflexes; the latent time of the 'total' reflex is shorter than that of either the initial or the incremental reflex.

Analysis of Latent Time

process which sets the synapse ready to conduct—a process of preparation for transmission as distinguished from a process of transmission. It argues that the delay is inherent in the process of transmission itself, and that therefore the actual nervous transmission at these points has, when the stimuli are weak, a different order of speed to that in nerve-fibres. The shorter latent time of the reflex induced by the stimulus delivered in full at the outset, is in harmony with the reflex being under that mode of excitation rather more intense (e.g. of greater amplitude) than when excited as an increment to a foregoing reflex of less strength. The shorter latent times given by intenser stimuli seem readily explicable by the minimal quantity of transmitted influence necessary to give detectible effect, being necessarily earlier reached with copious transmission than with weaker transmission.

The observations indicate, therefore, that the latent time belongs to some process which is the same in nature, both in initiating a reflex from a resting arc and in increasing a reflex through an arc already in submaximal activity—and probably therefore in maintaining a reflex in unaltered continuance in an arc. It argues that any 'setting' process in the nerve-centre, if it occur at all, is negligible in regard to the time it consumes. It suggests that even while at rest the reflex apparatus is just as prepared for immediately transmitting impulses as when actually engaged in reflex activity in the very direction the new impulses would require. It therefore suggests the greater need for active inhibition in the co-ordination of activity of arcs which have a final path in common and yet use that path to different effects. If resting paths all lie open for conduction, prevention of confusion must depend not on the path excited being the only one open for conduction, but on its excitation being accompanied by inhibition of others that, did they enter into action, would detrimentally confuse the issue of events.

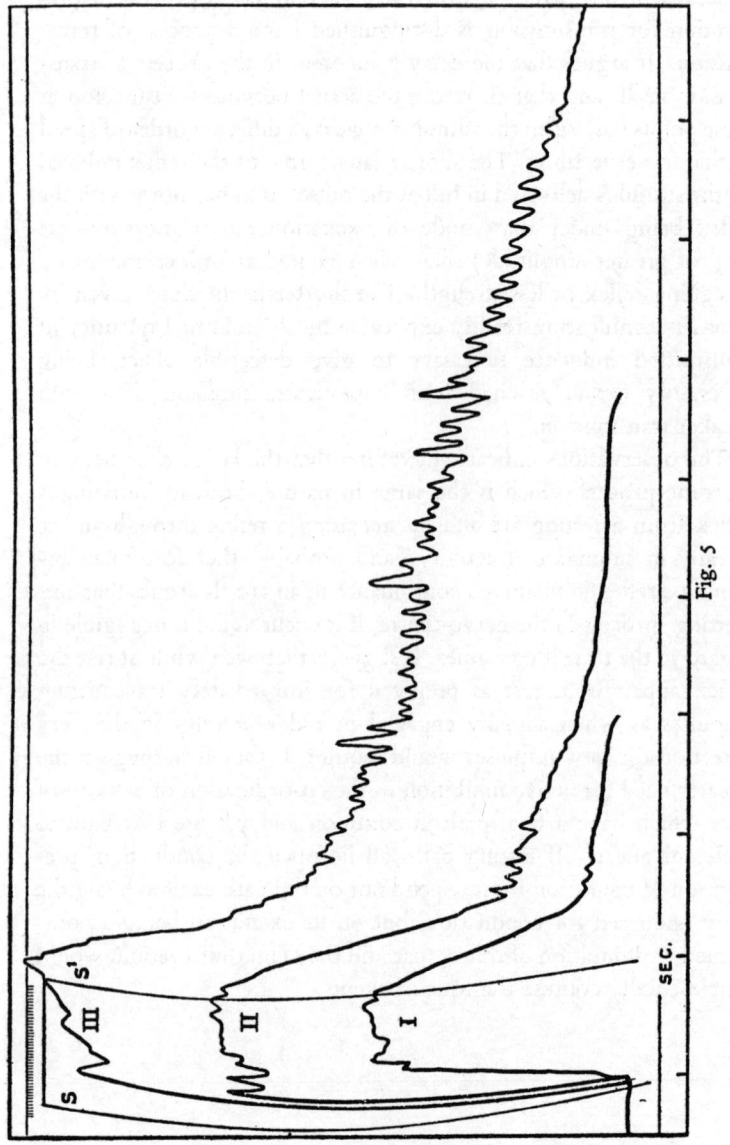

Fig. 5

After-Discharge

REFLEX AFTER-DISCHARGE

Another characteristic difference between conduction in nerve-trunks and in reflex-arcs is the less close correspondence in the latter between moment of cessation of stimulus and moment of cessation of end-effect. The reflex-arc shows marked 'after-discharge'; the nerve-trunk does not. Tetanic contraction of the knee-flexor muscles of the dog induced by brief faradization of the motor-nerve usually ceases within 150σ of the cessation of the stimulation of the nerve, if crude condition of fatigue, etc., be avoided. The contraction of those same muscles, when induced reflexly by a similar brief stimulation, often persists for 5000σ after cessation of the stimulus (Fig. 5).

We must subtract from the period of after-discharge a period equal to the latent time. But usually the latent time is quite insignificant in length as compared with the after-discharge. The after-discharge in flexion-reflex VI (Fig. 6) was more than five hundred times longer than the latent time.

The after-discharge increases with increase of intensity of the stimulus, not only absolutely, but relatively to the whole reflex—

Fig. 5. Flexion-reflex. Effect of intensity of stimulus on magnitude of response and on after-discharge

Records from above downwards:
  Period of stimulation: the stimulus consisted of 45 break shocks delivered at a frequency of 42 per sec. for each reflex; the interruptions of the electromagnet in the primary circuit are recorded.
  Myograph curves (I–III): the vertical arcs on the myograph curves show the onset (S) and cessation (S^1) of the stimulus.
    Time in sec.

	Intensity of stimulus	Measure of reflex	Measure of after-discharge
I	69	110	50
II	110	273	161
III	190	782	626
IV	300	1196	1016

Clonus is seen in the after-discharge. The measure of intensity of the stimulus is given from the units of the Kronecker coil; the measure of the reflex is from the area included between the myograph curve and the base line. Reflex IV is not shown in the figure.

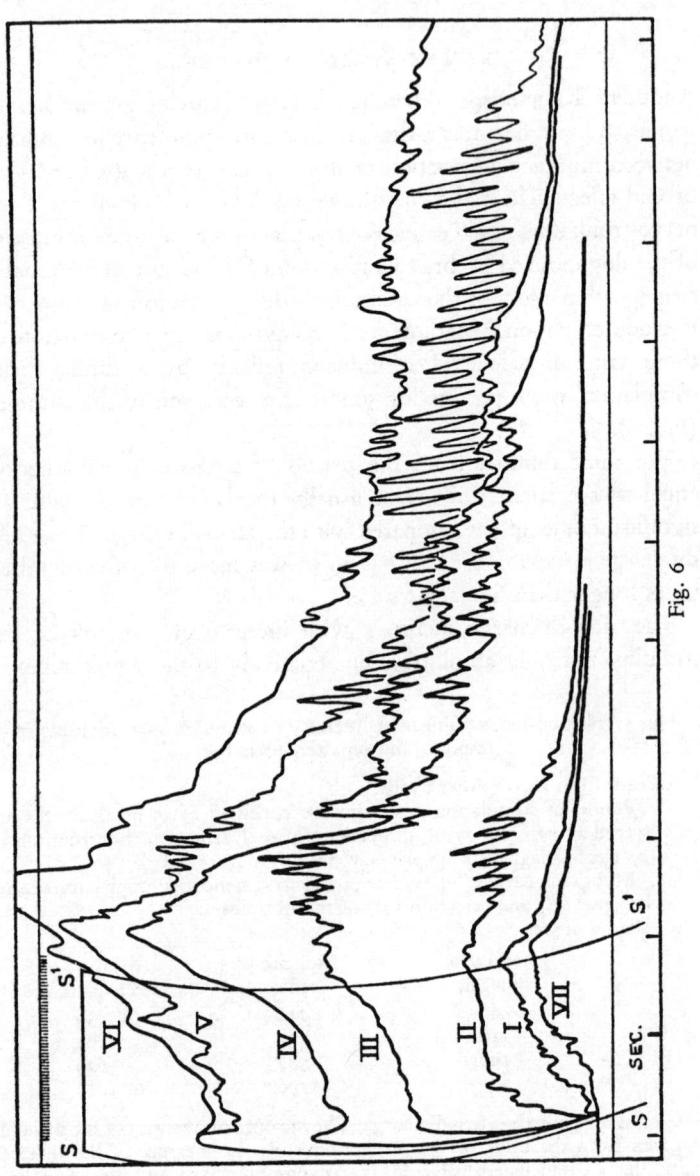

Fig. 6

Effect of Stimulus Strength on After-Discharge

when the stimulation is not long lasting. Taking the flexion-reflex for example, the increase of after-discharge with increasing intensity of stimulation is more marked than the increase of contraction-height (Fig. 7). With stimulation lasting not more than 1000σ the maximum amplitude of the reflex arrives, as the intensity of the stimulus is increased, later and later, so that with weaker stimuli it falls within the excitation period, but with stronger stimuli it is reached only *after* the application of the stimulus has ceased. Very marked in the after-discharge of this, the flexion-reflex, is a clonus (Figs. 5, 6) with a rate in my records varying between 7·5 and 12 per sec. Undulations of similar kinds are clear in the reflex movement even from the outset in weak intensities of the reflex.

Under short-lasting application of rather weak serial stimuli at slow frequency of repetition (break shocks at 20 per sec.), increase of the number of stimuli, without alteration of their intensity or rate, in other words mere prolongation of the stimulation, increases the after-discharge (Fig. 8). The reflex induced by nine stimuli has an after-discharge three times as great as the reflex from three similar stimuli. The maximum amplitude in this case may remain practically the

---

Fig. 6. Flexion-reflex. Effect of intensity of stimulus on magnitude of response and on after-discharge

Records from above downwards:
  Period of stimulation: the stimulus for each reflex was 72 break shocks at the rate of 40 per sec.; the interruptions of the electromagnet in the primary circuit are recorded.
  Myograph curves (I–VII): the vertical arcs on the myograph curves show the onset (S) and cessation (S^1) of the stimulus.
  Time in sec.

	Intensity of stimulus	Measure of reflex	Measure of after-discharge
I	350	94	51
II	475	200	119
III	690	666	509
IV	1100	913	692
V	1900	1277	964
VI	3000	1765	1432
VII	350	62	34

The clonus of the after-discharge is well seen.

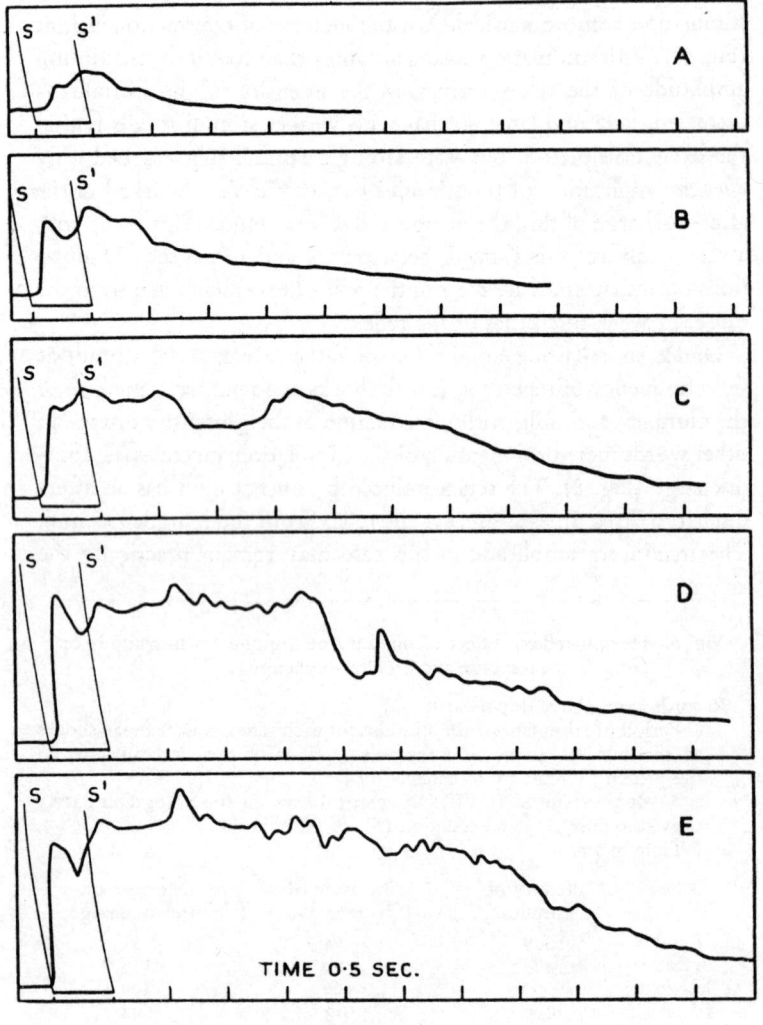

Fig. 7

After-Discharge in Crossed Extension-Reflex

same, the later stimuli simply prolonging the maximum without increasing it. They prolong it for a far greater time than their own delivery prolongs the stimulation time.

In the scratch-reflex, likewise, intensity increases the after-discharge (Fig. 9). Its after-discharge is rhythmic, a clonus like the rest of the reflex, with the slight lengthening of duration and sequence of the terminal beats that is characteristic of this reflex. The after-discharge from the scratch-reflex is not usually so prolonged as that from a flexion-reflex produced by a stimulus of like length and intensity (Fig. 10). Six to nine beats usually complete the after-discharge.

In the spinal dog there is a reflex of the hind-limb in which a movement of extension at knee, ankle, and hip is caused by stimulation of the skin of the contralateral hind-limb—the 'crossed extension-reflex'. When this reflex is provoked with more than a certain intensity its after-discharge becomes a feature of extraordinary prominence, both as regards degree of contraction and duration. This after-discharge may then be more intense than any other part of the reflex, and may persist, gradually declining for 10 or 15 sec. (Fig. 27). Wundt[69] and Biedermann[204] have noted that in the cooled frog the duration of the reflex after-discharge is prolonged.

Fig. 7. Flexion-reflex. Effect of increasing strength of stimulus on latent period, magnitude of response and after-discharge

The vertical arcs on the myograph curves show the onset (S) and cessation (S^1) of afferent stimulation.
Time in 0·5 sec.
Flexion-reflex elicited by 10 break shocks at rate of 20 per sec., i.e. stimulation lasting 0·5 sec. Intensity of stimuli increased by bringing secondary coil toward primary.

		Stimulus	Whole reflex	After-discharge
Top reflex	A	30	12	9
Next reflex	B	45	52	43
Next reflex	C	65	130	118
Next reflex	D	85	176	158
Bottom reflex	E	100	258	236

The intensity of stimulus is given in units of the Kronecker inductorium.
The amount of reflex is measured by the area between the myograph curve and the base-line.

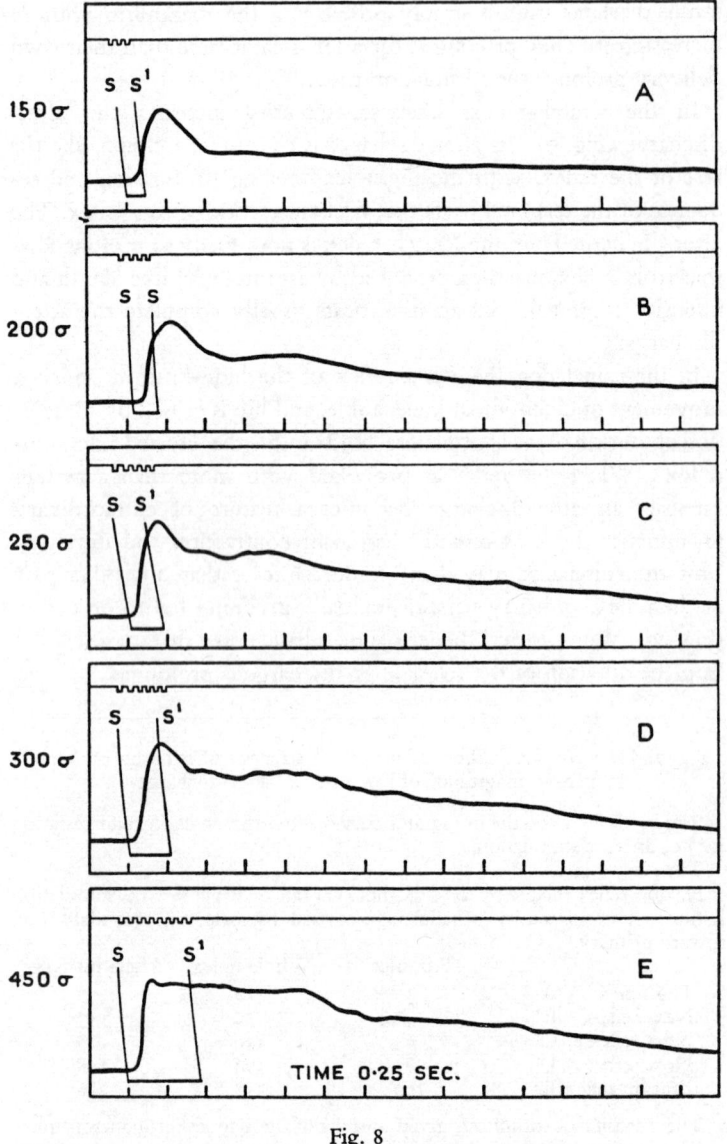

Fig. 8

After-Discharge

There is no feature of the conduction of a reflex-arc which distinguishes its mechanism more universally from that of a mere nerve-fibre tract or trunk than lengthy after-discharge. Richet[98] has paradoxically applied to this feature the old adage modified: "Sublata causa, non tollitur effectus." The after-discharge can, however, be cut short sharply by *inhibition*; it seems also to re-manifest itself sometimes after a passing interruption by inhibition.

The long latency and the marked after-discharge of reflex-conduction easily explain a phenomenon often met when studying reflexes provoked by stimuli that are brief, especially if they be also weak. The stimulus, though it may last for a good many sigmata, is over and past ere the reflex-response appears (Fig. 9). That response, when it appears, may nevertheless endure for 1000σ or more. There is nothing closely comparable with this in the conduction of nerve-trunks.

The after-discharge of a reflex may be considered analogous to a *positive* after-image left by a visual stimulus. The analogy is suggestive

---

Fig. 8. Flexion-reflex; 'spinal dog'. Effect of prolongation of exciting stimulation

Records from above downwards:
  Electromagnet recording the number of stimuli employed.
  Myograph curves: the vertical arcs show onset (S) and cessation (S^1) of afferent stimulation.
  Time in 0·25 sec.

The circular key rotating at constant speed interrupted the primary circuit of an inductorium, the break shocks of which were delivered through a needle electrode (kathode) to the plantar skin of the outermost digit. An adjustable spring rheotome allowed the desired number of interruptions in the primary, and therefore the desired number of break shocks in the exciting circuit when that was unshort-circuited. Three of the successive stimuli elicited the uppermost reflex, four the next, five the next, six the next, and nine the lowest. The 'after-discharge' is seen to be increased by mere prolongation of the stimulus within these limits. The frequency of the stimuli remained in all cases 20 per sec., and their intensity was the same for all the reflexes.

Duration of stimulus	Measure of reflex	Measure of after-discharge
A 150σ	20	19
B 200σ	37	34
C 250σ	53	47
D 300σ	58	49
E 450σ	70	58

The Simple Reflex

in connexion with others to be drawn between spinal and visual phenomena.

Conduction along reflex-arcs presents in contrast to that along nerve-trunks characters that may be figuratively described as indicating inertia and momentum. It is as though in the case of a weight to be pulled from a position of rest the tractive force were applied through a rigid rod in nerve-trunk conduction, but through a relatively yielding elastic band in reflex-arc conduction. But there are other differences between the two forms of conduction which this simple simile does not figure. We have to enter on such in our next lecture.

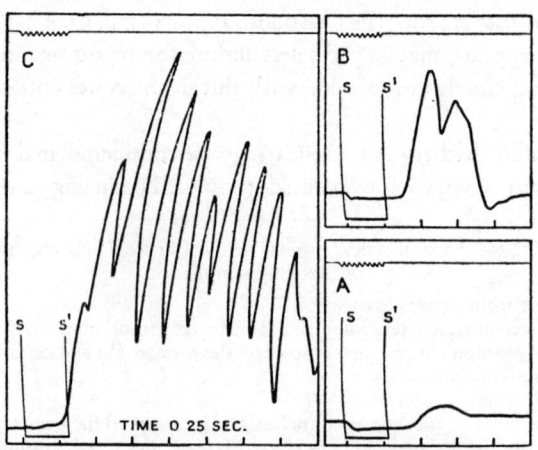

Fig. 9. Scratch-reflex. Effect of intensity of stimulus on response

Records from above downwards in A, B, C:

    Period of stimulation: the interruptions of the electromagnet in the primary circuit are recorded.

    Myograph curve: the onset (S) and cessation (S^1) of the stimulus are marked by the vertical arcs.

    Time in 0·25 sec.

Stimulus is 9 break shocks at rate of 25 per sec. delivered to a point in the scapular skin by unipolar faradization, the stigmatic electrode being the kathode. A, the stimulus is very weak: one small beat of characteristic slowness is evoked after a long latent period; B, increase in intensity of shocks with resulting shorter latent time and a reflex movement of two feeble beats; C, further increase of intensity of stimulus: the latent time is shorter, and a reflex of ten fairly quick and ample beats ensues. The stimulus lasted less than 0·5 sec.; the reflex is not completed for more than 2 sec. after cessation of the stimulus.

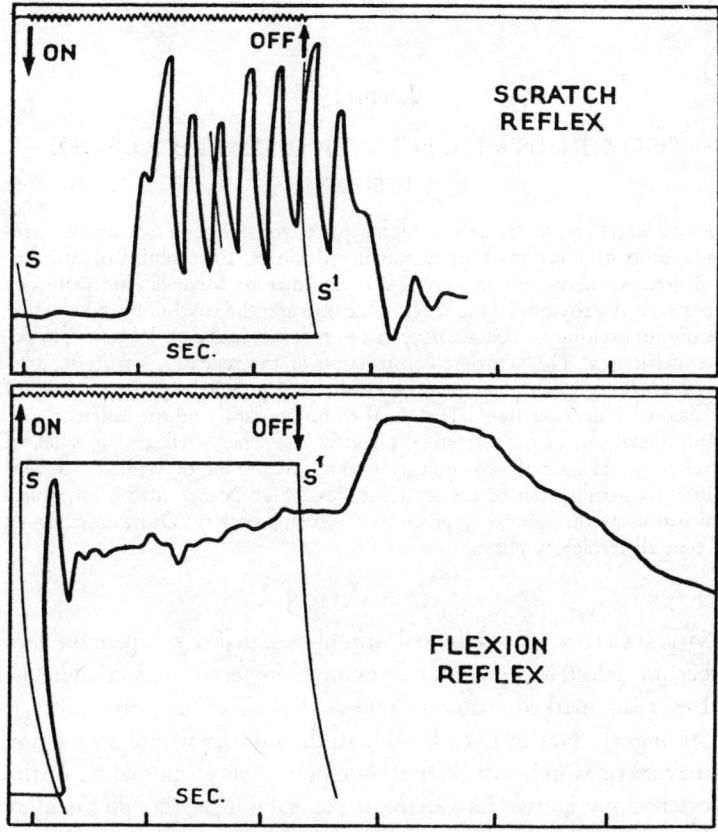

Fig. 10. Comparison of scratch-reflex and flexion-reflex provoked by similar stimulation in the same animal in quick succession

Records from above downwards for scratch-reflex (above) and flexion-reflex (below):
  Period of stimulation. An electromagnet in the primary circuit records the interruptions giving the shocks.
  Myograph curve: the vertical arcs show the onset (S) and cessation (S^1) of stimulation (also shown by the arrows ON and OFF).
  Time in sec.

Stimulation was unipolar faradization with 45 break shocks; the kathode was stigmatic and applied to the shoulder skin for scratch-reflex, to the fourth toe for flexion-reflex; diffuse electrode on fore-foot. Frequency of shocks, 18 per sec. The after-discharge of the scratch-reflex lasted barely 1 sec.; that of the flexion, nearly 8 sec.

Lecture II
CO-ORDINATION IN THE SIMPLE REFLEX
(continued)

ARGUMENT: Reflex-arcs show high capacity for summing excitations. Irreversibility of direction of conduction in reflex-arcs. Reversibility of direction of conduction in certain nerve-nets, e.g. that of Medusa. Independence between the rhythm of the reflex-discharge and the rhythm of the external stimulus exciting it. Refractory phase in reflexes; in the eyelid-reflex; in the scratch-reflex. The neuronic construction of the reflex-arc of the scratch-reflex. Long descending *proprio-spinal* tracts revealed by the method of 'successive degeneration'. The 'final common path' and the 'afferent arc'. Intraspinal seat of the refractory phase of the scratch-reflex. The value of refractory phase in the co-ordination of the swimming of Medusa. Its value in the co-ordination of the scratch-reflex. Significance of the intraspinal situation of the refractory phase of the scratch-reflex. Other instances of 'central' refractory phase.

SUMMATION

SUMMATION of subliminal stimuli so that by repetition they become effective is practically unknown in nerve-trunk conduction. But it is a marked feature of reflex-arc conduction (Setschenow,[31] Stirling[57]). Nor is it attributable to the muscles whose contraction may serve as index of the reflex-response, since summation of this extent is not known for vertebrate skeletal muscle, though found by Richet[98] in the claw-muscle of the crayfish.

We find striking instances of the summation of subliminal stimuli given by the scratch-reflex. The difficulty in exciting a reflex by a single-induction shock is well known. A scratch-reflex cannot in my experience be elicited by a single-induction shock, or even by two shocks, unless as physiological stimuli they are very intense and delivered less than 600σ apart. Although the strongest single-induction shock is therefore by itself a subliminal stimulus for this reflex, the summating power of this reflex mechanism is great. Very feeble shocks, each succeeding the other within a certain time—summation time—sum as stimuli and provoke a reflex. Thus long series of subliminal stimuli ultimately provoke the reflex. I have

Summation

records where the reflex appeared only after delivery of the fortieth successive double shock, the shocks having followed each other at a frequency of 11·3 per sec., and where the reflex appeared only after delivery of the forty-fourth successive make shock, the shocks having followed at 18 per sec. A momentary stimulus, e.g., a break shock of fair physiological strength applied by a stigmatic pole (needle point) to a skin-spot in the receptive field of this reflex, produces in the nervous arc a change which though, as just said, unable of itself alone to produce the reflex movement, shows its facilitating influence (*bahnung*) on a subsequent stimulus applied even 1400σ later. The duration of the excitatory change induced by a momentary stimulus is therefore in this mammalian arc (scratch-reflex) almost as long as that noted in the frog by Stirling, namely, 1500σ.

With serial stimuli of the same frequency of repetition the latent time of the scratch-reflex is shorter the more intense the individual stimuli. Stirling[57] conclusively traced length of latency to dependence on spinal summation of successive excitations. In accord with this in the 'scratch-reflex', when the serial stimuli follow slowly, the reflex *ceteris paribus* is prolonged. A single brief mechanical stimulation of the skin (rub, prick, or pull upon a hair) usually succeeds in exciting a scratch-reflex, though the reflex thus evoked is short; but there is nothing to show that these stimuli, though brief, are really simple and not essentially multiple. A striking dissimilarity, therefore, between reflex-arc conduction and nerve-trunk conduction is that in reflex-arc conduction considerable resistance is offered to the passage of a single nerve-impulse, but the resistance is easily forced by a succession of impulses; in other words, subliminal stimuli are summed.

It follows almost as a corollary from this that the threshold excitability of a reflex mechanism appears much more variable than that of a nerve-trunk, if the threshold excitability be measured in terms of the intensity of the liminal stimulus. The value will be more variable in the case of the reflex mechanism, because there the duration of the stimulus is a factor in its efficiency far more than in the case of the nerve-trunk. In the scratch-reflex a single stimulus which is far below threshold intensity is found, on its fortieth repetition and nearly 4 sec. after its first application, to become effective and provoke the reflex.

IRREVERSIBILITY OF DIRECTION OF CONDUCTION

Another remarkable difference between reflex-arc conduction and nerve-trunk conduction is the irreversibility of direction of the former and the reversibility of the latter. Double conduction, as it has been termed, is well established for nerve-trunks both afferent and efferent. It was shown by du Bois Reymond for the spinal nerve roots, for peripheral nerves by Kuhne's gracilis experiment, for the great single electric fibre of *Malapterurus* by Babuchin,[73] for sympathetic nerve-cords by Langley & Anderson,[150] and by myself[171] for certain fibres of the white tracts of the spinal cord. The nerve-fibres in all these cases, when excited anywhere in their course, conduct nerve-impulses in all directions from the point stimulated; that is, in their case both up and down, the only two directions open to them. Their substance may therefore be regarded as conductive in all directions along their extension.

From the Bell-Magendie law of the spinal nerve-roots we know that reflex-arcs conduct only in one direction. The stimulation of the central end of a motor-nerve remains without obvious effect. Bell[10] and Magendie[11] and their followers established that excitation of the spinal end of the severed motor root evokes no sign of reflex action or sensation. Evidently the central nexus between afferent channel and efferent is of a kind that, though it allows conduction from afferent to efferent, does not allow it from efferent to afferent. The path is patent in one direction only. This is the special case which forms the first foundation of the law that conduction in the neural system proceeds in one direction only, the 'law of forward direction' (W. James (1880)[82]). When the property of double conduction in nerve-fibres had been ascertained, the Bell-Magendie law of the spinal roots became more instructive. Gad[102] (1884) argued that the dendrites of the motor root-cell are capable of conduction in one direction only, namely, toward and not away from the axone. It

Reversibility of Conduction in Medusa

may, however, be that the irreciprocity of the conduction is referable to the synapse. The explanation of the valved condition of the reflex circuit may lie in a synaptic membrane more permeable in one direction than in the other. In other words, though intraneuronic conduction is reversible in direction, interneuronic may be irreversible.

Cell-chains of polarized conduction form the basis of the great majority of all the nervous reactions of the cerebrospinal system of higher animals. It appears, however, that not *all* pluricellular nervous circuits exhibit irreversible direction of conduction. The nerve-net of Medusa is a pluricellular conductor which exhibits reversibility of direction of conduction. In Medusa locomotion is effected by contraction of a sheet of muscle in the swimming-bell. When the swimming-bell, which resembles an inverted cup, contracts, its capacity is lessened, and some of the water embraced by it is expelled through the open end, the animal itself being propelled in the reverse direction by recoil. The mechanism is like that of the heart, but the heart propels its contents, the swimming-bell propels itself against its contents. The contractions of both recur rhythmically, though Medusa, unlike the heart, has periods of prolonged diastolic inactivity. At such a period an appropriate stimulus restarts the swimming-bell. The contractile beat begins from the point stimulated and spreads thence over the whole muscular sheet. 72 It spreads rapidly enough for the contraction not to have culminated at the initial point before it has set in at the most remote part. The beat is thus not only everywhere in progress at the same time, but is practically in the same phase of progress everywhere, and similarly synchronously passes off.72

The arrangement of the nervous system of Medusa, e.g. *Rhizostoma*, is, according to Bethe, of the following kind (Fig. 11). The nerve-cell has on one hand threadlike arms that extend to the surface of the sub-umbrella, and on the other hand others which stretch down to the sheet of contractile cells on the underside of the bell. Each nerve-cell has also long side threads which join similar side threads from other nerve-cells. By virtue of these lateral connexions the nerve-cells form a network of conductors spreading horizontally

The Simple Reflex

through the bell in a layer of tissue between a receptive sheet and a contractile sheet. From this nerve-net, throughout its extent, there pass nerve-threads to the adjacent muscle; it also receives at many

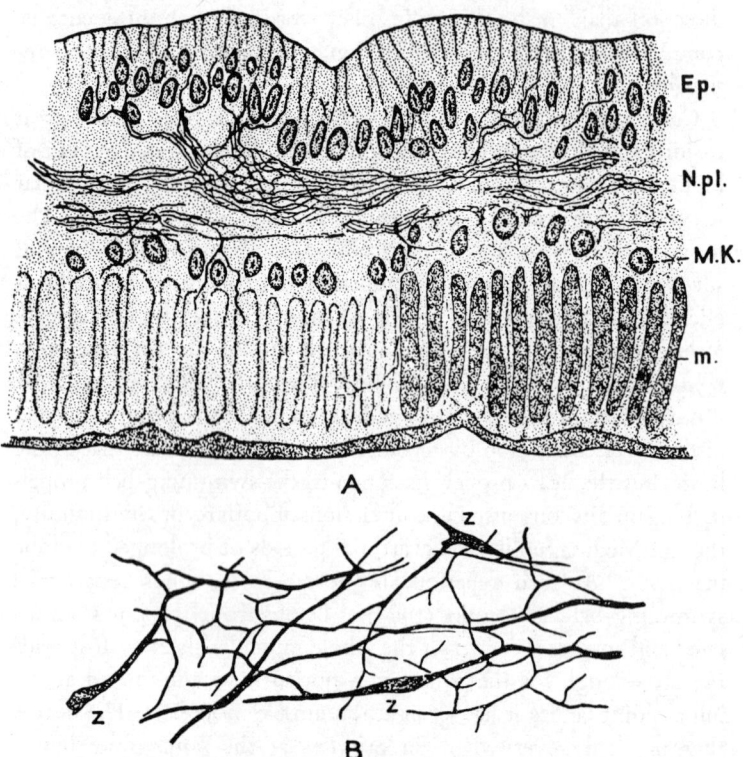

Fig. 11 (A. Bethe 268). Nerve-net of *Rhizostoma*

A, radial section through a muscular field of the sub-umbrella; *Ep*, epithelium; *m*, muscle-fibres in cross-section; *M.K.*, their nuclei; *N.pl.*, nerve-plexus with fibres running into the epithelium and to the muscles.

B, nerve-plexus with scattered cells, from a horizontal section.
Magnification 1200 in A, 200 in B.

points of its extent nerve-threads from specially receptive areas of surface.

The circularly arranged sheet of muscle does not form a continuous field toward the centre of the disk; there are wide radial gaps

Nerve-Net of Medusa

in it. Across these gaps the 'conduction' passes: the microscope reveals no muscular tissue in these gaps, but the nerve-net can be seen to spread across them.263 The presence of the nerve-net explains the conduction across them. It is therefore argued by Bethe that the spread of the contraction over the muscular sheet in *Rhizostoma* does not imply conduction of the contraction from one muscle-cell to another, but is the result of the spread of nervous action over the nerve-network. In its progress along the nerve-net, the nervous discharge, as it reaches each part of the nerve-net, spreads down the nerve-threads, descending thence to the underlying muscle-sheet. So long as the nerve-cell network is intact, *wherever* the point stimulated, the ensuing contraction is of the *whole* bell, that is, the nerve-impulses started at one point of the receptive surface, on entering the nerve-network, spread over it in all directions. When the bell-shaped disk is spirally cut into a long band, to whichever end of the band the stimulus be applied, the conduction spreads from that end to the other and over the whole strip (Romanes72). The nerve-net therefore conducts nerve-impulses in both directions along its length. Therefore it is not a polarized conductor, conductive in one direction only. In the chains of nerve-cells of higher animals, such as Arthropods and Vertebrates, although the conduction is reversible in each nerve-cell—at least along that piece of it which forms a nerve-fibre—the pluricellular chain *in toto* constitutes a polarized conductor, conductive in one direction only. In such cell-chains the individual nerve-cells are characterized morphologically by possessing two kinds of cell-branches, which differ one from another in microscopic form, the one kind *dendrites*, the other *axones*. The difference in appearance between *dendrites* and *axones* is marked enough for recognition by microscopical inspection. Since in many well-known instances the dendrites conduct impulses away from their free ends, while the axone conducts towards its free end, it is possible on mere microscopic inspection of nerve-cells of this type to infer by analogy the normal direction of the conduction through the nerve-cell. But in the nerve-cells forming the nerve-network of Medusa there seems no such distinct differentiation of their branches into two types. Their cell-processes are not distinguishable into dendrites and axones.

The Simple Reflex

Moreover, microscopic examination of the nerve-net of Medusa reveals another difference between it and the nerve-cell chains of higher animals. In these latter the neuro-fibrils of one nerve-cell are not found unbrokenly continuous with those of the next cell along the nerve-chain. Although the union may be close, there is not homogeneous continuity. The one nerve-cell joins another by synapsis. But in the nerve-net of Medusa the neuro-fibrils pass, according to Bethe, uninterruptedly across from one cell to another. Even if we admit the neuro-fibrils to be in a measure artifacts, the appearance of their continuity from one cell to another in one type, and of their discontinuity from one cell to another in the other type remains significant of a difference between the conduction-process from cell to cell in the two types. The nerve-net of Medusa appears an unbroken retiform continuum from end to end. Each nerve-cell in it joins its neighbours much as at a node in the myelinate nerve-fibre the axis-cylinder of each segment joins the next. Reversibility of conduction may be related to this apparent continuity of structure, and irreversibility to want of it. This points to the latter being referable to the synapse; if the *synaptic membrane* (Lect. I, p. 17) be permeable only in one direction to certain ions, that may explain the irreversibility of conduction. The polarized conduction of nerve-arcs would be related to the one-sided permeability of the intestinal wall, e.g. to NaCl (O. Cohnheim).

RHYTHM OF RESPONSE

One of the differences between nerve-trunk conduction and reflex-arc conduction is the less close correspondence in the latter between rhythm of stimulus and rhythm of end-effect. The number of separable excitatory states (impulses) engendered in a nerve-trunk by serially repeated stimuli corresponds closely with the stimuli in number and rhythm. Whether the stimuli follow each other once per sec. or 500 times per sec., the nervous responses follow the rhythm of stimulation. Using contraction of skeletal muscle as index of the response the correspondence at rhythms above 30 per sec. becomes difficult to trace, because the mechanical effects tend at

Stimulus Rhythm and Rhythm Response

rates beyond that to fuse indistinguishably. The electrical responses of the muscle can with ease be observed isolatedly up to faster rates: their rhythm is found to agree with that of stimulation; thus, at 80 per sec. their responses are 80 per sec. If the muscle note be accepted as an indication of the response of the muscle, its pitch follows *pari passu* the rate of stimulation of the nerve through a still greater range.

The case is quite different with reflex-arcs. Schäfer[206] noted undulations of a frequency of 10–12 per sec. on myograms of spinal reflexes evoked by excitation of the afferent nerve by faradic currents of frequency much above 10–12 per sec. In such a case we may assume the absence in the afferent nerve itself of any refractory period long enough to give a 10 per sec. rhythm to the response. The refractory period in nerve-trunk conduction seems to last not longer than 1σ. The rhythm of discharge from the motor-cell, as far as the undulations noted indicate rhythmic response, are totally different in rhythm from that of the action induced in the afferent cell by the stimulation applied. In the reflex centre the rhythm has been transmuted from one rate to another. Schäfer refers this change to the synapse.

Again, as noted above, undulations at rates varying between 7·5 and 12 per sec. are seen in the flexion-reflex both in its after-discharge and during the excitation and quite independently of the rate of delivery of the induction shocks used as stimuli (Figs. 6, 12), and even when the stimulus is a constant current. Again, reflexes of weak intensity, both in the case of the flexion-reflex and of the crossed extension-reflex, exhibit at their commencement a stepped form of myogram: the steps usually succeed each other at about 8 per sec., and their rate is independent of the rate of delivery of the electric stimuli (Fig. 12) exciting the reflex.

In such cases, therefore, the rhythm of the end-effect indicates that in transmission along the reflex-arc the impulses generated at the receptive end of the arc are not actually passed on from one cell element to another in the arc, but that new impulses with a different period are generated in the course of the reflex-conduction. This is confirmatory of a neurone-threshold as a feature in central conduction.

The Simple Reflex

REFRACTORY PHASE

A conductor which replies intermittently to a stimulus exhibits a refractory phase. It seems that even in nerve-trunk conduction a refractory phase must occur; otherwise, the conductor being capable of reversible direction of conduction, a backward propagation of the excited state as well as a forward would ensue from every point of the conductor reached by the nervous impulse. The excited state would then, when once excited, maintain itself in a tetanic manner along the whole length of the conductor. The propagation would thus lose undulatory character such as we know it has; it would merely have an initial wave-front. But this refractory phase in nerve-fibres seems of very brief duration, not longer than 1σ.

The reflex-discharge from nerve-cells seems to be rhythmic even under continuous stimulation; but the cases in which this has been examined are sparse. The existence of rhythm in nerve-cell discharge is presumptive evidence of a refractory phase in their reaction. Refractory phase was first called attention to by Kronecker and Stirling[55] in 1874, in the heart, and recognized by them as a fact of central importance for cardiac rhythm. In 1876 Marey[67] met the same phenomenon and gave it the name by which it is now known. A year later Romanes' fundamental work on Medusa demonstrated

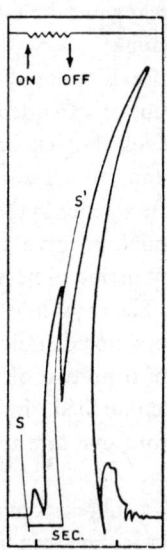

Fig. 12. Flexion-reflex showing imperfect fusion under excitation of the skin with break-shocks at the rate of 10 per sec.

Records from above downwards are:
  Period of stimulus showing six interruptions of the primary circuit (beginning and end of stimulation indicated by arrows ON and OFF).
  Myograph record: the vertical arcs show onset (S) and cessation (S^1) of stimulation.
  Time in sec.

Refractory Phase

the existence of the same phenomenon there.[72] The inconspicuous duration of the phase in nerve-trunk conduction and the progress of the view that regards the heart beat as of myogenic origin have contributed to delay recognition of refractory phase as a character of reflex-arc reactions. But in 1899 Zwaardemaker & Lans[198] showed the supervention of a refractory phase in reflex eyelid-closure. By refractory period was originally meant by Marey the time during which the heart was inexcitable to a stimulus however intense. But to-day by refractory phase is understood a state during which, apart from fatigue, the mechanism shows less than its full excitability. The cardiac refractory phase is absolute for a short time after commencement of systole, but excitability then returns gradually. In the eyelid-reflex for nearly a full second after initiation of a reflex, the chance that a second stimulus then delivered will, though otherwise appropriate, excite the reflex, is 50 per cent less than it is one second later. The refractory phase, therefore, is marked though not absolute: it operates longer for a visual stimulus than for a tactual or thermal.

Of the spinal reflexes of the dog's hind-limb, one, namely, the scratch-reflex, shows marked refractory phase.[287] When working originally with this reflex, I noticed (with Laslett)[251] that the rhythm of the scratching movement is in rate independent of the rhythm of the stimulus evoking it.

In the dog, when the spinal cord has been transected in the neck, the scratch or scalptor reflex becomes in a few months prominent. A stimulus applied at any point within a large saddle-shaped field of skin (Fig. 13) excites a scratching movement of the hind-leg. The movement is rhythmic alternate flexion and extension at hip, knee, and ankle. Each flexion recurs at a frequency of about four times per sec. The stimuli provocative[252] of it are mechanical, such as tickling the skin or pulling lightly on a hair. The receptive nerve-endings which generate the reflex lie in the surface layer of the skin, about the roots of the hairs. A convenient way of exciting the reflex is by feeble faradization, such as applied to one's own tongue is felt as a tickling sensation. For exciting the reflex electrically, I place a broad diffuse electrode on some indifferent part of the surface outside the receptive field of skin, and apply a stigmatic electrode to some

The Simple Reflex

point in the saddle-shaped area of dorsal skin. This electrode may consist of a minute needle, or a gilt entomological pin; it is inserted

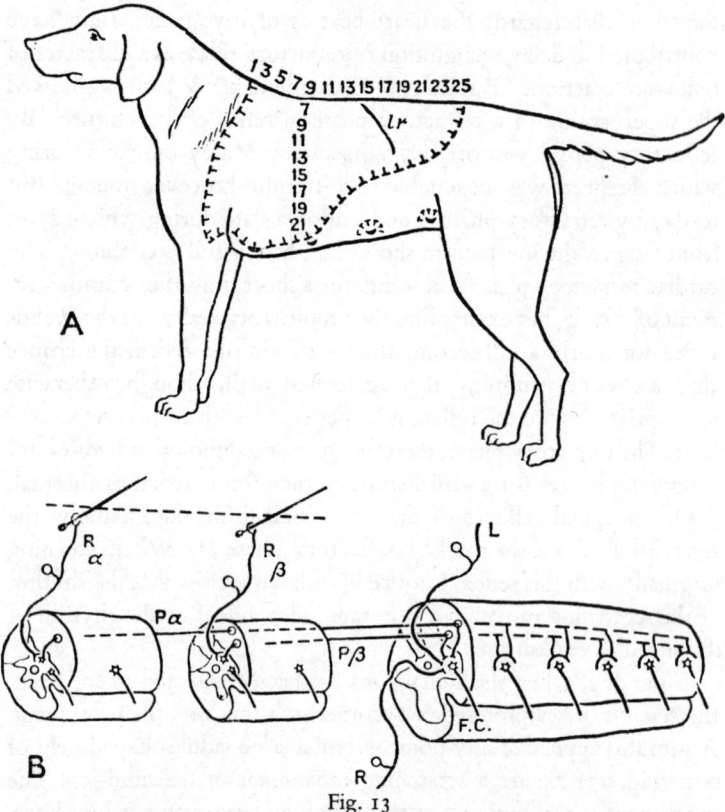

Fig. 13

A. The 'receptive field', as revealed after low cervical transection, a saddle-shaped area of dorsal skin, whence the scratch-reflex of the left hind-limb can be evoked. *lr* marks the position of the last rib.

B. Diagram of the spinal arcs involved. *L*, receptive or afferent nerve-path from the left foot; *R*, receptive nerve-path from the opposite foot; *Rα, Rβ*, receptive nerve-paths from hairs in the dorsal skin of the left side; *FC*, the final common path, in this case the motor neurone to a flexor muscle of the hip; *Pα, Pβ*, proprio-spinal neurones.

in the skin so lightly that its point just lies among the hair bulbs. If it be pushed further, other types of reflex may be produced and the scratch-reflex be inhibited. Prominent among the muscles active in

Refractory Phase in Scratch-Reflex

this reflex are the dorsi-flexors of the ankle, the flexors of the knee, and the flexors of the hip. If the rhythm of the last is recorded graphically, tracings,[300] as in Fig. 14, are obtained. It is then demonstrable that the series of brief contractions succeed one another at a rate the frequency of which is independent of that of the stimulation. Thus, the rhythmic reflex is elicitable by the application of a heat-beam or a constant current. The make and break of the current are especially able to excite it (Fig. 15), but it is for a time maintained even by the continued passage of the current, though it lapses in intensity until the current is broken, when it appears temporarily with renewed vigour. At make and break of the voltaic current the reflex-response is a short series of rhythmic flexions.

The reflex is still more easily evoked by unipolar application of high frequency currents; it can be evoked with great vigour and long duration by this mode of stimulation. Double-induction shocks applied at frequencies from once per sec. to 512 times per sec. and at various intermediate rates all evoke it easily; so likewise do single break or make shocks applied at rates varying in my experiments between 1·33 times per sec. and 40 times per sec.

Under all these various methods of excitation (heat-beam, constant current, double and single induced currents, high frequency currents, and mechanical stimuli) the rhythm of the flexor response remains—so long as the internal conditions of the reflex remain unaltered—almost the same.[287] It remains so also when, instead of a regular succession, a grouped succession of stimuli is used for excitation, e.g. stimuli grouped in twos and threes. It is obvious that this reflex exhibits *a refractory phase*. Take the instance where the stimulus applied consists of double-induction shocks, succeeding each other at a frequency of 100 per sec. The reflex-arc in response produces flexion at hip about four times per sec. So few as three successive double-induction shocks will suffice to excite the reflex, but since in the instance taken about twenty such shocks correspond in time with each flexor beat, and each such beat is divisible into about equal periods of contraction and relaxation, let us make the assumption—a liberal one—that ten out of the twenty available shocks are serving as stimuli. The arc, while the following ten are being applied, fails in

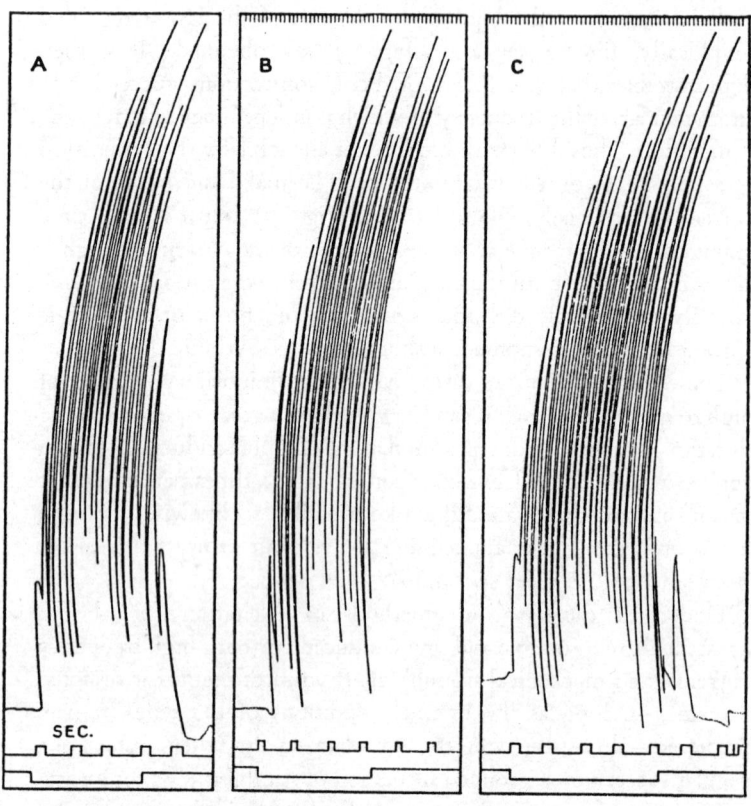

Fig. 14. Flexion of the hip in the 'scratch-reflex' of a 'spinal dog'

Records from above downwards:
    An electric signal marks (in B and C only) the double induction shocks delivered.
    Myographic curve.
    Time in sec.
    Signal line: descent of the signal marks onset of application of the stimulus.

In A the reflex is evoked by lightly rubbing the skin at a point behind the shoulder, in B and C by unipolar faradization with weak double-induction shocks applied to the same point of skin through a needle point lightly inserted among the hair roots.

Rhythm of Scratch-Reflex

spite of them to excite the flexor muscles. To those ten it does not respond at all.

Nor can this refractory state be overcome by simply increasing the intensity of the stimuli. The reflex remains as perfectly rhythmic and clonic under the strongest stimuli as under weaker (Fig. 16). The frequency of the beats is under strong stimulation often somewhat

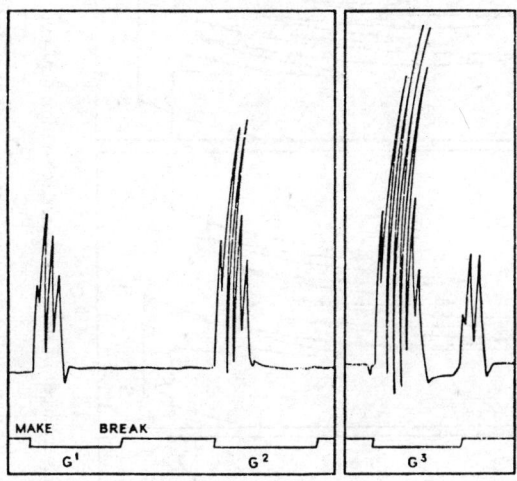

Fig. 15. Scratch-reflex evoked by a galvanic current with the kathode at a spot of skin behind the shoulder and a diffuse anode applied to the forepaw

Records from above downwards:
    Myograph curve.
    Signal line: the descent of the signal represents the 'make' and the ascent the 'break' of the stimulating galvanic current.

The make of the current excites a stronger reflex than the break; the break with the two weaker strengths of current G^1 and G^2 did not suffice to excite the reflex at all; but in G^3 it did. Current in G^3 was 1·5 mA.

higher than under quite weak, especially at outset of the reflex, but the difference is small, e.g. 5·8 beats per sec. instead of 4·5 beats per sec. No mode or intensity of stimulation to which I have had recourse converts rhythmic clonic beat into a maintained steady contraction. In this respect, as in certain others, the scalptor reflex-arc closely resembles in its behaviour the mechanism of the Medusa

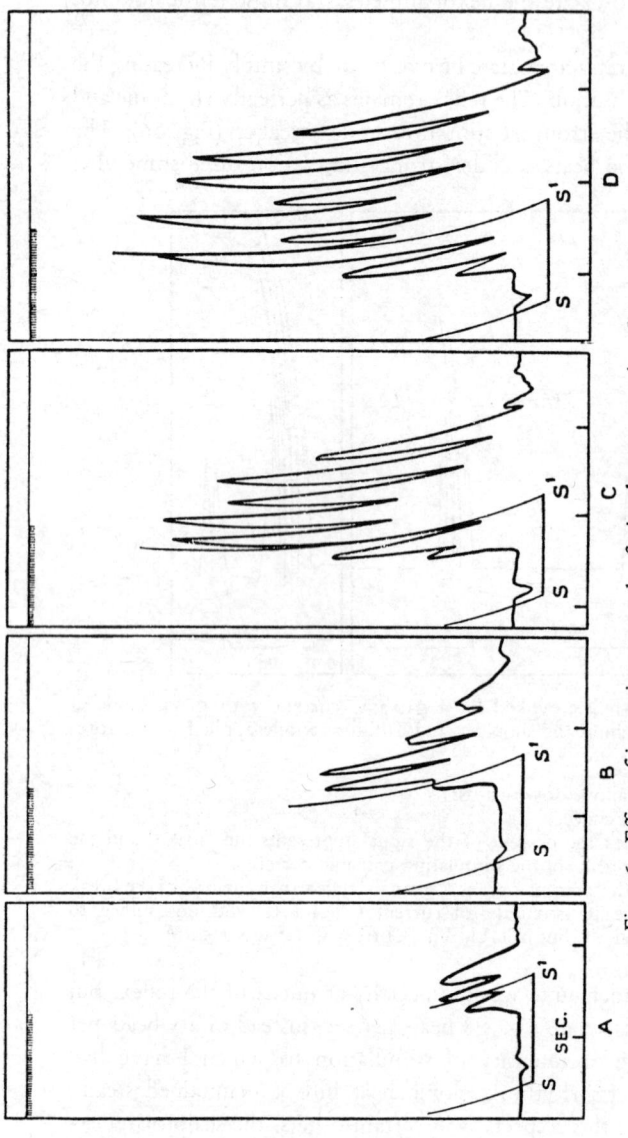

Fig. 16. Effect of increasing strength of stimulus on scratch-reflex response

Records from above downwards:

Signal line: the interruptions in the primary circuit of the stimulating current are recorded by an electromagnet.
Myograph curve. The onset (S) and cessation (S') of the stimulus are indicated by the vertical arcs.
Time in sec.

Scratch-reflex, provoked by 42 break shocks delivered at the rate of 40 per sec. As the stimulus is without other change rendered more and more intense at 690, 1100, 1900 and 3000 units of the Kronecker scale respectively, the reflexes A, B, C, D show the differences seen. Instead of one beat during the stimulus and two afterwards, as in A, the reflex gives three beats during the stimulus and six beats afterwards, as in D.

Neurone Arc of Scratch-Reflex

bell and heart-wall. It resembles these more closely than it resembles the mammalian respiratory reflex-arc, which can under several circumstances be made to produce from the diaphragm an enduring tetanic contraction.

I refer to the contraction of the flexor muscles in the sculptor-reflex as a 'beat', not implying that it is a single twitch, but rather because the term denotes a short-lasting phase of action in a rhythmic series, and because of its close analogy to the beat of Medusa and of the heart.

What is the neuronic construction of the arc in the sculptor-reflex? The reflex is in a sense unilateral; stimulation of the left shoulder evokes scratching by the left leg, not the right. Search in the spinal cord[251] for the paths of the reflex demonstrates that a lesion breaking through one lateral half of the cord anywhere between shoulder and leg abolishes the ability of the skin of that shoulder to excite the scratch-reflex, but leaves intact the reflex of the opposite shoulder. In the lateral half of the spinal cord which the reflex-path descends, severance of the dorsal column does not obviously interfere with the reflex; nor does the severance of the ventral and the dorsal columns together of that side; no more does severance of the grey matter in addition. But severance of the lateral part of the lateral column itself permanently abolishes the conduction of the reflex; and it does so even if all the other parts of the transverse extent of the cord remain intact. The paths of the reflex, therefore, descend the lateral part of the lateral column. These details help towards construction of the reflex-arc involved. For in the lateral part of the lateral column, as shown by the method of *successive degeneration*, lie long *proprio-spinal* fibres which directly connect the grey matter of the spinal segments of the shoulder with the spinal segments containing the motor neurones for the flexor muscles of the hip, and knee, and ankle. The course of the descending *proprio-spinal* fibres can be traced and their number counted. The method of 'successive degeneration'[251] enables one to unravel them from descending fibres of other sources, such as cerebral, mesencephalic, or bulbar, and from proprio-spinal fibres descending from the foremost segments of the neck. This is done—as the term 'successive degeneration' implies—in a preliminary

The Simple Reflex

lesion by severing that part of the spinal cord it is desired to examine for the particular proprio-spinal fibres sought, from all the central nervous system lying farther forward. To determine the propriospinal fibres descending from the third and fourth thoracic segments, the first step is to transect the cord between the second and third thoracic segments. There then ensues throughout the length of the cord behind that transection degeneration of all the fibres that enter it from the brain, mid-brain, bulb, and cervical and first two thoracic segments. This heavy degeneration, after developing, reaches a maximum and gradually passes away, all the debris of the degenerated nerve-fibres being in time removed. For this a period of a year suffices in a dog. The spinal cord is then ripe for determination of the proprio-spinal fibres it is desired to examine. It becomes once more a clean slate on which a new degeneration can be written. The proprio-spinal fibres are revealed by making a transection between the fourth and fifth thoracic segments. Four weeks after this second lesion the proprio-spinal fibres descending from the third and fourth thoracic segments are degenerate. They can be studied (Fig. 17) throughout their course from the fourth thoracic segments backwards along the cord by any of the ordinary methods, such as the Marchi method, for studying degenerate fibres. Many of these proprio-spinal fibres pass from the shoulder segments to end in the hind-limb segments. The existence of the neuroglial scar, left by old degeneration that has cleared up, far from complicating the tracing of the new degeneration assists by forming a contrast background to it, the sharpness of which leaves nothing to be desired.

From the results obtained by this method the following reflex-chain can be inferred[251] as possible and probable for the scratch-reflex.

1. The receptive neurone (Fig. 13, B, $R\alpha$) from the skin to the spinal grey matter of the corresponding spinal segment in the shoulder.

2. The long descending proprio-spinal neurone (Fig. 13, B, $P\alpha$) from shoulder segment to the grey matter of the leg segments.

3. The motor neurone (Fig. 13, B, FC) from the spinal segment of the leg to a flexor muscle.

Locus of Refractory State

This chain thus consists of three neurones. It enters the grey matter twice; that is, it has two neuronic junctions, two synapses. It is a *disynaptic* arc.

In venturing to thus schematically express the construction of this arc as disynaptic, I am influenced by the desire to express its construction as simply as possible so far as consistent with the ascertained data of the case. I therefore omit from the scheme the possible Schalt-Zellen (v. Monakow) between $R\alpha$ and $P\alpha$, and between $P\alpha$ and FC. Much of what I intend to express by 'disynaptic' would be as clearly though not as concisely expressed by saying that grey matter is intercalated in the arc twice i.e. at two separate places. That, however, is not expressible by a single adjective, and since synapses occur so far as we know only in grey matter, disynaptic does include that idea. But it also implies somewhat more. I venture upon it in spite of the assumptions it includes because, in my opinion, much in those further assumptions seems justifiable and useful as a working hypothesis, and because it lays stress on the importance of the synapse in reflex conduction—an importance which for reasons given before seems considerable.

The reflex-arc consists, therefore, of at least three neurones. It is convenient to have a term distinguishing the ultimate neurone FC from the rest of the arc. For reasons to be given later it may be spoken of as the *final common path*.300 The rest of the arc leading up to the final common path is conveniently termed *the afferent arc*.

The morphological components of this reflex mechanism include, in addition to the above neural elements, the muscle-fibres of the flexor muscle at one end, and possibly a receptive cutaneous organ at the other end probably in the root-sheath of a hair. Somewhere in this chain of structures the property of refractory phase has its seat, and refractory phase is a pivot on which the whole co-ordinating mechanism of this reflex turns.

In attempting to locate the seat of the refractory state, considerations that arise are the following. The muscle involved is one which neither when excited directly nor through its motor-nerve exhibits this refractory period. We can exclude the phenomenon, therefore, from it, and from its motor-nerve, and from the link between it and

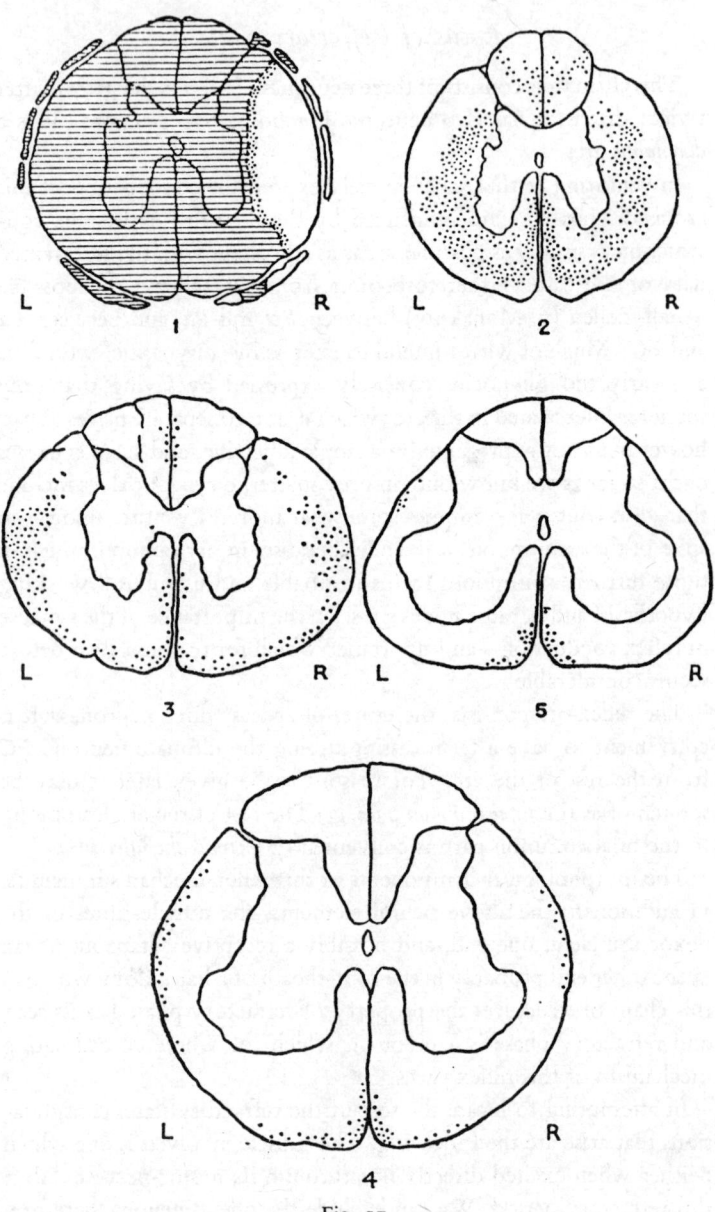

Fig. 17

Refractory State in Scratch-Reflex

its motor-nerve—the end-plate. Further, this refractory state is not exhibited when the motor neurones of this muscle are excited to activity by various other channels; for instance, by the afferent neurones coming in from the receptive organs of the leg itself, or by the pallio-spinal pyramidal neurones descending to them from the cortex of the cerebral hemisphere. We are free, therefore, to exclude the motor neurone FC supplying the flexor muscle itself as the source of the refractory state characterizing the scalptor-reflex. Again, the elicitation of the reflex typically (Fig. 14) by all the various above-mentioned forms of artificial (electrical) stimuli applied through a needle electrode inserted in the skin suggests that it is the commencement of the receptive nerve-fibres in the skin rather than any specialized cutaneous sense-organ therein that are the seat of stimulation when the reflex is thus artificially excited. We have no knowledge of the existence of a refractory phase of such duration as this as a property of any afferent fibre passing from the skin to the spinal cord. There is indeed conclusive evidence that the seat of this refractory phase lies neither in the skin nor in the afferent neurone itself. When the reflex is in progress under stimulation of the skin at one point, e.g. $R\alpha$ (Fig. 13, B), stimulation at some other, even remote, point also producing the reflex—as can be proved in various ways—does not break the rhythm of the reflex[287, 300] or complicate

---

Fig. 17. Cross-sections of the spinal cord of the dog, revealing the position of the nerve-tracts descending to the hind-limb region from origin in the foremost three thoracic segments, by the method of 'successive degeneration'. The eighth cervical segment had been exsected, and 568 days later a cross-cut was made at the hindmost level of the third thoracic segment. The transverse extent of this lesion, as determined by microscopical sections afterwards, is shown in diagram 1 of the figure. The greater part of the right lateral column is seen to have been spared from injury. Three weeks subsequent to this second lesion the animal was sacrificed. Preparations made with the Marchi method for revealing degenerate nerve-fibres showed the degeneration indicated by diagrams 2, 3, 4 and 5 in the figure. After the second injury to the cord the scratch-reflex remained elicitable from the right shoulder, but was lost from the left shoulder in its anterior scapular region. The degeneration of these proprio-spinal fibres descending from the shoulder segments went, therefore, hand in hand with disappearance of the scratch-reflex from a region of skin of the shoulder whence it was elicitable previously.

The Simple Reflex

it in any way. The reflex elicited from spot $R\beta$ may be initiated while that elicited from $R\alpha$ is in progress, and may then be carried on while A is allowed to cease, or vice versa; but *in neither case is the rhythm of the reflex broken or reduplicated.* And this although, from other evidence, we know that the flexor muscle and the motor neurone *FC* can respond rhythmically to stimuli with a rate of rhythm more than twice as high as that of the stimuli applied to produce the reflex. Or the reflex from a spot B may be introduced into the middle of one from a spot A, and although its reflex (B) impresses characters of its own as to amplitude, direction of the foot, etc., it does not reduplicate or break up the already existing rhythm. The result does not differ whether the individual stimuli of the two series of stimulations at spots A and B are alternate or not. Figs. 18, 19, 20, 21 illustrate these points. The refractory phases obtaining in the reflex arising from spot A are respected by the stimuli delivered at B also and are not broken down by them.

There is evidently some part of the reflex mechanism which is common to impulses started both at A and at B. And this holds when spots A and B lie even 10 cm. apart. It is against what we know of the receptive neurones to suppose that there is between them any collateral nexus beyond their impingement directly or indirectly on *other neurones* more or less *common* to them both. The seat of the refractory phase seems therefore to lie somewhere central to the receptive neurones in the afferent arcs. The refractory phase induced in some element of the arc by the reflex from A extends to some element which is also concerned in the conduction of the reflex induced from B. This element must be some neurone common to the two arcs from A and B respectively. Neurone *FC* (Fig. 13), the final common path, is such an element. But neurone *FC* as tested by other reflexes, e.g. the flexion-reflex, shows no such refractory period. The common mechanism sought for seems therefore to lie somewhere between *FC* and $R\alpha$, $R\beta$. It may well be that neurone $P\alpha$ is partly common to $R\alpha$ and $R\beta$, for these *R* neurones are well known to split intraspinally into headward and tailward stem-fibres, each carrying many collaterals, and probably by them connected with the grey matter in not only one spinal segment but in a series of segments.

Swimming-Beat of Medusa

Collaterals from $R\beta$ as well as from $R\alpha$ may reach $P\alpha$, therefore; and similarly with $P\beta$.

The scratch-reflex has instructive points of likeness to that of the swimming-beat of Medusa. The arrangement of its response is quite like that of the muscular response of the swimming-bell of Medusa under stimulation of two points of the subumbrella or two of the marginal receptor organs. We can compare each lateral half of the saddle-shaped receptive area of the dog's back in regard to the scratch-reflex quite strictly to the marginal surface of *Rhizostoma* in regard to its swimming-beat reflex.

In Medusa a second stimulus following close upon a first does not prolong the contraction;[72] it finds the bell in refractory phase. The beat induced by the first stimulus has no second contraction fused with it in consequence of the second stimulus. The principles of the co-ordination thus obtained in the relatively simple swimming of Medusa seem as follows.

One condition of the co-ordination of the swimming-beat, as said above, is the unpolarized nature of the nerve-channels allowing free flow of nervous impulses in either direction from conductor to conductor along the nerve-net. Another condition is the continuity mediate or immediate of every conductor with every other. These conditions of the nervous system allow a single stimulus given at any single point to evoke a co-ordinate contraction of the whole musculature, to evoke, in short, a full and perfect swimming stroke or beat. But they do not insure that, under a series of stimuli delivered in irregular and varied sequence and at various points in perhaps rapid succession, a series of co-ordinate strokes or beats shall result.

Romanes[72] showed that the receptor organs at the edge of the bell were the source of the natural beats of the bell, and that, so long as even one of these remained, the swimming-bell continued to beat spontaneously. There therefore exist in this case quite a number of points which all tend under natural circumstances to initiate the beats of the bell.

Suppose that shortly after a stimulus has occurred at A, and before the contraction induced by it has passed off, another stimulus is delivered at B, and then similarly at C. All these stimuli are, taken

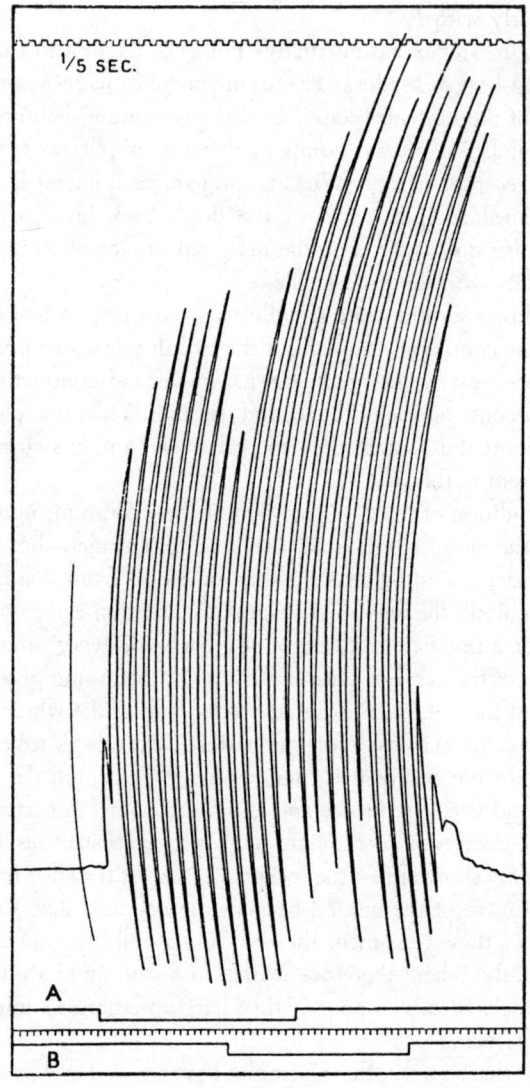

Fig. 18

Refractory Phase in Medusa

singly, similarly provocative of locomotion, and the only locomotive act of the creature is the systolic stroke of its bell. Each reaction is therefore aimed at incitement of locomotion only for a propulsive movement of the bell. But the two conditions, i.e. unpolarized conduction and end-to-end continuity obtaining in the nerve-net, though they insure that result for one stimulus, defeat it in the case of a series of stimuli quickly following either at one and the same point or at several—and for the following reason. The series of stimuli would, were those two conditions all, merely immobilize the bell. The second stimulus following during the contraction excited by the first would be conducted, as was the former, to all the musculature of the movement, and would simply accentuate and prolong the systolic condition already in progress. But that would interrupt locomotion, nôt promote it. The contraction of the muscular disk to produce the stroke must be immediately preceded by diastole, enabling it to embrace the proper volume of water for re-expulsion.

An essential feature of the co-ordination is therefore due to alternation of the two converse phases of contraction and relaxation in the one muscle; these execute the locomotion of this simple animal. This necessary condition is insured, even under irregular series of stimuli, by refractory phase.

When the bell is replying or has just replied to a stimulus, it remains inexcitable to further stimuli for a period which outlasts its phase of

---

Fig. 18. Tracing of the flexion of the hip in the 'scratch-reflex'

The reflex is evoked by two separate stimulations (unipolar faradization) at points 10 cm. apart on the skin surface.

Records from above downwards:

Time in $\frac{1}{5}$ sec.

Myograph curve: the vertical arc indicates onset of first stimulation to point A.

Signal A: descent of the signal shows the time of application of the first stimulation (to point A).

Frequency of repetition of double induction shocks of stimulation of A.

Signal B: descent of the signal shows the time of application of the second stimulation (to point B). The frequency of repetition of the double shocks in this stimulation was much greater than in the case of A and is not shown.

The periods of the two separate stimulations overlap, the second beginning a full second before the first ends, but no interruption or increase of the rate of rhythmic reflex-response appears.

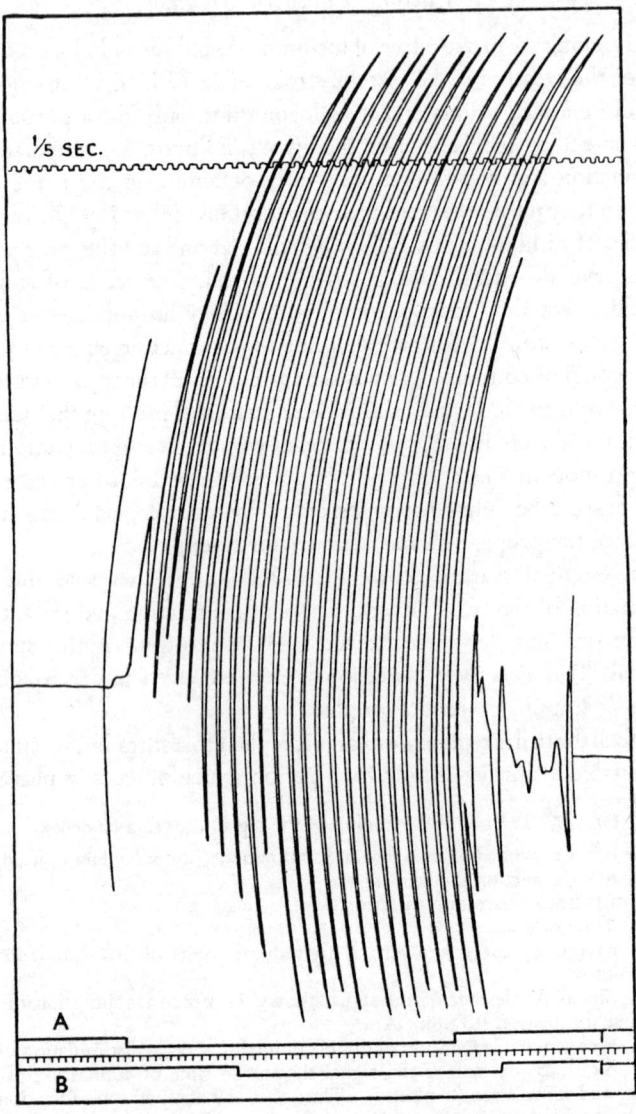

Fig. 19. Tracing of flexion of the hip in the scratch-reflex

Records from above downwards are as in Fig. 18 but with different points of stimulation and with longer overlapping in time of the two separate stimulations.

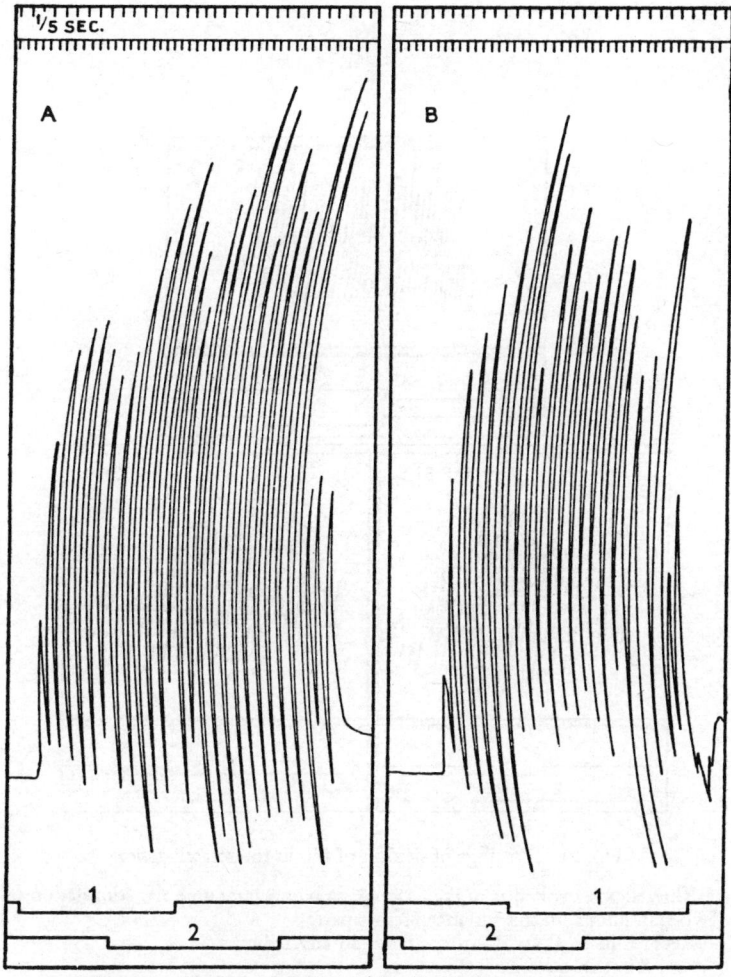

Fig. 20. Tracing of flexion of the hip in the scratch-reflex

The reflex is evoked by two separate stimulations (unipolar faradization) on the skin surface as in Figs. 18 and 19 but with different skin points and slower series of induction shocks; the moments of delivery of the shocks at one skin point being midway between those of delivery at the other.

Records from above downwards:
    Time in $\frac{1}{5}$ sec.
    Frequency of repetition of the weak double shocks, the rate being the same for both stimuli.
    Myograph curves.
    Signals 1 and 2 showing (descent) the time of application of each of the two separate stimulations.

The sequence of stimulation at the two skin points in B is the reverse of that in A.

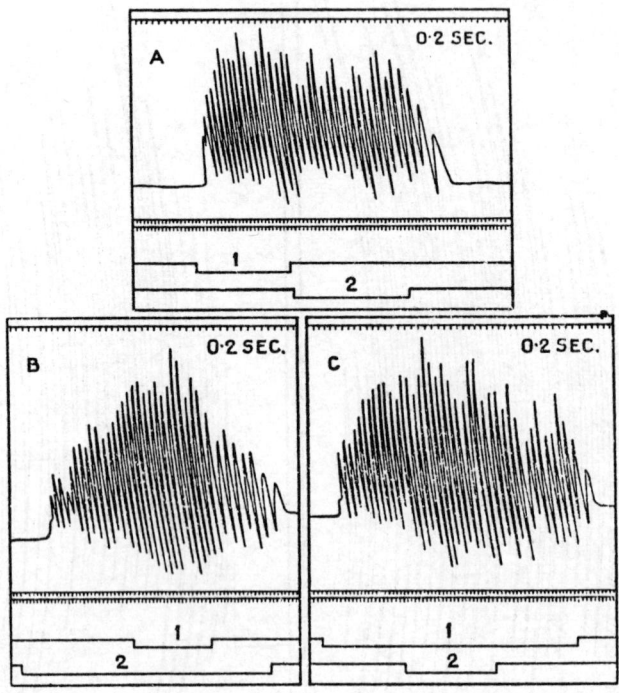

Fig. 21. Tracings of flexion of hip in the scratch-reflex

The reflex is evoked as in Figs. 18, 19, 20 by separate unipolar stimulation of two skin points, in this instance 8 cm. apart.

Records in A, B and C from above downwards:
Time in 0·2 sec.
Myograph curve.
Rate of delivery of double induction shocks in stimulus 1 and 2.
Signals 1 and 2.

In A the second stimulation commences during the after-discharge of the first reflex and causes no interruption or alteration in the rhythm of the reflex response. In B the stimulation of the second of the above pair (stimulus 2) evokes the reflex, and during its progress the stimulation which comes first in A (stimulus 1) is introduced; and conversely in C. In none of the three cases is there interruption of or alteration in rate of the rhythmic reflex response.

contraction. This prevents disharmony occurring in the rhythmic movement under multiple stimulation.

It is on conditions like these governing Medusa's swimming-bell that the co-ordination of the heart's action is based, except that in the heart there is but one *initiatory* spot, prepotent permanently, as in Vertebrates, or temporarily, as in Tunicates. In Medusa presumably any one of various specialized points (border organs) becomes prepotent at different times, by reason of stimulation from the environment. In this Medusa more closely resembles the scratch-reflex, where any one of many points in a large receptive field becomes temporarily prepotent under stimulation, e.g. puncture by a flea or other parasite, and then initiates and leads a series of beats which can be prolonged or intensified by concurrent stimulation by parasites at other points, but cannot by their concurrence be upset as regards rhythm. In the action of scratching it is as necessary as in the swimming of Medusa, or the beating of the heart, that relaxation follow contraction.

Refractory phase is obviously an essential condition in the co-ordination of the scalptor-reflex. The scratching-reflex, in order to secure its aim, must evidently consist of a succession of movements repeated in the same direction, and intervening between the several members of that series there must be a complemental series of movements in the opposite direction. Whether these two series involve reflex contractions of two antagonistic muscle-groups respectively in alternate time, I would leave for the present. The muscle-groups or their reflex-arcs must show phases of refractory state during which stimuli cannot excite, alternating with phases in which such stimuli easily excite. Evidently this is fundamental for securing return to the initial position whence the next stroke shall start. The refractory phase secures this. By its extension through the whole series of arcs it prevents that confusion which would result were refractory phase in some of the arcs allowed to concur with excitatory phase in others.

But there is one significant difference between refractory state in the scratch-reflex and in the swimming mechanism of Medusa. In the latter, as in the heart, the refractory state is a property not relegated to a central nervous organ remote from the peripheral tissue in whose function it finds expression. It is located in intimate connexion

The Simple Reflex

with the peripheral organ itself. From observations of Bethe it seems likely that refractory phase in Medusa is a function of the nerve-net. Magnus[268] has recently shown that the refractory phase of the beat of the isolated intestine is referable to the local nerve-plexus (Auerbach's) lying in the gut-wall. In these cases the refractory state seems to belong to the nervous elements, but to nervous elements diffused through the peripheral tissue. But in the scratch-reflex the site of the refractory state is central, intraspinal.

The centrality of seat of the refractory state of the scratch-reflex is significant of the difference of the conditions under which the scratch-reflex and the swimming of Medusa respectively go forward. In the case of the locomotor action of the swimming-bell of Medusa, we have a simple musculature which can execute practically but one movement. It is in fact a single muscle, that is to say, comparable with what in the more complex musculature of higher organisms— e.g. Vertebrates—is regarded as a unit of musculature, a single muscle, such as the *gastrocnemius*, *tibialis*, etc., in the frog. Each and every receptor organ which under stimulation produces locomotion is therefore connected by nerve with that single muscle of locomotion, and when impelled by each or any of them, the muscle effects practically the same action as it does when impelled by any other of the sister receptor organs. The movement of locomotion which is provoked through each receptor is practically the same as that provoked through any of the rest. The mechanical organ in this case can perform but one movement, and its performance of that movement is, so to say, the one purpose demanded from it by each of all the receptor channels playing upon it.

But with the mechanical organ which the scratch-reflex employs the case is different. That organ is the hind-limb, a complex structure built of parts, many of them spatially opposed, and able as a whole to execute movements of various kinds. Thus it can reflexly not only scratch, but stand, walk, run, or gallop, squat in defecation, abduct and flex in micturition, etc. In the swimming-bell of Medusa there is no opportunity for antagonism between the motor end-results of the reflexes that employ it, save in respect to the possible confusion of successive contractions which would destroy the rhythmic pulse, and

Seat of Refractory Phase

that confusion is avoided by refractory phase. The swimming-bell of Medusa is at the behest of but one type-reflex. The scratch-reflex possesses the same safeguard against destruction of its rhythmic character. But in the case of the scratch-reflex that reflex is but one of several reflexes that share in a condominium over the effector organ—the limb. It must therefore be possible for the scratch-reflex, taken as a whole, to be, as occasion demands, replaced in exercise of its use of the limb by other reflexes, and many of these do not require clonic action from the limb—indeed, would be defeated by clonic action. It would not do, then, for the peripheral organ itself to be a clonic mechanism. The clonic mechanism must lie at some place where other kinds of reflex can preclude the clonic actuator from affecting the peripheral organ. Now such a place is obviously the central organ itself; for that organ is, as its name implies, a nodal point of meeting to which converge all the nervous arcs of the body, and among others all those which for their several ends have to employ the same mechanical organ as does the scratch-reflex itself. It is therefore only in accord with expectation that the seat of the refractory phase of the scratch-reflex lies where we traced it, in the central nervous organ itself, and somewhere between the motor neurone to the muscle and the receptive neurone from the skin. For it is upon the motor neurone that other arcs impinge.

The refractory state is obviously akin to a state of inhibition, and just as there are well-known examples in which the inhibitory state is peripheral (e.g. the heart), and others in which the inhibition is central, so undoubtedly phases of refractory state are in some instances peripheral, but also in numerous instances are central—and this is so in certain reflex actions.

The reflexes of which refractory phase constitutes a prominent feature are those concerned with cyclic actions occurring in rhythmic series; such as the scratch-reflex, reflexes of swallowing and blinking, and probably the rhythmically recurring reflexes concerned in the stepping of the limbs.

Nothnagel (1870),[48] following up an observation by Setschenow,[31] studied a periodic and rhythmic reflex of the crossed hind-limb in the spinal frog. He found that if some days after the

The Simple Reflex

frog's cord had been transected at the fourth vertebra, the central end of the sciatic is faradized, a rhythmic alternating flexion and extension of the opposite hind limb is evoked. He noted that no intensity of stimulation makes the rhythmic movement alter from clonic to tonic. A reflex of this kind is, I find, elicitable in the spinal

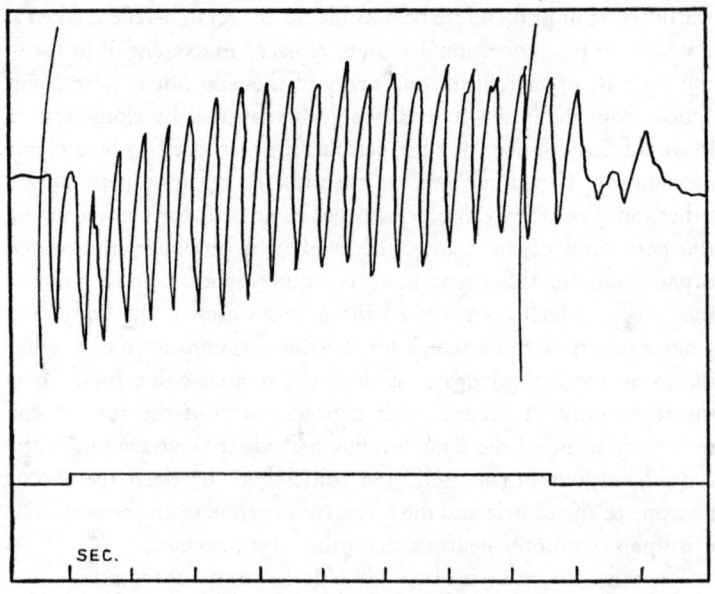

Fig. 22. Crossed stepping-reflex in the spinal dog

Records from above downwards:
  Myograph curve.
  Signal line: ascent shows the period of application of the stimulus.
  Time in sec.

The reflex was elicited by unipolar faradization of the opposite foot. The flexions of the limb succeed each other at a rate of about five times in 2 sec.—about half the frequence they exhibit in the scratch-reflex. The 'after-discharge' of the reflex includes four 'steps', the last being of small amplitude and slow, as with the final beats of the scratch-reflex.

dog's hind-leg by unipolar faradization of the opposite foot, and, as Nothnagel noted in the frog, no mere increase of intensity of stimulation converts its clonic character into maintained tonic. It is rhythmic (Fig. 22), and has a refractory period which no ordinary increase of intensity of stimulation suffices to break down. The

The Extensor-Thrust

frequency of its rhythm averages 2·3 per sec., but varies somewhat in different observations. This is about twice as slow as the frequency of the scratch-reflex, which averages 4·5 per sec. The average rhythm of the scratch-reflex is almost exactly the same as that ascertained by Gotch & Burch[164] for reflex-discharge from the electric cell of *Malapterurus*, but the rate in *Malapterurus* appears to vary much more than that of the scratch-reflex.

There is a peculiar brief extension-reflex of the dog's hind leg which I term[304] the 'extensor-thrust'. Baglioni[288] has more recently noted an analogous reflex in the frog. This reflex is elicited by mechanical stimuli applied to the planta. In the spinal dog, where well marked, it is often elicitable by even lightly stroking with the edge of a piece of paper the skin behind the plantar cushion. It is more certainly evoked by pushing the finger-tip between the plantar cushion and the toe-pads, especially when the hip and knee, not necessarily the ankle, are resting, passively flexed.

The 'extensor-thrust' I have never succeeded in prolonging to a full half-second—none of my records exhibits it as long as that. Usually the duration as recorded is about a fifth of a second (Fig. 23). Possibly its muscular contraction may be a simple twitch, though reflexly excited. Its muscular field involves the muscles of the 'knee-jerk'. The myogram of the extensor thrust is shorter than that of tetanic contraction of the diaphragm (Head's slip[118]) caused by two successive stimuli to the phrenic nerve when the muscular responses of the two just fuse (Fig. 24).

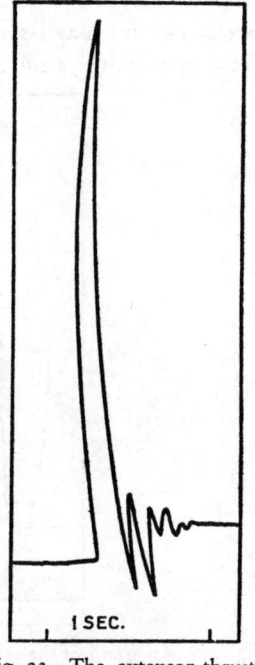

Fig. 23. The extensor-thrust; spinal dog
Time in sec.
The application of the stimulus is not indicated but the latent period of the response is very brief.

The Simple Reflex

Immediately after its elicitation this reflex, in my experience, remains in the spinal dog for nearly a second relatively inelicitable. Its reflex-arc exhibits after its phase of activity a refractory phase. The refractory phase is here far longer than that of the scalptor-reflex. It may last six times as long as the period of activity; thus the extensor-thrust may last only 170σ while the succeeding refractory phase may endure a full second.

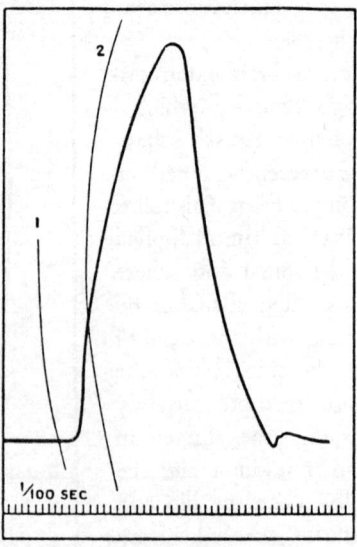

Fig. 24. Myogram of the contraction of the diaphragm of the rabbit (Head's slip) elicited by two break shocks applied to the phrenic nerve

The moments of application of the two shocks are indicated by the vertical arcs on the myograph curve.

Time in $\frac{1}{100}$ sec. (Macdonald & Sherrington).

The extensor-thrust is probably an important element in the reflex mechanism of the dog's locomotion.* One peculiarity it has as compared with other spinal reflexes of the limb is the considerable force which it exerts. In the locomotion of the animal it provides much of the propulsive power required. Bearing these points in mind, it is obvious that as an element in locomotion its repetition is

* Compare the paper by M. Philippson.[309]

The Extensor-Thrust

required only at intervals considerably longer than the duration of the thrust itself, namely, at a particular phase of each successive step taken in the progression of the animal. After the extensor-thrust, the limb has to be given over to the flexor muscles in order, without touching the ground, to swing forward in preparation for the next step by the limb. It is reasonable to suppose that part of the means by which selective adaptation has secured this result is the evolution of the long refractory phase following the activity in the reflex-arc of the extensor-thrust. Zwaardemaker[272] has shown that the reflex movement of swallowing in the narcotized cat is followed by a refractory period,* lasting half a second or longer. This refractory state is central, for when the reflex swallow has been elicited by the superior laryngeal nerve of one side, the after-lasting refractory period holds good also for excitation of the opposite superior laryngeal nerve.

Variation of the external stimulus has comparatively little effect upon the length of the refractory period. But internal conditions, such as blood supply, fatigue, narcosis, etc., do influence it greatly. For reflexes which exhibit a refractory phase, a certain duration of that phase, subject to some variations, is characteristic. The duration of the phase varies considerably in different types of these reflexes.

It is clear that an essential part of many reflexes is a more or less prolonged refractory phase succeeding nervous discharge.

Refractory phase appears therefore at the one end and at the other of the animal scale as a factor of fundamental importance in the co-ordination of certain motile actions. In the lowly animal form (Medusa) it attaches locally to the neuro-muscular organ, and so also in the visceral and blood-vascular tubes of Vertebrates. But in higher forms (dog) refractory phase occurs as regards the taxis of the skeletal musculature, not in the peripheral neuro-muscular organ, but in the centres of the nervous system itself.

* Baglioni[285] has pointed out refractory phase in a-reflex in the frog.

Lecture III

CO-ORDINATION IN THE SIMPLE REFLEX
(*concluded*)

ARGUMENT: Correspondence between intensity of stimulus and intensity of reflex reaction. Differences between different reflexes in this respect. Functional solidarity of the intraspinal group of elements composing a reflex 'centre'. Sensitivity of reflexes, as compared with nerve-trunks, to asphyxial and anaemic conditions, and to anaesthetic and certain other drugs. Functional significance of the neural perikarya. Reflexes of double-sign. Reflexes of successive double-sign, and of simultaneous double-sign. Evidence of reciprocal innervation in reflexes. Reflex inhibition of the tonus of skeletal muscles. Reflex inhibition of the knee-jerk. Time-relations and other characters of reflex inhibition as exemplified by the flexion-reflex. Other examples of inhibition as part of reflex reciprocal innervation. The seat of this reflex inhibition is intraspinal. Conversion of reflex inhibition into reflex excitation by strychnine and by tetanus toxin. Significance of the 'central' situation of reflex inhibition in the cases here dealt with.

GRADING OF INTENSITY

A FURTHER difference between the reaction of a reflex-arc and that of a nerve-trunk lies in the greater ease with which in the latter the intensity of effect can be graded by grading the intensity of the stimulus. In the nerve-trunk this has been examined both with the action-current (Waller[163]) and for motor-nerves by the muscular contraction (Fick, Cybulski & Zanietowski[145]). The accuracy of grading within a certain range of stimulus-intensity is so remarkable that the ratio between stimulus-intensity and response-intensity has by some observers been assigned mathematical expression. Waller finds the response in a nerve-trunk, directly stimulated, increase in much closer direct proportion to the increment of external stimulus than does the response of muscle to indirect stimulation, or the response of the optic nerve when the retina is adequately stimulated. The correspondence between intensity of external stimulus and reflex end-effect is again less close still; indeed it is often stated that reflex reactions resemble as to intensity the 'all-or-nothing' principle of the cardiac beat (Wundt). Biedermann remarks of reflexes

Grading of Intensity of Reflex

evoked by single-induction shocks in the cooled frog, that there is practically no grading of intensity: they are all maximal. Baglioni makes the same remark for other reflexes in the frog.

Yet graded intensity of reflex-effect does occur. Walton[91] noted as one of the features of strychnine poisoning, that at a certain stage the grading of intensity is lost and all reflexes become maximal. Merzbacher[210] and Pari[294] have supplied some measurements of the increment in amplitude of the reflex movements of the frog's leg under increase of intensity of stimulation.

The flexion-reflex of the hind-limb of the spinal dog increases in amplitude in correspondence with increase of intensity of stimulus—alterations of time-relations of stimulus being excluded. Increase of intensity of stimulus heightens the reflex contraction both in power and amplitude. Fig. 25 shows a successive series of these reflexes, each elicited by a series of break shocks delivered at the same skin-spot by a stigmatic kathode. The increments of the reflex run fairly steadily with the up-gradient of intensity of stimulus.

In the scratch-reflex a grading of the intensity of the reflex is easily obtainable by grading the intensity of the stimulus. By a suitably weak stimulus a scratch-reflex can be elicited which exhibits but a single beat. Increase of intensity of the reaction does not show itself in increase in frequency of the rhythm of this reflex, or shows itself very slightly in that form, the refractory period being hardly curtailed at all. The increase reveals itself as greater amplitude of the individual beats of the rhythmic contraction. By simply bringing the secondary coil nearer to the primary in a dozen successive steps, it is easy to obtain a dozen grades of amplitude in a dozen successive examples of this reflex (Fig. 26). The beats in response to a strong stimulus may have six times the amplitude of those evoked by a weak. The single beat that can be obtained by a suitably feeble stimulus (Fig. 9) is not only small but slow; it resembles the last beat the reflex gives as it dies out after cessation of an ordinary stimulus. The feeble, slow character of the terminal beat of the ordinary reflex is not therefore due to fatigue, but simply to weak intensity of excitatory process at the moment.

The scratch-reflex, though it resembles the heart beat in relative

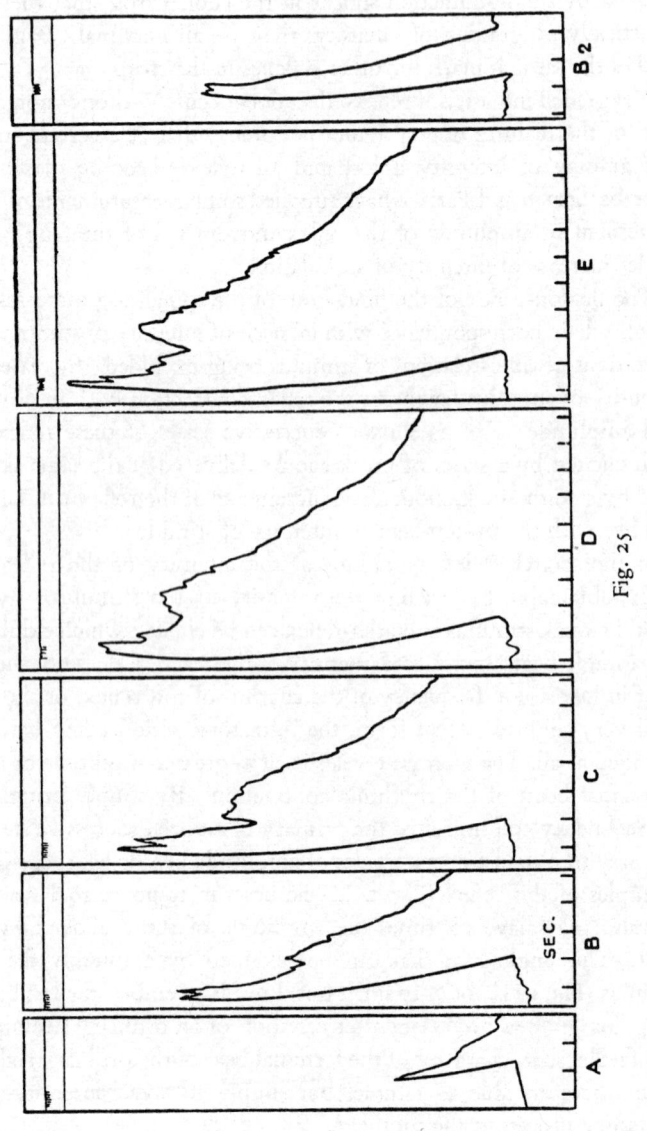

Fig. 25

Grading of Intensity of Reflex

immutability of rhythm under change of intensity of stimulation, differs from it in the change of intensity of its beat, which follows change in intensity of stimulus. It does not observe the 'all-or-nothing' principle. It is obvious that in the heart beat the object is to put a pressure on the contents of the ventricle higher than that obtaining in the aorta, and that aim reached, any further excess of pressure is useless or harmful, for it subjects the heart and the arterial wall to an unnecessary strain. Clifford Allbutt[180] remarks: "It is the function of a healthy heart and arteries to promote the maximum of blood displacement with the minimal alteration of pressures." The stress under which the heart is driven is less closely associated with intensities of stimulus than with conditions internal to itself, e.g. distension, etc. But with the scratching movement it is obvious that a strong scratching movement may remove an irritation more quickly and more effectually than weak movement.

On the crossed extension-reflex the effect of increase of intensity of stimulus shows, in my experience, somewhat differently. After a relatively slow and gradual increase of reflex-response, there appears

---

Fig. 25. The flexion-reflex, showing grading of intensity due to graded intensities of stimulus (spinal dog)

Records from above downwards:
  Signal line recording time of the stimulus: the stimulus consisted in each case of twelve break shocks delivered at the rate of 25 per sec., applied by unipolar method with kathode needle point in skin of a digit, the diffuse pole lying headward of the spinal transection.
  Myograph curve.
  Time in sec.
The interval between commencement of each reflex was 2 min.

	Intensity of stimulus	Measure of reflex
A	690	8·5
B	3000	59
C	5200	110
D	9800	168
E	12500	213
B2	3000	29

Intensity is given in units of the Kronecker scale.

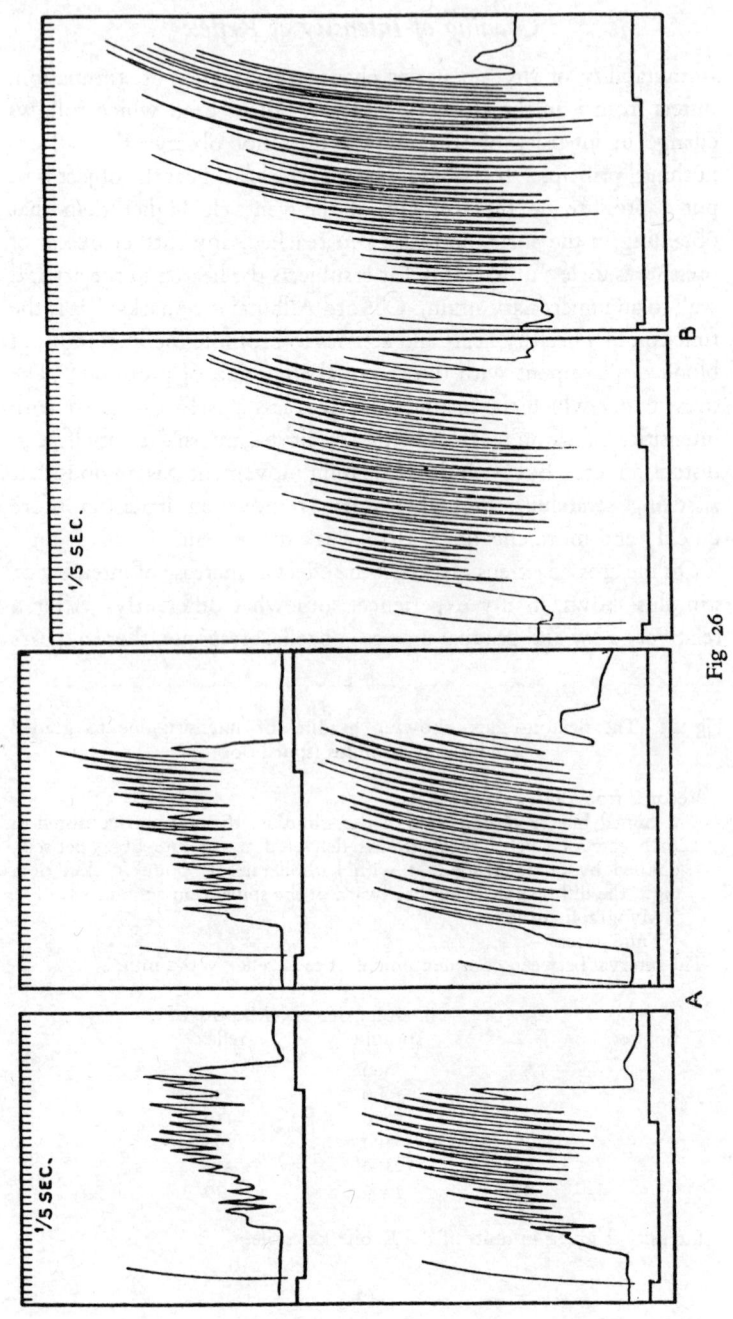

Fig 26

Grading of Intensity of Reflex

at a certain intensity of stimulation a sudden relatively large increase of the response. This augmentation is chiefly in the form of 'after-discharge' (Fig. 27). This reflex shows well that internal conditions play a greater role as compared with external in reflex conductions than in nerve-trunk conduction. Under strong stimuli the augmentation of the reaction by after-discharge becomes enormous.

The 'extensor-thrust' I have failed to evoke by any stimulus easy to grade or record a measure of. But my experience of it under the particular form of mechanical stimulation it appears to require, leads me to think that strength of external stimulus affects the reflex-response but little, and that this reflex much resembles the heart in responding either not at all or fully. Its graphic record in a series of stimulations repeats itself time after time with very little difference of character.

Therefore, from the reflexes of the limb of the spinal dog, it would appear that in respect to ability to be graded in intensity in accordance with grading of intensity of stimulus, there exist great *differences* between the various type-reflexes. Some reflexes—e.g. the flexion-reflex and the scratch-reflex—easily exhibit grading, while others do not. The difference between reflex-conduction in various reflexes in this respect may explain the discrepancies between various observers on this point.

A factor in the grading of submaximal effects in muscle and nerve by weak stimuli may well be limitation to certain of the

---

Fig. 26 A, B. Scratch-reflex graded by intensity of stimulus (spinal dog)

Records from above downwards:
  Time in $\frac{1}{5}$ sec.
  Myograph curve.
  Signal line (descent indicates time of application of the stimulation).

The reflexes were elicited by unipolar faradization with needle as kathode to shoulder skin. Double shocks at rate of 17 per sec. were used. The examples are taken from a series of twelve, exhibiting twelve grades of amplitude. The twelve grades of intensity of stimulus used were, reckoned in units of the Kronecker inductorium scale, 250, 350, 475, 690, 1100, 1900, 3000, 4000, 5200, 6300, 7500. The examples in the figure were the second, fourth, sixth, eighth, tenth, and twelfth of the series. Intervals of 1 min. elapsed between commencement of each reflex. The needle-point kathode remained unmoved throughout.

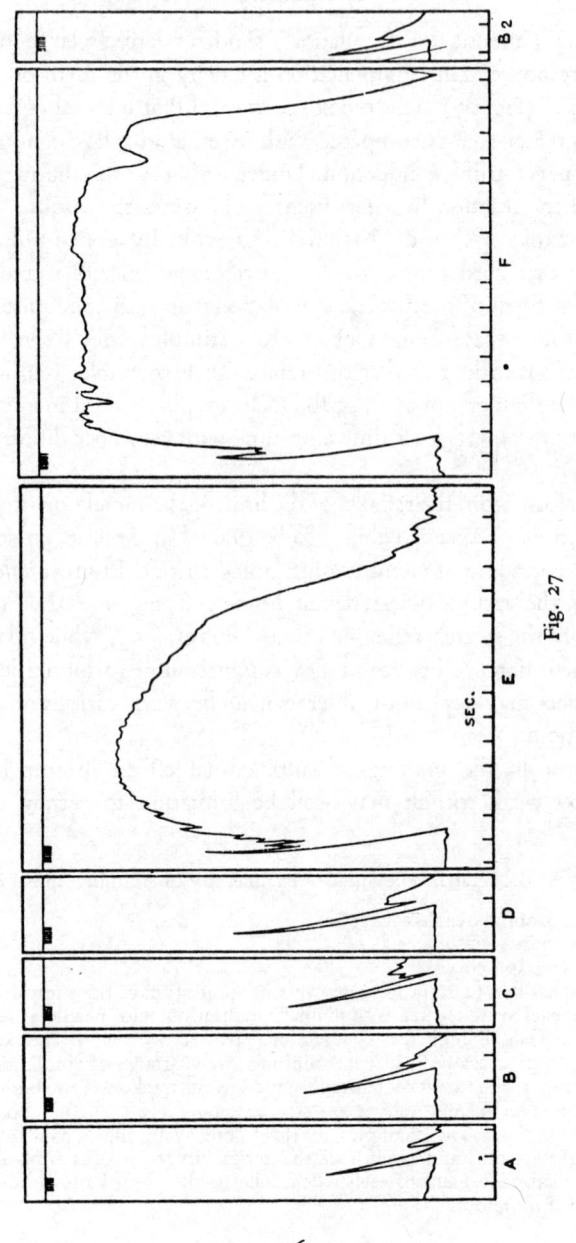

Fig. 27

Grading of Intensity of Reflex

component fibres, whereas a maximal stimulus excites them all. It is a matter of interest how far this numerical factor explains submaximal responses from a spinal centre. If its elements are functionally separate, partial responses are open to occur in such a mechanism since it is multiple as regards its physiological components. Gotch[244] has recently raised this question in an interesting way. He points out that in the electrical organ of *Malapterurus*, where the whole organ is innervated by a *single nerve-fibre*, the reflex-response is little variable in its intensity in comparison with the wide range of response to increasing stimulus-intensities exhibited by stimulation of the electric nerve of *Torpedo*—a structure containing many nerve-fibres. Concerning the grading of motor discharges from the central nervous system he asks: "Is it not possible that these grades are largely dependent on the number of central elements involved, and are only incidentally associated with variations in the intensity of the nervous process in any one neurone?"

That in spinal reflexes increase of the intensity of the exciting stimulus causes increase in the number of motor neurones excited is clearly shown by the wider field of musculature seen to be engaged

---

Fig. 27. The crossed extension-reflex showing grading of intensity corresponding with grading of intensity of stimulus (spinal dog)

Records from above downwards:
  Signal line showing time of stimulation which in each case consisted of twelve break shocks delivered at the rate of 25 per sec. applied by a needle-point kathode to the skin of a digit of the opposite foot; the other electrode was diffuse and applied headward of the spinal transection. An interval of 2 min. elapsed between each succeeding observation.
  Myograph curve.
  Time in sec.

	Intensity of stimulus	Measure of reflex
A	475	3·5
B	560	5
C	690	7
D	890	9
E	1100	355
F	1400	459
B2	560	4·5

Intensity is given in units of the Kronecker scale. The record is from the same animal as yielded those of preceding Fig. 25.

The Simple Reflex

as the reflex irradiates under intenser stimulation. This is the well-known spread which Pflüger[24] endeavoured to formulate rules to express. Within one and the same muscle-groups, and even within one and the same individual muscle, grading of intensity of reflex contraction by this numerical implication of more or fewer motor-cells seems not only possible but probable. It is perhaps one object of their multiplicity. The want of difference between the latent time of the incremental and initial reflexes mentioned above (Lect. I, p. 22) might be explicable thus.

With very feeble stimuli, or under spinal shock, when only feeble reflex reactions can be evoked, it is easy to see *partial* contractions of muscles, e.g. in the tibialis anticus, sartorius, and semimembranosus. Under like circumstances the scratch-reflex may have the form of simply a feeble rhythmic dorsiflexion at ankle and toes, or even of the toes alone. We have referred to such phenomena before, and they harmonize well with the view of a fractional activity of the motor centre of the scratch and other reflexes.

Yet we must not lose sight of the physiological solidarity of the action of the group of elements that compose a 'reflex centre' in its reflex activity. 'Immediate spinal induction' (vide infra, Lect. IV) and the spatial spread of the refractory phase in scratch-reflexes evoked from separate points show (Lect. II, p. 53) that, intraspinally, the various component arcs of the type-reflex are interconnected to something like a unitary mechanism. Further, the evidence that when the scratch-reflex is being elicited from one point the refractory period obtains practically throughout its intraspinal centre indicates the same functional unity. The nerve-cells building the centre seem combined like those of the nerve-net of Medusa. The elements seem incapable of isolated excitation. Such an intraspinal group as that involved in the scratch-reflex must extend through a considerable length of the cord. And yet though interconnected, like the web of Medusa's nerve-net, there is evidence that in the various reflex forms which the scratching movement takes according as elicited from one point or another, one part of the centre is the more active in one form of the reflex and another in another form of the reflex. The mechanism is not therefore always equally affected throughout,

Irradiation and After-Discharge

and in this inequality numerical proportion of active to inactive elements may play a part. The mechanism, nevertheless, although anatomically an assemblage of units, is functionally itself a unit. And a comparable solidarity obtains in other reflex mechanisms. Even the irradiation which suggests extension to new units itself gives evidence of the welding of the unit elements of centres together into functional unit groups possessing solidarity. When in the flexion-reflex the response spreads from the knee to the hip, the spread is not gradual, but the hip flexion suddenly comes in, marking a sharp step-like rise on the record (Fig. 45, p. 154). It is not as though the irradiation gradually reached the motor elements of the hip-flexion centre cell by cell: the irradiation on involving that centre forthwith evokes discharge from it which, judging from its powerful effect, represents discharge from the centre practically as a whole. The reaction as it irradiates treats the centre as a unit.

The great *prolongation* of the reflex-discharge produced by intensifying, apart from prolonging, the external stimulus is also against the increase of discharge being explicable merely or chiefly by implication of a greater number of motor elements. In the flexion-reflex, the period of discharge may be lengthened tenfold by increasing simply the intensity of the stimulus without lengthening it. In the 'crossed-extension reflex' I have seen the period of discharge lengthened more than twentyfold. This argues that the grading of the motor discharge in these reflexes is in important measure due to graded intensities of discharge from the unit elements themselves, of which the reflex centres are compounded. The functional unity of a reflex centre seems also evident from the fact that it is the instrument of a number of receptive organs scattered over a relatively wide field—a field which for the flexion-reflex is almost co-extensive with the whole skin surface of the limb—and nevertheless an *intense* stimulus from any limited part of that field can elicit a reflex of full strength. This it can only attain if the whole centre of the reflex be at its disposal. Therefore, as we saw in the scratch-reflex, the *whole* motor centre potentially belongs to all and each of the groups of receptive organs proper to the reflex. The centre, although consisting of anatomical units which are individual, seems knitted

The Simple Reflex

together functionally. It is not necessarily the motor cells which conjoin—were that so one hardly sees how stimulation of the central end of a motor root could fail to excite discharge from other motor roots, which the Bell-Magendie law shows that it does actually fail to do.

REFLEX CONDUCTION LESS RESISTANT THAN NERVE CONDUCTION

THE differences traced thus far between reflex-arc conduction and nerve-trunk conduction have been differences brought out by variations of stimulus and other external conditions. Differences no less notable appear under changes of internal kind. Without entering on these fully, a glance at them is helpful for the understanding of reflex-arc conduction.

Conduction by nerve-trunks is but slowly affected by interference with blood-supply; reflexes are nevertheless among the earliest reactions to alter or fail under asphyxial conditions. v. Baeyer[239] found the sciatic nerve of the frog retains excitability and conductivity for 3-5 hr. in nitrogen, and on readmission of oxygen regain its powers in a few minutes. Bergmann (cited by Biedermann) found interruption of the circulation in the frog extinguishes reflexes in 30 min. Verworn has shown that the spinal centres of a strychnized frog, if unsupplied with oxygen, fail to react in about an hour's time, but are promptly restored by resupply of oxygen. Baglioni[293] has shown that the spinal centres of the frog, deprived of circulation and immersed in nitrogen, fail to give reflexes in about 45 min., but in an atmosphere of oxygen continue to react for 20 hr.

Again, the dosage of chloroform or ether required to depress and abolish nerve-trunk conduction is much greater than is required to depress and abolish the cerebro-spinal reflexes. In Waller's observations on extinction of action-current in nerve-trunks a 3 per cent dose of chloroform in air was required. Using in the cat indirect contraction of the gastrocnemius as an index of sciatic nerve-conduction, Miss Sowton and myself found that 0·3 per cent chloroform in diluted blood at 36° C. was required to abolish the reaction (Fig. 28). This is a much higher percentage than suffices to depress the heart's

Chloroform and Reflex Conduction

action. Since many reflexes are abolished by doses which do not markedly depress the heart, reflex conduction is abolished by doses *a fortiori* smaller than those which set aside nerve-trunk conduction.

Again, a number of agents, e.g. strychnine, tetanus toxin, etc., that do not appreciably affect nerve-trunk conduction enormously alter reflex-arc conduction. All these seem to exert their influence on some part of the reflex conductor which lies in grey matter. It is interesting to ask whether they, e.g. strychnine, have an effect similar to their spinal effect when exhibited in Bethe's preparation of the second antenna ganglion of *Carcinus*, whence the motor perikarya have been removed. If these agents have their locus of incidence at the synapse, it must be conceded that they act with very different intensities at different synapses.

From this rehearsal of the differences between nerve-trunk conduction and reflex-arc conduction it seems evident that certain elements of co-ordination of 'the simple reflex' are to be found in the qualities of conduction of the reflex-arc. Each of the various types of simple reflex possesses to a large extent its own peculiarities of conduction. Though there are differences between conduction in various nerve-trunks, e.g. in speed of transmission of impulses, etc., these differences sink to insignificance when contrasted with the extent and variety of the conductive differences exhibited by different reflex-arcs. And in the case of each reflex-arc its idiosyncrasies of conduction form an obvious basis for the co-ordination exhibited by its reflex-act.

FUNCTIONS OF THE PERIKARYON

It may appear that our tendency is to attribute the distinctive characters of reflex-arc conduction so liberally to the synapse that the perikaryon is stripped of all functions and only equivalent to a piece of nerve-fibre. But it is to be remembered that two functions of great importance certainly belong to the perikaryon. In the first place, even if the conductive process in it be wholly similar to that of a nerve-fibre, it is at least a place where the conductor branches, often to such an extent as occurs nowhere else, so that it is a nodal

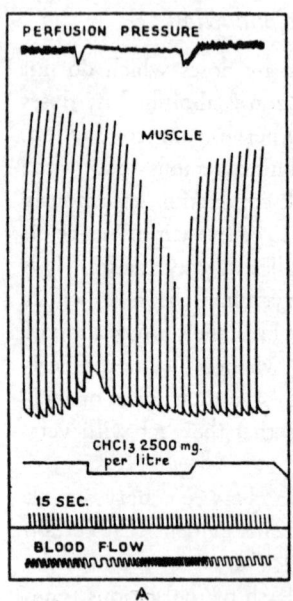 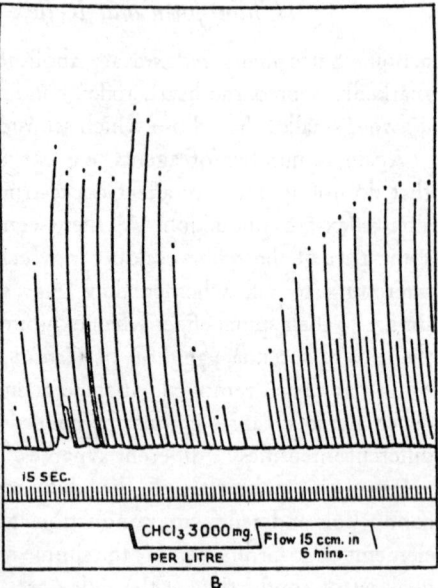

Fig. 28

A. Effect of chloroform (0·25 per cent) on contractions of gastrocnemius muscle stimulated through its nerve. Hind-limb of cat.

Records from above downwards:
Pressure of delivery of the perfused blood at the entrant cannula.
Response of muscle to motor-nerve stimulation.
Signal: descent indicates the time of perfusion of blood containing $CHCl_3$ 0·25 per cent; similar blood but free from $CHCl_3$ being perfused before and after.
Time in 15 sec.
Blood flow: each notch indicates one emptying of the Schäfer 'tilter' receiving the blood at outflow from the limb.

The chloroform reduces the contractions of the muscle stimulated through its nerve by more than a half. The blood flow shows a diminution at first, then a marked decrease.

B. Effect of chloroform (0·3 per cent) on the contractions of the gastrocnemius muscle stimulated alternatively through its nerve (dot above curve) and directly.

Records from above downwards:
Response of muscle to stimulation.
Time in 15 sec.
Signal: descent of line indicates period of perfusion with chloroform 0·3 per cent.

The nerve was inexcitable before the perfusing fluid was turned on, and the record which begins immediately after perfusion had been started shows the gradual recovery of excitability. $CHCl_3$ at 0·3 per cent abolishes the response of the muscle to indirect stimulation, and reduces its direct response almost to zero. The second, fourth, sixth, etc., are direct responses of the muscle; the first, third, fifth, etc., are responses to stimulation through the nerve-trunk. (Sowton & Sherrington.)

Reciprocal Inhibition

point in the spatial distribution of the conductive lines. In the second place, there seems no valid reason yet to doubt the long-held view that regards the perikaryon as the nutritive centre of the neurone to which it belongs.

Certain features mentioned already as saliently distinguishing reflex-conduction from nerve-trunk conduction still remain for consideration. Among these are fatigability, facilitation, inhibitory interference, spinal induction. These will, however, be better taken under the compounding of reflexes. One feature that we have not considered may, however, with advantage be considered at once. This feature is inhibition.

RECIPROCAL INHIBITION

In the end-effect of certain reflexes, for instance the scratch-reflex, there supervenes on a phase of excitatory state a state refractory to excitation—a refractory phase. This refractory phase, if we seek to put it into the class of physiological phenomena to which it must obviously belong, is a state of inhibition. In the scratch-reflex we have therefore a reflex in which an external stimulus evokes as its end-effect an excitatory phase, succeeded by an inhibitory phase, and this succession in this reflex, the stimuli being continued, is repeated many times. If we denote excitation as an end-effect by the sign *plus* (+), and inhibition as end-effect by the sign *minus* (−), such a reflex as the scratch-reflex can be termed a reflex of double-sign, for it develops excitatory end-effect and then inhibitory end-effect even during the duration of the exciting stimulus.

There is a further numerous class of reflexes in which the end-effect consists both in excitatory state and in inhibitory state, but the inhibitory state does not supervene on the excitatory or have the same locus of incidence as the excitatory; it occurs simultaneously with it at another interrelated locus. The ordinary flexion-reflex of the hind-limb of the spinal cat and dog is a reflex of this type. The end-effect of the reflex is expressed by two groups of muscles whose contractions act in opposed direction at the same joints. This opposition is obviated in the end-effect of the reflex by the end-

The Simple Reflex

effect having the form of excitatory state as regards the motor-nerve to the flexor muscle, but suppression or withholding of excitatory state (central inhibition) as regards the motor neurone of the extensor. Such reflex is a reflex of double-sign, but whereas the scratch-reflex and the eyelid-reflex, etc., are reflexes with *successive* double-sign, the flexion-reflex and reflexes of that type, e.g. the crossed extension-reflex, are reflexes with *simultaneous* double-sign.

The form in which this central inhibition occurs may be best gathered from illustrative examples.

The simple reflex mechanism examined in the swimming-bell of Medusa gives little evidence of an arrangement for a form of spatial co-ordination which is very prevalent in more complex mechanisms. In many cases the body, or some part of it, can be actively moved, not merely in one direction but in two or more, opposed or partially opposed. The musculature is then usually divided into various discrete pieces called 'muscles'. The contraction of one muscle, or set of muscles, produces movement in one direction; the contraction of another produces movement in another direction. Instances of this are common in the limbs, neck, tail, etc., of vertebrates and arthropods.

Reflex co-ordination makes separate muscles whose contractions act harmoniously, e.g. on a lever, contract together, although at separate places, so that they assist toward the same end. In other words, it excites synergic muscles. But in many cases it does more than that. Where two muscles would antagonize each other's action the reflex-arc, instead of activating merely one of the two, when it activates the one causes depression of the activity (tonic or rhythmic contraction) of the other. The latter is an inhibitory effect.

Classical examples of inhibition are those of the vagus nerve on the heart, and of the chorda tympani on the blood-vessels of the submaxillary region. In these cases the stimulation of the distal end of a peripheral nerve quells the existing contraction of the muscles of the heart and blood-vessels respectively. When the submaxillary gland is called into activity reflexly, depression of the tonic contraction of the muscular coat of its arteries accompanies the heightened secretory activity of gland cells simultaneously evoked. The two reflex

Peripheral Inhibition

actions—the one depressing the activity of one tissue, the other heightening that of the other tissue—are mutually co-operative, and are combined in the one reflex action, and are instances of a reflex co-ordination quite comparable with that in which one muscle of an antagonistic couple is thrown out of action when the other is brought into action. And as in this case, so in *some* cases of mutual co-operation of inhibition with pressor action in the nervous regulation of antagonistic muscles, the inhibition is *peripheral*; that is to say, stimulation of the distal piece of the divided peripheral nerve itself suffices to produce it. Instances of this occur in the claw of *Astacus*, and in the muscles opening the shell of the bivalve *Anodon*. In *Astacus*, as is well known (Richet,[98] Biedermann,[109] Piotrowski[141]), stimulation of the distal end of the cut peripheral nerve, under suitable conditions, causes relaxation of the closing muscle at the same time as contraction of the opening muscle. This is comparable with the stimulation of the distal end of the cut chorda tympani, which produces relaxation of the muscular coat of the arteries of the submaxillary gland at the same time as it causes secretion by the gland cells.

The muscles of the claw of *Astacus* are striated, and the case is interesting as one in which the co-ordination of action of two antagonistic muscles of skeletal type is effected by peripheral inhibition of one through the same nerve-trunk that induces active contraction of the other. But the similar co-ordination in the taxis of the skeletal musculature of vertebrates exerts its inhibition not at the periphery but in the nerve-centres. It occurs within the grey matter of the central nervous system.

When the spinal cord has been transected headward of the lumbar region, reflex movements of the hind-limb can, after the period of shock has passed, be studied with much uniformity of result. Electric stimuli applied to the skin of the limb, especially of the foot, evoke practically uniformly a drawing up of the limb. This flexion-reflex, as presented by the spinal dog, consists in flexion at knee, hip, and ankle.

The afferent fibres from each (even small) area of the skin of the foot do not enter together as a tiny group into the spinal cord in any

The Simple Reflex

single filament of a single afferent root, but scatter and make their entrance into the cord via a number of rootlets,[139] belonging not merely to one but to two or even three adjacent afferent spinal roots. These afferent fibres, having entered the cord, severally subdivide in the manner well known since the researches of Nansen, Ramon, Van Gehuchten, v. Lenhossek, and others; and their collaterals and terminals must, as it were, seek out the motor cells of the above-cited flexor muscles, and, as it might appear from the above evidence, leave the motor cells of other muscles, for instance, of the extensors, alone. Increase of intensity of the stimulation of the plantar skin does not in my experience make the spinal reflex action flow over, so to say, from the flexor muscles to the extensors. As the strength of the stimulus is increased from minimal, the number of the flexor muscles obviously thrown into action in the limb is increased, and the reaction irradiates to other regions of the body; for instance, to the extensor muscles of the contra-lateral hind leg. In the muscles already implicated in the weaker response the contraction becomes, as the stimulus is increased, stronger, but I have not found it involve the muscles, causing extension of the homolateral hind-limb itself. This flexor-reflex of the limb therefore, although able to excite to various degrees of activity the flexor musculature of the limb, appears unable to excite the extensor musculature.

It would be a mistake, however, to suppose that it is without any direct influence on the latter musculature. It might appear from the statement that the distribution of the afferent conductors of the reflex was to the motor neurones of flexion only, and not to those of the extensor muscles. But the motor neurones of the extensor muscles are not inaccessible to impulses arriving by this afferent path. On the contrary, they can be shown to be easily and habitually accessible to them.

To examine this we may turn to the 'knee-jerk', and to the tonus of the extensor muscles of the knee. In the spinal animal, for instance in the dog and cat, after transection of the spinal cord in the thoracic region, it is easy to satisfy one's self that, after the shock has passed off the extensor muscles of the knee still possess considerable tonus. The spinal tonus is reflex, and it has been shown[304] that in the crureus and

Reciprocal Inhibition

vastus medialis muscles of the cat, the reflex tonus of those muscles is traceable to afferent nerves arising in those very muscles themselves.

The reflex-arc through which the tonus is produced and maintained arises in those muscles themselves and returns to them again. The knee-jerk is easily elicited in the spinal cat and dog. The muscles which contract when the patellar tendon is struck are in these animals the vastus medialis and crureus.[136] The knee-jerk seems, however, only obtainable in them when their reflex spinal tonus is present. Its briskness varies *pari passu* with the degree of this tonus. Severance of the afferent nerves of these muscles destroys their tonus, and renders at the same time the knee-jerk inelicitable, just as also does the severance of their motor-nerves.

The knee-jerk is, therefore, like the spinal tonus itself, dependent on the integrity of the reflex spinal arc of the muscles. But it is customary to regard the knee-jerk not as a reflex action (Westphal, Waller, and others); hence it is termed 'knee-phenomenon', 'knee-jerk', etc. The main ground for denying its claim to be really reflex is that its latent period is shorter than that of other indubitable reflexes. The latency for the knee-jerk has been shown (Waller,[131] Gotch,[167] and others) to be about 10σ, whereas the shortest latency found by Exner[59] for reflex eyelid-closure was 45σ and by Fr. Franck[111] for a spinal reflex about 17σ. The latency for the knee-jerk is but little longer than that for direct excitation of the extensor muscle itself.

If we regard the knee-jerk not as a true reflex but as a 'direct' response of the muscle, we have to suppose that the reflex tonus of the muscle, which is admittedly a *conditio sine qua non* for the jerk, so raises the direct excitability of the muscle that the muscle responds by a contraction to a sudden slight stretch of itself due to a tap on its tendon. No experimenter has, however, satisfactorily succeeded by artificial stimulation of the motor-nerve in similarly raising the direct excitability of the muscle. Moreover, Gotch[167] found the muscle in its state of tonus gave no other indication of increased excitability than simply that it then yielded 'the jerk'. It has been urged against the reflex nature of the jerk that the contraction given by the muscle to the jerk is a simple twitch. The 'jerk' contraction

The Simple Reflex

lasts no longer, or hardly longer, than the twitch given by the muscle in response to a single stimulus, e.g. an induction shock. All reflex contractions are usually considered as tetanic. That is in the main doubtless true. It is what might be inferred from the great part played by summation of stimuli in the elicitation of reflexes. Yet the extensor-thrust reflex, which is undoubtedly a true reflex, appears on measurement (p. 67) to be as brief as the knee-jerk. Its time-relations have been referred to. It is interesting that this brief-lasting reflex also has, as has the knee-jerk itself, the extensor muscles of the hind limb for its seat of expression. The mere brevity of the period of contraction of the knee-jerk is therefore no good evidence that it is not reflex.

The knee-jerk, whether reflex or not, since it is an index of the reflex tonus of the extensor muscles, furnishes a gauge for the effect, if any, exerted by the flexion-reflex on the extensor muscles of the limb. It was said above that the extensors are not thrown into contraction by this flexion-reflex. The reflex reaction may therefore either be neutral to them and leave them and their condition untouched, or it may inhibit them and depress their reflex activity, even if that activity should have at the time only the form of tonus.

If the hamstring muscles (flexors of the knee) be separated from their attachments at their distal (knee) end, and then while the knee joint is passively held in approximate or full extension the flexor-reflex be elicited, e.g. by electric stimulation of the foot, the extensor muscles above the knee are easily felt by palpation to lose at once their tonus and relax.[304] At the same moment the exposed and freed flexor muscles are seen to enter contraction. That is to say, the same exciting stimulus that reflexly throws the flexors into contraction interrupts reflexly the reflex tonus of the extensor muscles. If the knee-jerk be elicited at regular short intervals, signalled for instance by a metronome, and while it is in progress the flexor-reflex be elicited after the flexor muscles have been detached from their knee attachments and the knee thus left free, the knee-jerk is found inelicitable or much diminished directly the reflex contraction of the hamstring muscles sets in (Fig. 29). This inhibition of the jerk sometimes seems to set in even before the reflex contraction of the flexors

Inhibition of Knee-jerk

is apparent. It occurs sometimes when the stimulus is not even strong enough to evoke obvious contraction of the flexors. In the 'flexion-reflex', therefore, the reflex excitation of the flexor muscles is accompanied by reflex inhibition of the antagonistic extensor muscles both as regards their reflex tonus which is in progress when the

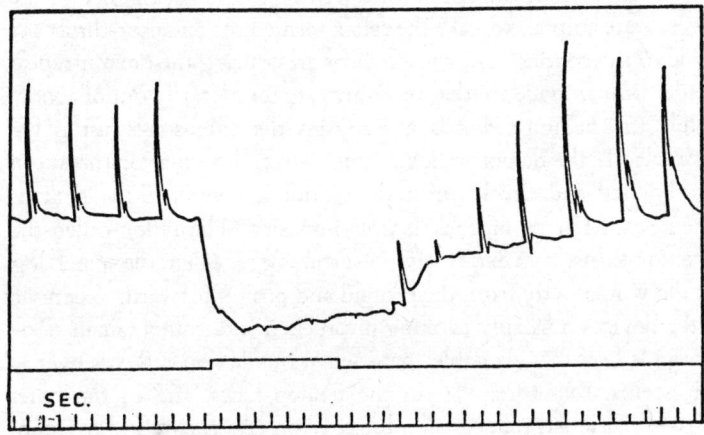

Fig. 29. Reflex inhibition of the knee-jerk

Records from above downwards:
   Tracing from preparation of the extensor muscles of the knee, recording a series of knee-jerks elicited at each alternate beat of a metronome.
   Signal line: weak faradization of the central end of the hamstring nerve was applied during the time marked by the rise of the signal.
   Time in sec.
At onset of stimulation the tonus of the extensor muscles at once fell and with it the knee-jerk was temporarily abolished. After cessation of the inhibiting stimulus the tonus and the knee-jerk quickly returned, and the latter became more brisk than previous to the inhibition.

flexor-reflex is excited, and as regards their response to a stimulus (tap on tendon or muscle) that otherwise excites them.

A corresponding reaction is seen also after ablation of the cerebral hemispheres and thalamencephalon. After removal of those organs, there ensues 'decerebrate rigidity'.[304,182] One feature of this condition is a heightened tonus of the extensor muscles of the knee. The knee is maintained rigidly extended. At the same time the knee-

The Simple Reflex

jerk is elicitable in unusual degree. When the knee is under these circumstances freed from the flexor muscles, and the flexor-reflex is then induced by appropriate excitation, e.g. of the plantar skin, the knee joint at once drops loose, and if the knee-jerk be tested, it is found to be inelicitable, or elicitable only very faintly (Fig. 29).

Similarly, if instead of the knee-jerk or the reflex rigidity of the decerebrate animal, we take the reflex termed the extensor-thrust as a guide to the condition of the extensor arcs during the flexion-reflex, we get similar evidence that those arcs are temporarily out of action. While the flexion-reflex is in progress the extensor-thrust is less elicitable. If the flexion-reflex is quite weak, the extensor-thrust can be obtained and breaks through it; but it cannot if the flexion-reflex be of fair or of considerable intensity. The reflex called the extensor-thrust is an extremely powerful one; it can in the spinal dog lift the whole body from the ground and push it forward. Yet none of the devices normally evoking it can elicit it during a fair flexion-reflex. It becomes elicitable again when the flexion-reflex is over.

It seems, therefore, that in the flexion-reflex and in the other above-mentioned reflexes an inhibitory process is part and parcel of the reflex reaction, so that the inhibition goes on side by side with excitation of other muscles opposed to those which are inhibited. This view, that the inhibition process in these reflexes is a simultaneous counterpart to the excitatory, is supported by the following evidence from the flexion-reflex.

A salient feature of this reflex is flexion at the knee. For comparison of the inhibition and excitation respectively, both hind-limbs are taken and so prepared that in one leg only the knee-flexors can act, in the other leg only the knee-extensors. The stimuli to provoke the reflex are applied either to symmetrical skin points or to symmetrical afferent nerves, as far as practicable, at symmetrical places in their course. For comparison, the stimuli are made as far as possible equal on the two sides. This being arranged, certain characteristic features of the reflex have been examined on the two sides respectively.

(α) The flexion-reflex has a 'receptive skin-field' which though extensive is characteristic for it. Examined by the above preparation

Reciprocal Inhibition

the skin-field whence the excitation (contraction) is elicitable and that whence the inhibition is elicitable has proved in my observations to be one and the same. Thus, stigmatic unipolar faradization of a point in the skin of a right pedal digit provokes in the homonymous limb contraction of the flexors of the knee, and similar stimulation of the corresponding left digit provokes in its own limb inhibition of the extensors of the knee. Again, similar stimulation of the skin of the fore-foot (in my experience that of the crossed fore-foot acts more readily than that of the homonymous) induces excitation (contraction) of the flexors of the crossed knee; and the corresponding skin-region of the opposite fore-limb induces inhibition (relaxation) of the extensors of the knee contralateral to it.

(β) Turning to stimuli other than electrical, it is not, as I have pointed out, *every* form of stimulus that can excite it, when applied within the skin-field appropriate for the direct flexion-reflex. The kinds of skin-stimuli which excite it are those which may be termed 'nocuous',[252] e.g. a prick, strong squeeze, harmful heat (the heat-beam), and chemical agents. Touches, innocuous pressures, rubbing, etc., though effective for various reflexes, e.g. for the extensor-thrust, scratch-reflex, pinna-reflex, etc., do not in my experience excite this reflex. The stimuli which do excite it, for instance, from the *planta*, excite, when applied on the side where the flexor muscles alone remain intact, contraction of those muscles, and when applied correspondingly on the opposite side, where the extensors alone remain intact, inhibit them (relaxation).

(γ) The nerve-twig, similar to that which under faradization on the 'flexors' side excites the flexors (contraction), when faradized on the 'extensors' side inhibits the extensors (relaxation). This comparison has been made not only with skin nerves, but with muscular nerves, notably with the nerves of the hamstring muscles and of the gastrocnemius.

(δ) The flexion-reflex, although it exhibits well the potency of summation of successive stimuli as a factor in its initiation, differs in my experience from various other reflexes, e.g. extensor-thrust, scratch-reflex, pinna-reflex, in being elicitable fairly easily by a single-induction shock. The shock may be applied either to the skin

The Simple Reflex

in the receptive skin-field of the reflex or to an appropriate afferent nerve either cutaneous or muscular. When this is done in the prepared limbs the single-induction shock applied on the 'flexors' side excites a brief reflex contraction of those muscles, correspondingly applied on the 'extensors' side it provokes a brief reflex inhibition of those muscles.

(ϵ) The flexion-reflex, unlike extensor-thrust, pinna-reflex, etc., can be well evoked in my experience by make or break of a galvanic current. This make or break reflex is shown in the 'extensor' preparation by inhibition, just as it is shown in the 'flexor' preparation by contraction. With suitable strength of stimulus the break of a descending current is more effective for the reflex inhibition than the make, and vice versa for an ascending current, just as with contraction. The flexion-reflex can also be maintained by passage of the constant current to a much greater extent than can the scratch-reflex. In this respect it resembles the vasomotor and respiratory reflexes examined by Grützner,[77] and by Langendorff & Oldag,[147] and also the sensual reaction which similar stimulation excites in ourselves—a point of interest when the connexion between *nociceptive* reflexes and dolorous sensation is remembered. When the constant current is thus applied to the limb in which the extensors have been prepared, inhibition proceeds in them as does contraction in the flexors when that current is similarly applied to the limb in which the flexors have been prepared.

(ζ) The latent time of the flexion-reflex is short. This feature is revealed in the inhibition of the extensors just as in the contraction of the flexors. Great differences of latency in the flexion-reflex as in other reflexes can be obtained, apart from variance in intrinsic condition of the reflex preparation, by variance in the external stimuli in intensity, suddenness, frequency of repetition, etc. The effect of such variations is the same in kind, and, in my experience, in extent, when tested by the reflex inhibition as when tested by the reflex contraction. Thus, with strong stimuli I have found as short a latency as 32σ for the inhibition, which is slightly shorter than the shortest for contraction that I have yet met with under like circumstances. With weak stimuli I have occasionally met with a latency as long as 400σ for each effect.

Reciprocal Inhibition

(η) A good criterion of comparison between the reflex inhibition and the reflex contraction in the flexion-reflex under excitation by an intermittent stimulus is the number of stimuli summed for initiation of the reflex as exhibited on the one hand in contraction of the flexors, on the other hand in relaxation of the extensors. The number of successive single stimuli summed for the initiation is less as their individual intensity is greater.[57]

When the summation is compared in the same reflex preparation, in the reflex exhibited as inhibition (relaxation) in the knee-extensors of one limb and in the reflex exhibited as contraction in the knee-flexors of the other limb, good agreement is found; the number has been often actually the same, though the observations are made alternately, first one on one limb, then one on the other limb. Figs. 30A and 30B, and 31A and 31B are such pairs, and illustrate the kind of agreement.

(θ) The course of the flexion-reflex as shown in myograms differs much from that of certain other reflexes of the limb, notably from the extensor-thrust and from the scratch-reflex. Its duration follows more closely that of the eliciting stimulus. If the stimulus is quite

---

Fig. 30 A, B. The 'flexion-reflex' observed as reflex contraction (excitation) of the flexor muscle of the knee (Fig. 30A) and as reflex relaxation (inhibition) of the extensor muscle of the knee (Fig. 30B). The afferent nerve stimulated is a twig of the internal saphenous below the knee

Records from above downwards:
    Time in 0·1 sec.
    Time in $\frac{1}{100}$ sec.
    Signal line: the stimulation is by a series of break induction currents, the number and frequency of which are shown by the electromagnet record of the breaks and makes of the constant current feeding the primary spiral of the inductorium through a rotating key. The distance of the secondary coil from the primary remained the same in the two observations (Figs. 30A and B).
    Myograph curve: the vertical arcs S and S^1 indicate the onset and cessation of stimulation. Vertical arcs also indicate the delivery of the first six stimuli following on S.
    Time in 1 sec.

The observation of Fig. 30B was made from the same preparation as Fig. 30A and about 4 min. later. In Fig. 30A six stimuli were delivered before the reflex contraction set in; similarly in Fig. 30B, six stimuli were delivered before the reflex relaxation set in. The intensity of the stimulating shocks was feeble, hence the relatively long latent period.

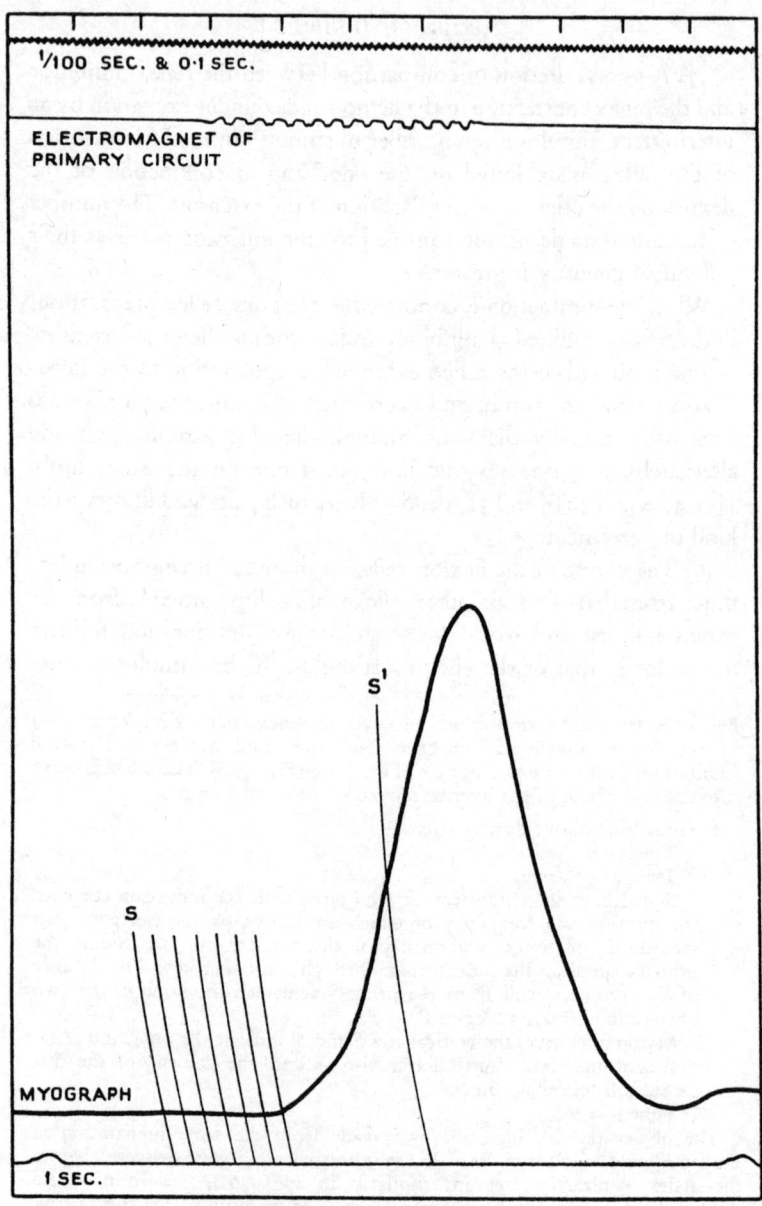

Fig. 30A (For description see p. 93)

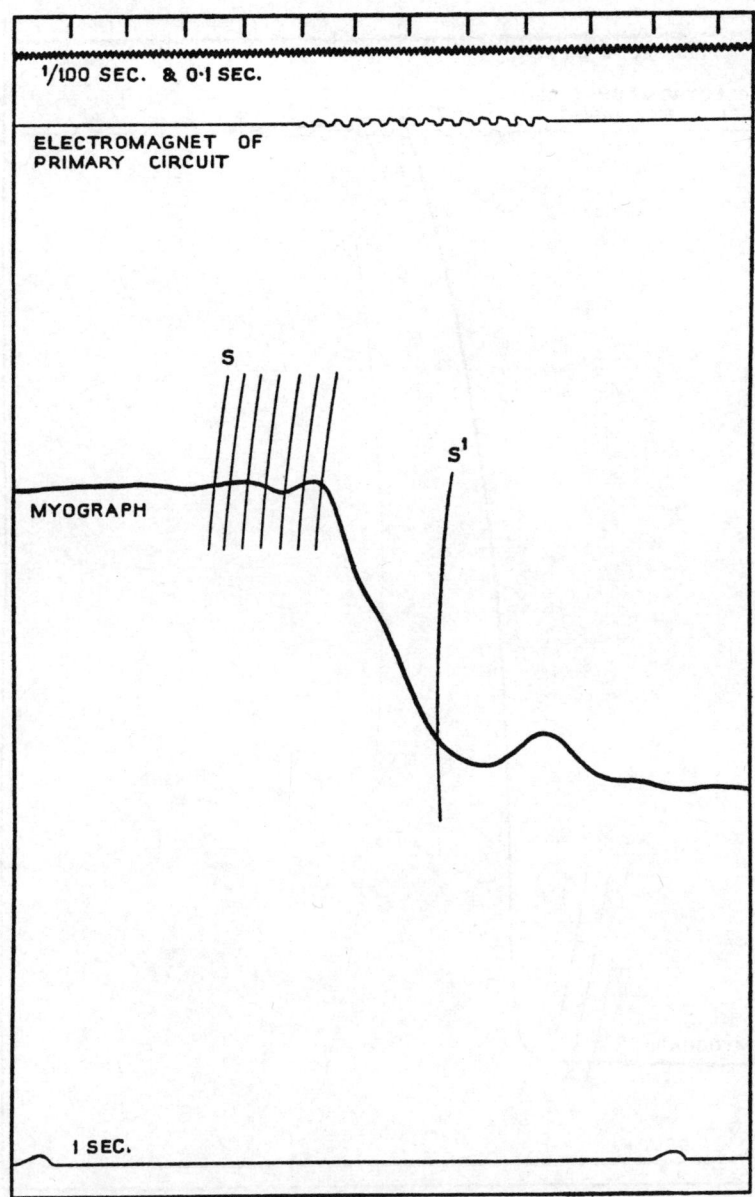

Fig. 30 B (For description see p. 93)

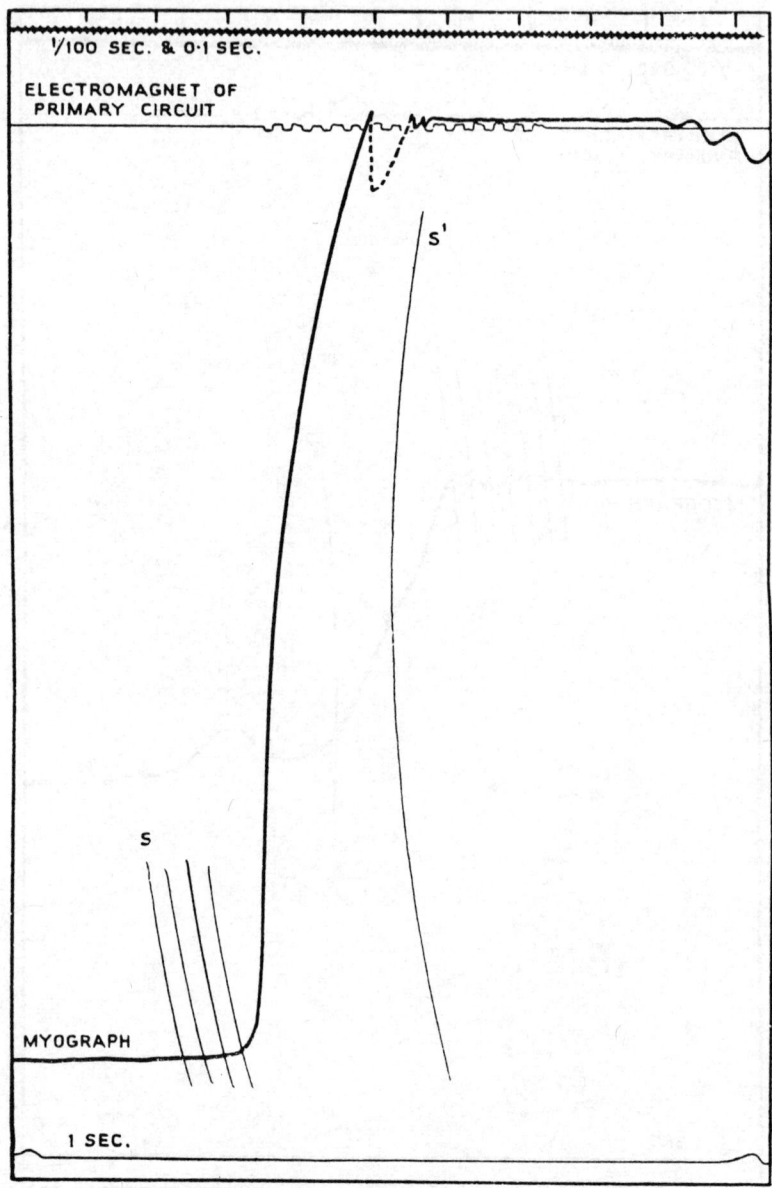

Fig. 31 A (For description see p. 98)

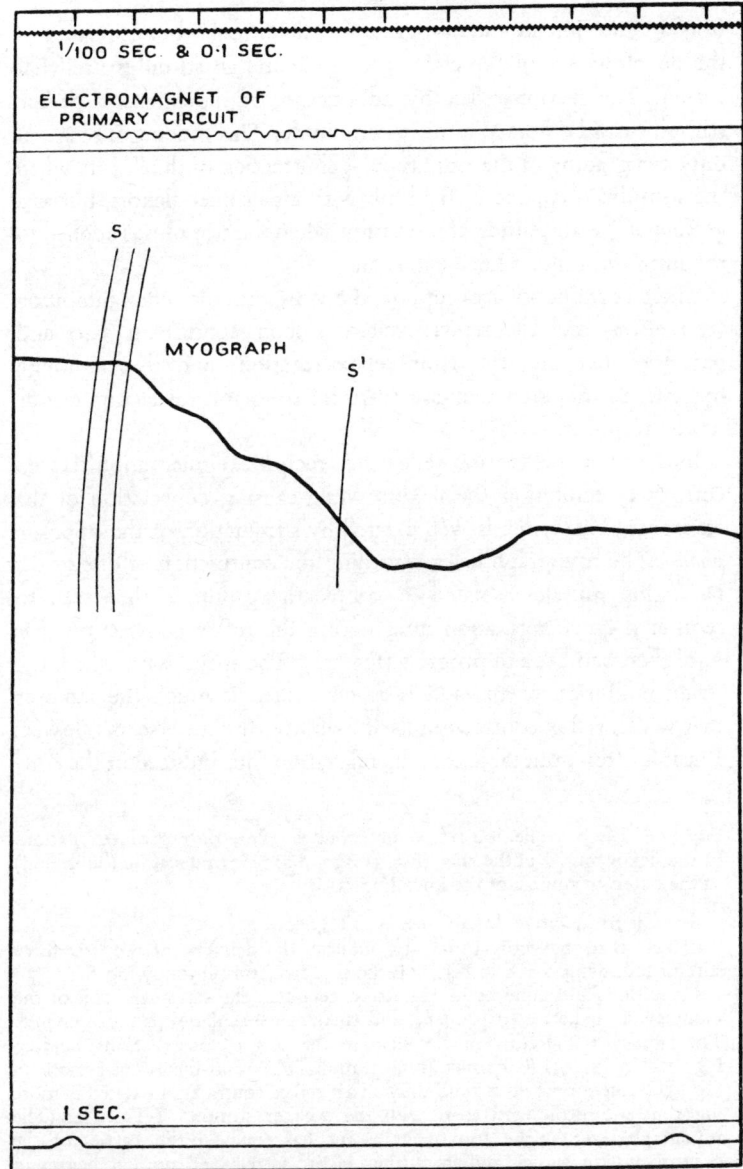

Fig. 31 B (For description see p. 98)

The Simple Reflex

brief and not intense the myogram shows but a short continuance of the development of the effect after the external stimulus itself has ceased. The flexion-reflex by adjustment of the intensity of the stimulus can be graded as to its amplitude. This grading is seen not only as a grading of the amplitude of contraction of the flexors when the stimulus is applied to the limb with intact knee-flexors, but as a *grading* of the amplitude of relaxation when the stimulus is applied to the limb with intact knee-extensors.

These correspondences support the view that the reflex inhibition (relaxation) and the reflex excitation (contraction) are part and parcel of one and the same reflex reaction; and that although opposite in direction they are co-ordinate reciprocal factors in one united response.

In the crossed extension-reflex this 'reciprocal innervation' is seen conversely inhibiting the flexors while causing contraction of the extensors. This reflex is well excited by stimulation of the opposite *planta*. The myograph lever recording the contraction of one of the hamstring muscles, isolated to sample the group, is then seen to register a quick relaxation interrupting the reflex contraction that until then had been in progress (Fig. 32). The speed with which the reflex inhibition occurs and is accomplished is much the same as that which reflex contraction itself exhibits. It hardly seems slower. But it is often noticeable that the relaxation thus induced in the con-

---

Fig. 31 A, B. The 'flexion-reflex' observed as reflex contraction (excitation) of the flexor muscle of the knee (Fig. 31 A) and as reflex relaxation (inhibition) of the extensor muscle of the knee (Fig. 31 B).

Records from above downwards as in Fig. 30.

In Fig. 31 A the vertical arcs also indicate the delivery of the first three stimuli following S and in Fig. 31 B the first two stimuli following S.

Conditions the same as in Fig. 30, except that the secondary coil of the inductorium is nearer to primary, and therefore stimulation is more intense. The latency is therefore shorter than in the pair of observations yielding Fig. 30. In Fig. 31 A the first three stimuli fall within the latent period; in Fig. 31 B the first two stimuli only. The reflex contraction excited is more vigorous and prolonged than with the weaker stimuli of Fig. 30. (The myograph lever at the top of its ascent has touched the carrier of the electromagnetic signal, and its further record is retarded until it begins to descend.)

Reciprocal Inhibition

traction does not reduce the contraction to zero (Fig. 32). The relaxation ensues down to another grade of contraction, at which grade the inhibition often continues to hold it; at least, the muscle continues to remain at that length. In such cases the contraction is

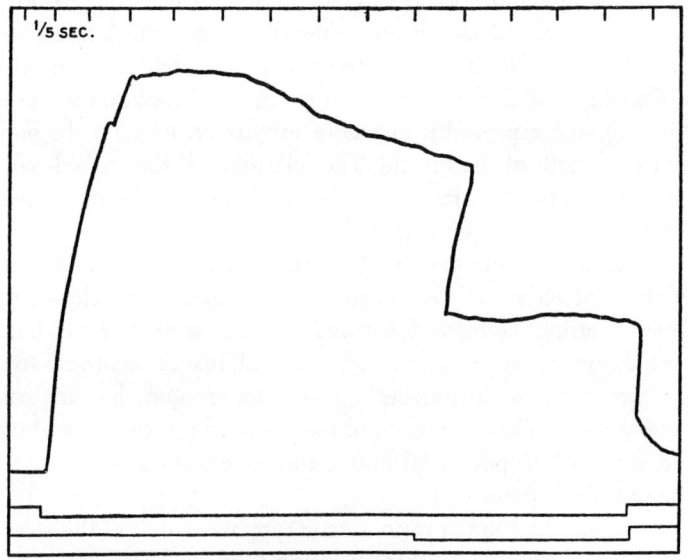

Fig. 32. Inhibition of flexor reflex

Records from above downwards:
 Time in $\frac{1}{5}$ sec.
 Myograph curve recording reflex contraction of semimembranosus induced by stimulation (unipolar faradization) of the skin of the homonymous foot.
 Upper signal line: descent records stimulation described above.
 Lower signal line: descent marks the time of application of a stimulation (unipolar faradization) of the skin of the contralateral foot: this stimulation caused immediate relaxation of the contracting hamstring muscle, but the relaxation did not proceed beyond a certain grade.

reduced suddenly from a high level of intensity to a lower level, but a remainder of contraction persists. It may be that this lower grade represents another functional act in which the muscle is simply adjuvant towards steadying the levers for other muscles which replace itself in its previous role of principal actor. The condition

The Simple Reflex

under which I have most frequently met it has been when the exposed and freed tendon of the semitendinosus (dog) has been attached to the myograph.

It is interesting that when (Fig. 33) the inhibiting stimulus is strong the relaxation of the extensor muscles is actually to a point beyond their initial length obtaining at the time the 'crossed extension-reflex' began. The pre-existent 'decerebrate' tonus is inhibited as well as the intercurrent reflex. The relaxation is indeed down to, as I expressed it in one of my earlier notes,[304] the post-mortem length of the muscle. The relaxation, if the crossed-reflex stimulus continues, is rapidly recovered from, and the interrupted reflex reasserts itself (Figs. 33 and 34).

Concordantly with these results examination with the myograph of the contractions of the pre-tibial and post-tibial muscles of the frog[136] during alternate flexor and extensor strokes of the hind-limb shows in many cases, though not in all, that the contractions of the two antagonistic muscles are not synchronous, but are conversely timed. The contraction of the pre-tibial muscle breaks down just as that of the post-tibial ensues, and the post-tibial relaxes just as the pre-tibial contracts.

An early noted and in various ways typical example of this role of reflex 'inhibition' was that discovered by E. Hering[43] and J. Breuer[44] (1868) in the 'self-regulating' respiratory vagus action. Distension of the lung by exciting afferent fibres in the pulmonary vagus inhibits inspiration and excites expiration. I reverted to this as a fundamental instance in my first note[304] on the subject. If we regard the heart and ring-musculature of the arteries as two antagonistic muscles, v. Cyon's[41] still earlier discovery (1866) that the afferent nerve of the heart and aorta (A. Tschermak & Koster[230])—the latter from this point of view, a tendon of the heart muscle—evokes reflex inhibition of the arterial ring musculature, is another instance. The suggestiveness of these facts for the co-ordination of skeletal muscles was not recognized generally. But Meltzer, the discoverer with Kronecker[89] of the role of inhibition in normal deglutition, wrote in 1883[100]: "Of a purposeful arrangement we could expect that a nerve, the stimulation of which causes flexion, ought to contain also

Central Inhibition

inhibitory fibres for the extensors. Now such an arrangement is indeed present—at least in the respiratory mechanism. Of the superior laryngeal nerve, of the second branch of the trigeminus, and of the splanchnics, we know that stimulation of their central end causes inhibition of the inspiratory and contraction of the expiratory muscles."

Now in the case of the skeletal muscles of the mammalian limb, no efferent nerve-fibres appear to be supplied to them which under stimulation produce inhibition of their contraction. Such have been sought for by various observers, but without success. I have myself looked for them and obtained no unequivocal evidence of their existence. Moreover, Verworn[207] has shown that during the inhibitory relaxation produced by the reflex induced from the nerve of the antagonistic muscles the excitability of the relaxed muscle and its motor-nerve to electrical stimuli remains undiminished.

Moreover, in the condition of decerebrate rigidity, when the elbow is being kept in extension by the heightened tonic action of the extensor muscles, their contraction can be inhibited not only by stimulation of the crossed hind-foot, but by direct electrical stimulation of a point in the lateral column of the transected spinal cord in the hind thoracic region, as has been shown by A. Fröhlich and myself.[222] The inhibition reflexly produced has therefore its seat in the spinal part of the reflex-arcs. It is therefore a *central* inhibition.

This central inhibition appears more than equivalent to merely arresting the play of an excited afferent channel upon the motor centre. Were that all, the phenomenon should resemble the effect of suddenly stopping the stimulation of the afferent nerve causing the reflex. What happens is often not like that; the arrest is more rapid. The 'after-discharge', whatever its seat, can be at once arrested by the inhibition (Fig. 35). The 'after-discharge' of a centre, with its concomitant persistence of contraction of muscles, might well be disadvantageous to the organism. That it is rapidly arrested by the inhibitory side of a succeeding reflex, is an adaptation which facilitates the successive interchange of reflexes. The inhibition can arrest some forms of clonic spasm arising during experimentation (Fig. 36).

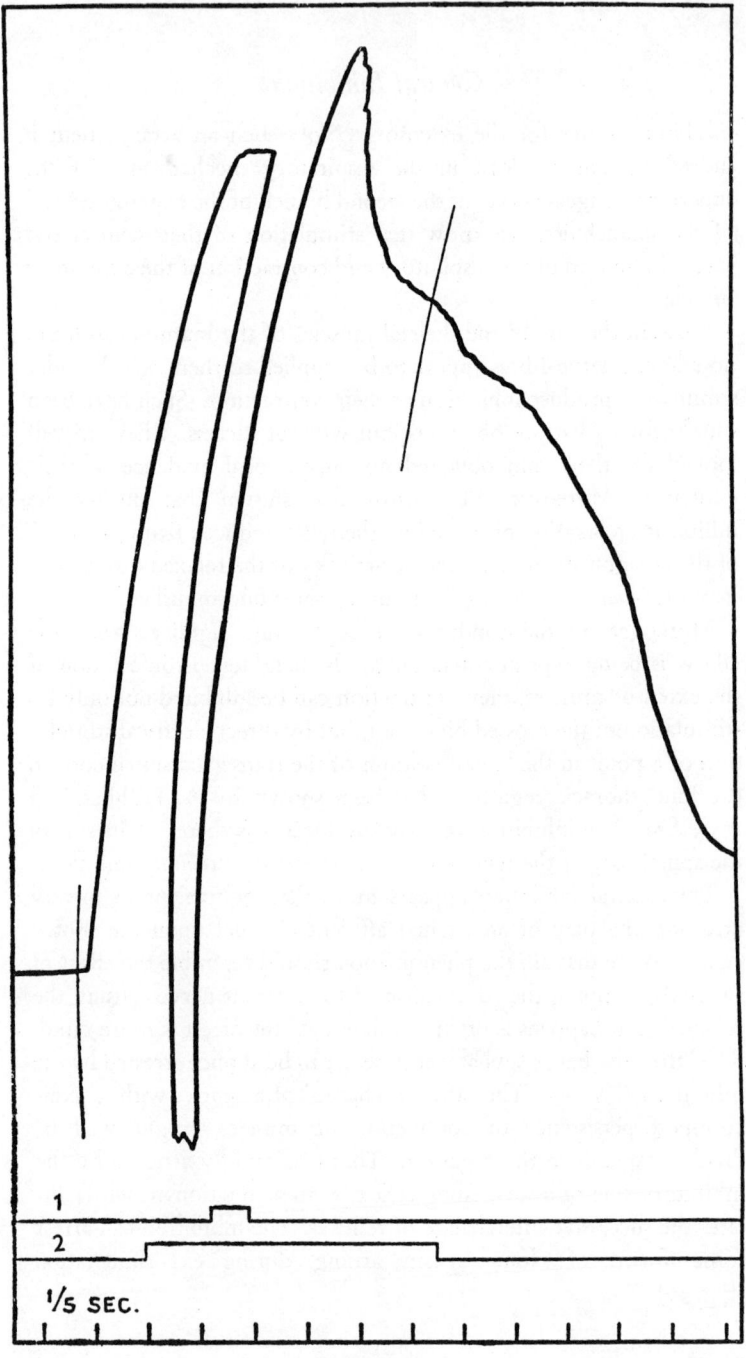

Fig. 33

Inhibition of Internuncial Neurone

The motor neurones of the flexor muscles of the hind-limb can be excited to the clonic discharge characteristic of the scratch-reflex at a time when the flexion-reflex is inhibited from employing them. When the scratch-reflex is in progress it is more difficult to excite a 'flexion-reflex', and vice versa. One reflex seems to be precluded from acting on a motor neurone at a time when another and different reflex is employing it.300 The preclusion of the motor neurone from *one* reflex while it is still left open to it to respond to other reflexes appears to be one of the services of inhibition to the organism. The motor neurone itself seems not to be the actual seat of the inhibition, for if so, it would be inhibited for all reflexes; unless the motor neurone is functionally divisible, and one part of it, e.g. one set of dendrites, can be inhibited at a time when another is not. The seat of the inhibition appears, therefore, with some likelihood, to lie neither in the afferent neurone proper nor in the efferent neurone proper, but in an internuncial mechanism—synapse or neurone—between them. I say 'neurone proper', meaning to exclude from that term the synapse, although in a synapse the neurone terminals are included.

The striking correspondence observed (*vide supra*) between the reflex inhibition and the reflex contraction, when examined in one

---

Fig. 33. Inhibition of crossed extensor-reflex and of muscle tone

Records from above downwards:
   Myograph curve recording reflex contraction of extensor of knee (beginning and end of stimulation are indicated by vertical arcs), interrupted by a reflex inhibition (relaxation).
   Upper signal line (1): Ascent indicates stimulation producing reflex inhibition.
   Lower signal line (2): Ascent indicates stimulation producing crossed extensor-reflex.
   Both signal lines are displaced somewhat to the right.
   Time in $\frac{1}{5}$ sec.

The reflex contraction (crossed extensor-reflex) was induced by stimulation (unipolar faradization) of the skin of the opposite foot during the period indicated by the vertical arcs and lower signal (2). Towards the height of the reflex contraction a brief stimulation (unipolar faradization) was applied to the skin of the foot homonymous with the knee extensor yielding the myogram: the duration of this inhibiting stimulus is marked by upper signal (1). The knee extensor at outset was in some tonic contraction due to 'decerebrate rigidity'. The reflex inhibition relaxes this in addition to inhibiting the current reflex from the crossed foot.

The Simple Reflex

and the same type-reflex, allows the inference that the nerve-fibres from the receptive field of the reflex each divide in the spinal cord into end-branches (e.g. collaterals), one set of which, when the

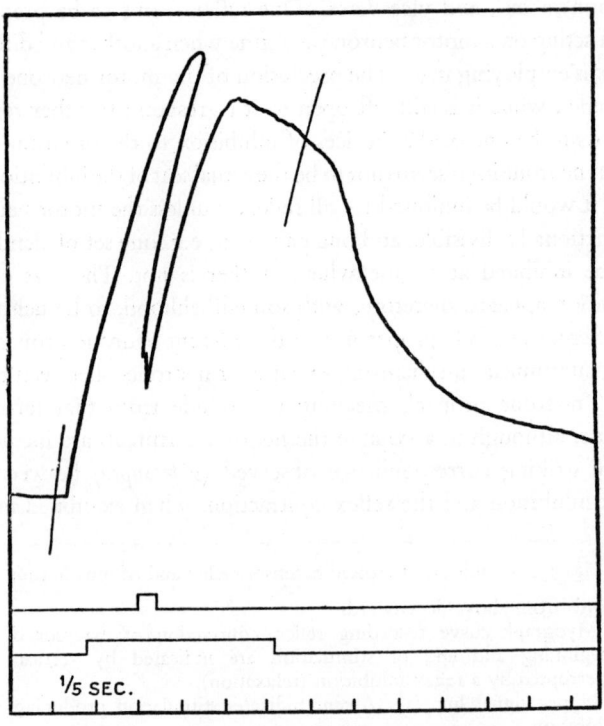

Fig. 34. Inhibition of crossed extensor-reflex

Records and procedures as in Fig. 33: lower signal and vertical arcs indicate contralateral stimulation producing crossed extensor-reflex.

The inhibiting stimulus (upper signal) in this instance was weak faradization applied to the proximal end of the severed 'hamstring nerve'.

nerve-fibre is active, produces excitation, while another set, when the nerve-fibre is active, produces inhibition.[205, 304] The single afferent nerve-fibre would therefore in regard to one set of its terminal branches be *specifically excitor*, and in regard to another set of

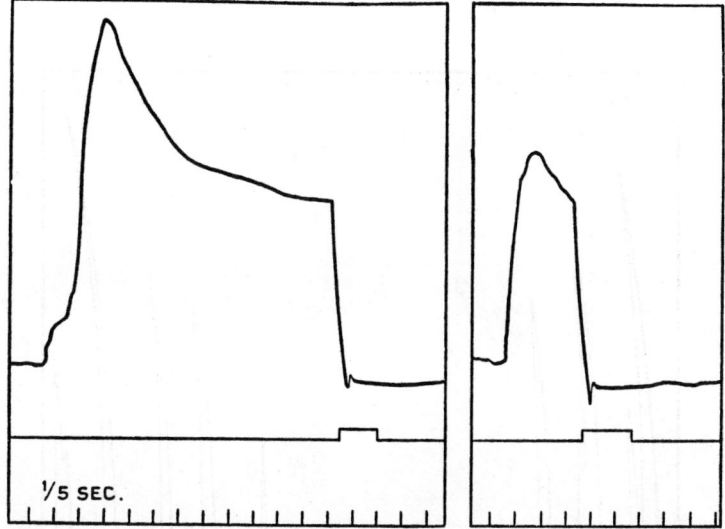

Fig. 35. Inhibition of after-discharge of extensor thrust and of crossed extensor-reflex

Records from above downwards:
  Myograph curve: left, extensor thrust; right, crossed extensor-reflex.
  Signal line: ascent indicates application of inhibitory stimulus.
  Time in $\frac{1}{5}$ sec.

Myograph records of reflex contractions of the extensor of the knee in 'decerebrate' cat. The exciting stimulus was, in the observation reproduced on the left of the figure, a brief compression—lasting less than a second—of a digit of the contralateral foot. After this stimulus had been given and discontinued, and while the after-discharge of the reflex was still in progress, the proximal end of a branch of the severed hamstring nerve was stimulated by faradization for about $\frac{1}{4}$ sec. The time of this inhibiting stimulus is marked by the signal. The reflex after-discharge is seen to have been at once inhibited and in this case not to have returned.

The observation reproduced on the right was from the same experiment, but later; in it the stimulation exciting the reflex contraction (crossed extensor-reflex) was faradization of the proximal end of a twig of the internal saphenous of the contralateral leg. This stimulation lasted about $\frac{2}{5}$ sec. or less. Its cessation was quickly succeeded by faradization of the proximal end of a branch of the severed hamstring nerve as in the previous observation. The after-discharge of the contraction reflex is cut short as before.

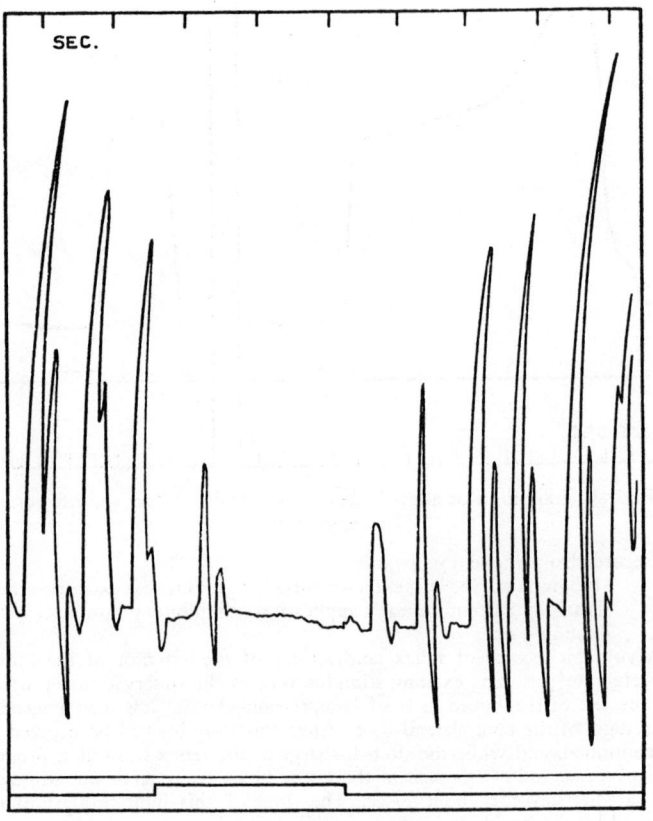

Fig. 36. Reflex inhibition of clonic spasm of semitendinosus

Records from above downwards:
 Time in sec.
 Myograph curve of convulsive twitching of semitendinosus in a spinal dog.
 Signal line: ascent indicates application of inhibitory stimulus.
The spasms are reduced and temporarily suspended by stimulation (faradization) of the proximal end of a branch of the internal saphenous nerve of the contralateral leg.

Reciprocal Inhibition

its central endings be *specifically inhibitory*. It would, in this respect, be duplex centrally (Fig. 37). There is analogy between the structural arrangement for reflex reciprocal innervation and that of *Astacus* claw, if it be supposed that the individual nerve-fibres of the crayfish-claw preparation dichotomize, one division of the nerve-fibre passing to the closing muscle, the other to the opening muscle; so that one division of the fibre exerts the excitor action, the other the well-known inhibitory, studied by Richet,[98] Biedermann,[109] Piotrowski,[141] and others.

In denoting one set of central terminations of an afferent arc *specifically inhibitory*, it is here meant that by no mere change in intensity or mode of stimulation can they be brought to yield any other effect than inhibition. But the fact that stimulation of a single set of afferent arcs, namely a single small afferent nerve, excites frequently a reflex movement of alternating direction in which, for instance at the knee, extension succeeds primary flexion, shows that a change of internal conditions may presumably convert an intraspinal connexion that under the primary conditions is inhibitory into one that under later supervening conditions becomes excitatory. The fact that under certain forms of cerebral action true antagonistic muscles can be thrown synchronously into contraction, points to the same limitation of the term 'specific' in this connexion. Further, there is the intraspinal action of strychnine.

There is the long recognized fact that under strychnine practically all the skeletal muscles of the body may be reflexly thrown into contraction simultaneously, and this is obviously inclusive of, and was proved for, antagonistic muscles.[136] Evidently strychnine in some way must alter or obscure reciprocal innervation. I have furnished (1892) tracings showing that the pre-tibial and post-tibial muscles of the frog, although in normal reflex movements so frequently exhibiting concurrent contraction and relaxation in the two groups reciprocally, under strychnine reveal in the double myogram perfectly synchronous contraction in both groups.[136]

Such a result may be explicable in several ways. In order to discover what the nature of the change wrought by strychnine really is, there have to be fulfilled in the test experiments certain conditions

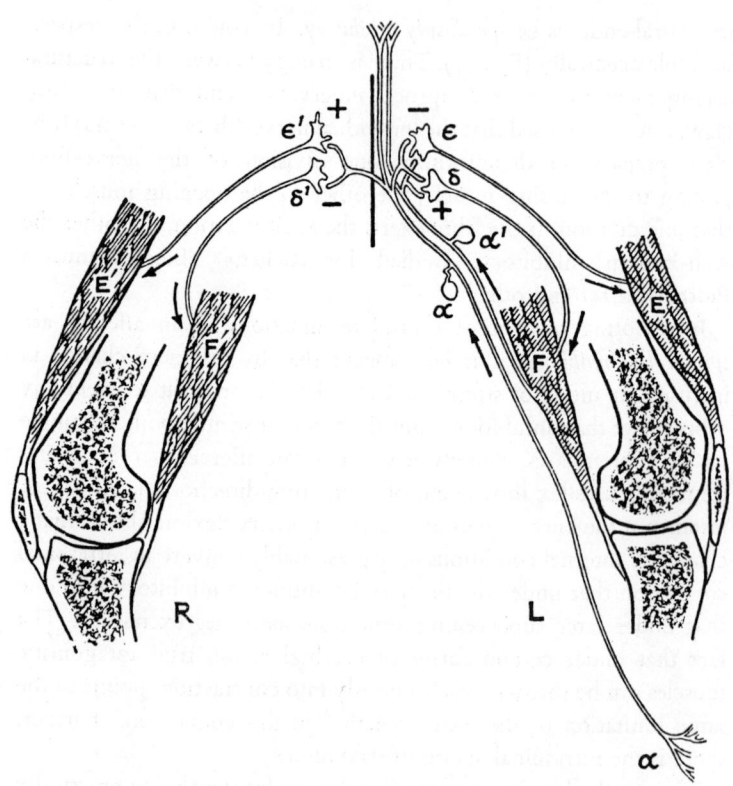

Fig. 37. Diagram indicating connexions and actions of two afferent spinal root-cells, α and α^1, in regard to their reflex influence on the extensor and flexor muscles of the two knees

α, Root-cell afferent from skin below knee; α^1, root-cell afferent from flexor muscle of knee, i.e. in hamstring nerve; ϵ and ϵ^1, efferent neurones to the extensor muscles of the knee, left and right; δ and δ^1, efferent neurones to the flexor muscles; E and E^1, extensor muscles; F and F^1, flexor muscles. The 'schalt-zellen' (v. Monakow) probable between the afferent and efferent root-cells are for simplicity omitted. The sign + indicates that at the synapse which it marks the afferent fibre α (and α^1) excites the motor neurone to discharging activity, whereas the sign − indicates that at the synapse which it marks the afferent fibre α (and α^1) inhibits the discharging activity of the motor neurones. The effect of strychnine and of tetanus toxin is to convert the *minus* sign into *plus* sign.

Action of Strychnine

which not every preparation of antagonistic muscles can supply. Muscles acting over two joints are to be avoided in such a test. Thus the gastrocnemius of the frog extends the ankle but flexes the knee; it antagonizes the action of the pre-tibial muscles which flex the ankle, but since flexion of the knee so commonly accompanies flexion of the ankle, it is synergic with the pre-tibial muscles in the great flexion-reflex that draws up the limb. If it acts synchronously with pre-tibial muscles under strychnine, we are still left in a dilemma as to whether the co-ordinate reciprocal action at the ankle is essentially destroyed, or whether a reflex attempt to flex the knee has not been simply added to it under a lowering of the intraspinal resistances. And this dilemma is the greater in that the afferent nerves and surfaces used for exciting reflexes contain admixed afferent channels, some exciting contraction in one group of the opposed muscles, and some exciting contraction in the other. Thus in the afferent nerves from the foot, both in the dog[304] and the frog,[288] there are commingled with fibres which excite the flexor muscles those which excite the extensor muscles—witness the extensor-thrust and flexion-reflex, both elicitable from the dog's foot, and Baglioni's extension-reflex of the leg and the flexion-reflex, both elicitable from the frog's leg. That the extensor muscles of the limb should under strychnine be thrown into contraction synchronously with the flexors in these cases might be due either to the two reflexes being elicited together when spinal resistance has been lowered, or to a conversion of the inhibition part of one reflex into an excitation. And in this latter case it is still left undecided whether the extension under strychnine is due to prepotent extensor-reflex with its accompanying flexor inhibition changed into excitation, or whether it is the flexion-reflex which is changed conversely.

On similar grounds the 'spontaneous' convulsions due to strychnine afford no deeper insight into the problem. These 'spontaneous' convulsions are really reflex (Stannius, Cl. Bernard, H. E. Hering, and others) in the sense that they originate in the afferent arcs; and in the convulsive movements antagonistic muscles contract simultaneously. But the difficulty here again is, that the reflex source may and probably does, operate in many afferent arcs concurrently. Some

The Simple Reflex

of these arcs excite extensor muscles normally, while others excite flexors. The simultaneous contraction of both flexors and extensors might thus be naturally explicable by lowered spinal resistance, both sets of reflexes being equally induced together, or the explanation might be of an alternative kind, such as suggested above. On the former view the reciprocal innervation of antagonistic muscles would merely be obscured by a simultaneous double reflex; on the latter a more profound alteration would have taken place. The occurrence and form of the convulsion fail to decide among these possibilities.

Conditions for determining the nature of the action that really occurs seem offered, however, in certain instances. Thus, in the hind-limb of the cat we have two afferent nerves which never, under any normal conditions[304] in my experience, yield as their primary reflex in the vasti-crureus muscle any action but relaxation; in other words, they, without exception, produce reflex inhibition of that muscle. To suppose that these nerves contain afferent fibres which evoke reflexly at the knee any action other than flexion would be mere hypothesis. These two nerves are the internal saphenous in its course below the knee, and the hamstring nerve, coming from the flexor muscles of the knee. Further, the vasti-crureus is a single-joint muscle, and unlike the rest of the quadriceps extensor of the thigh is not a flexor of the hip; therefore contraction in it cannot mean merely its participation in the synergy of the flexion-reflex itself, which includes flexion at the hip. A reflex preparation suited for examining the action of strychnine on reciprocal innervation can, therefore, be obtained in the hind-limb by severing, in the decerebrate animal for instance, the following nerves: the external popliteal, the internal popliteal, the obturator and pudic in the pelvis, the superior gluteal, the external and cutaneous divisions of the anterior crural and the hamstring nerve. The last named is ligated and cut close to its entrance in the muscles, so that its central end can be stimulated. A branch of the internal saphenous nerve below the knee is also prepared for stimulation of its central end. When this is done it is found that no change in intensity or other conditions of excitation of the afferent nerve ever provokes anything but inhibition of the extensor of the knee, but a small dose of strychnine at once

Action of Strychnine

transmutes the inhibitory effect into an excitation effect.304 Reflex contraction is obtained in place of reflex relaxation. If small doses are carefully graded it is possible to see a state in which the reflex relaxation is diminished but is not replaced by excitation. This phenomenon shows well how little competent is the view of lowered spinal resistance to really explain the action of strychnine; for at this stage the stimulated arc that normally acts on the extensor muscle by inhibition is less able to affect it than before, so that on the spinal resistance view the resistance at this stage is actually heightened.

A similar conversion of inhibitory effect into excitatory is produced more gradually but not less potently by tetanus toxin.304

This conversion sets in before and under smaller doses of strychnine or toxin than are required to produce the convulsive seizures characteristic of strychnine poisoning, or general tetanus.

The transformation of effect by strychnine holds good not only for the nerves above mentioned but for skin-stimuli, and also for those skin points remote from the hind-limb itself, which provoke reflex inhibition of the test muscle; for instance, in the case of the knee-extensor as test muscle, the skin of the fore-paws.

The conversion of inhibitory effect into excitation effect by strychnine is more easily obtained in the case of some nerves than of others. In the instances of the nerves above mentioned the conversion is least facile, i.e. requires larger doses or longer time for development, in the case of the hamstring nerve, than in the others. The inhibitory effect belonging to that nerve is readily lessened by the strychnine, but its actual replacement by excitation effect, e.g. contraction of knee-extensor, not only requires larger doses of strychnine, but is even then phasic rather than continuous. When this nerve is tested by stimulation at regular short intervals during one of these phasic periods, it can be seen that, starting from the phase in which it still evokes inhibition little, or perhaps not at all, less obviously than in the normal state, its inhibitory effect then becomes progressively less, until it is replaced by excitation effect (contraction), at first mild, later violent. This periodic phase will repeat itself many times.

The conversion of inhibition effect as thus tested on the knee-extensor might be attributable to the afferent nerves stimulated

The Simple Reflex

containing *two* kinds of afferent fibres admixed, one kind causing reflex contraction of the muscle, the other kind reflex inhibition. Strychnine might, by augmenting the action of the former or by depressing the action of the latter, change the effect of stimulation of the mixed nerve. But the latter fibres would be expected to be associated in their action with—or, as urged above, to be even the selfsame fibres which evoke—contraction of the flexor muscles. Now there is at the stage of strychnization, at which the change of inhibitory into excitatory effect occurs, no trace of any paralysis or even depression of the flexor contractions. The protagonist and the antagonist muscles are thrown together into synchronous contraction as an effect of strychnine. This and other considerations appear to me to weigh against explaining the conversion of inhibition effect into excitation effect by the hypothesis of reflex antagonistic sets of fibres, oppositely poisoned centrally, commingled in these afferent nerves. Moreover, when a hamstring muscle is taken as the test muscle, a similar conversion of inhibition into excitation (contraction) by strychnine is seen under the crossed extension-reflex. This reflex, elicitable through the skin or various afferent nerves of the contra-lateral hind-limb, normally excites the knee-extensor to contraction and inhibits the hamstrings, the knee-flexors. Under strychnine its reflex inhibition of the hamstring muscle is converted into reflex excitation (contraction) of that muscle. The observations, as they stand at present, incline me to the inference that the action of the alkaloid is to convert in the spinal cord the process of inhibition—whatever that may essentially be—into the process of excitation—whatever that may essentially be.* The reflex nexus was pre-existent,

* From the predominance of extension as a reflex in the hind-limb of the 'spinal' frog under strychnine, flexion predominating normally, Cushny has recently (*Textbook of Pharmacology and Therapeutics*, 3rd ed. Philadelphia, 1903) argued much as I did (*Journ. Physiol.*, vol. XIII, 1892), also from experiments on the frog, that strychnine acts as a destroyer of reciprocal innervation. The hind-limb of the frog, owing to the number of double-joint muscles, is, as said in the text, not a preparation wherewith it seems possible to definitely test this argument or inference. But the evidence obtained from more suitable preparations fully bears out, as the text shows, the earlier inferences drawn by Cushny and myself regarding the frog.

[October, 1905. C.S.S.]

Action of Strychnine

but the effect across it was signalized by a different sign, namely *minus*, prior to the strychnine or tetanus toxin, instead of *plus*, as afterward (see Fig. 37).

The action of the toxin in respect to inhibition resembles that of strychnine closely in several ways. Thus, in the stages of the disease in which the tetanus is still 'local' and manifested in one limb, namely that (e.g. the hind-limb) which received the toxin injection, the toxin early converts into excitation the reflex inhibition of the extensor muscles, normally obtainable from the internal saphenous nerve, but that obtainable from the peroneal and popliteal nerves, and from the hamstring nerve, remains unreversed, though the strength of the inhibitory effect of these nerves may be very distinctly less than normal. Later, as the condition progresses, the inhibitory effect normally belonging to the peroneal and popliteal nerves becomes actually reversed into excitation. Finally, even that of the hamstring nerve itself is reversed. This is the same sequence of effect pursued by progressive increase of dosage of strychnine.

One difference that seems apparent between the action of the tetanus toxin and of strychnine in these observations is that in the relatively slow progress of the tetanus toxin it is easy to note the stage in which the conversion of the inhibition effect into excitation effect has occurred, while there is yet none of that obvious lowering of the threshold of reflex reaction which early marks the course of strychnine poisoning, and has been drawn attention to by many observers.

In experiments on the hind-limb, I have usually introduced the toxin into the sciatic trunk well below the hamstring branch, more rarely into the hamstring nerve as well, or alone. I have found the inhibitory effect of the internal saphenous nerve (stimulated in its course below the knee) converted to excitation in 48 hours from the time of inoculation. In the gradual progress of the condition, I have several times found the hamstring nerve produce slight inhibition of the extensor if the initial posture taken at the knee be extension, and yet produce distinct excitation of the extensor if the initial posture taken at the knee be flexion. This recalls the results of v. Uexküll in *Ophioglypha* and *Echinus*.1922

The Simple Reflex

The conversion of inhibition into excitation by tetanus toxin is demonstrable, as is that by strychnine, with the reflexes of the fore-limb as well as with those of the hind-limb, and in the 'decerebrate' animal as well as in the merely 'spinal'.

We can understand what havoc such a change must work in the co-ordinative mechanisms.304 The observed difference between the facility with which strychnine and tetanus toxin convert the inhibition by the hamstring nerve into excitation, and that with which they convert the inhibition of the other limb-nerves mentioned, does not seem referable to a different action on muscular afferents and cutaneous afferents respectively. Stimulation of the central end of the vasto-crureus nerve evokes normally inhibition of the hamstrings of the opposite limb, but under strychnine it evokes their contraction. In that case, therefore, the strychnine converts with facility the inhibition by a muscular afferent into excitation, just as with the skin nerves mentioned.

That strychnine and tetanus toxin can convert a central inhibition into an excitation, and that the various normal reflex spinal inhibitions show differences one from another in the ease with which they undergo conversion into excitation makes the synchronous excitation of antagonistic muscles in certain willed actions less difficult to understand. Vasodepressor reflexes under chloral (v. Cyon), chloroform (Bayliss),144 etc., change into vasoconstrictor under curare, morphia, etc. But the reversal does not appear to occur with equal facility in all afferent nerves alike. It is stated to be impossible to obtain any vascular reflex but a depressant one from the 'depressor' nerve. This nerve, arising in the heart (v. Cyon)41 and aorta (Tschermak & Köster),230 may in a sense be considered the afferent nerve of the muscle antagonistic to the ring musculature of the arteries, namely, the muscle whose tonus it reflexly depresses. It is in that way comparable with the afferent nerve of the hamstring muscles in relation to the extensors of the knee. The depressor action of the hamstring nerve on the knee-extensor seems, as just said, in my experience, particularly resistant to conversion from inhibition into excitation by strychnine.

In examples of reciprocal innervation drawn from lowlier

Action of Strychnine

organisms and visceral organs we find the inhibition a peripheral phenomenon, that is, with its seat outside the central nervous system. On the other hand, in examples drawn from higher organisms and skeletal movements, the inhibition is a central phenomenon, e.g. intraspinal. The same considerations which traced the line of adaptation in placing the seat of the refractory phase of spinal reflexes intraspinally between the ending of receptive neurone and the commencement of motor neurone, apply here to central inhibition. The significance of the centralization of these processes of refractory phase and reciprocal inhibition seems the same as we may infer for the centrality of the central nervous system itself (vide infra, Lect. IX).

Lecture IV

INTERACTION BETWEEN REFLEXES

ARGUMENT: The 'simple reflex' a convenient but artificial abstraction. Compounding of reflexes. The principle of the common path. Relative aperiodicity of the final common path. Afferent arcs which use the same final common path to different effect have successive but not simultaneous use of it. 'Allied' reflexes. Allied reflexes act harmoniously, are capable of simultaneous combination, and in many cases reinforce one another's action on the final common path. 'Antagonistic' reflexes. Alliance or coalition occurs between (1) individual reflexes belonging to the same 'type-reflex', (2) certain reflexes originated by receptors of different species but situate in the same region of surface, (3) certain reflexes belonging to proprio-ceptive organs secondarily excited by reflexes initiated at the body-surface (the three fields of reception, extero-ceptive, intero-ceptive, and proprio-ceptive), (4) certain reflexes initiated from widely separate but functionally interconnected body-regions. Alliance between reflexes exemplified in inhibitory actions as well as in excitatory. Antagonistic reflexes interfere, one reflex deferring, interrupting, or cutting short another, or precluding the latter altogether from taking effect on the final common path. Intraspinal seat of the interference. Compound reflexes may interfere in part. The place (? synapse) where convergent afferent paths impinge on a common path constitutes a mechanism of co-ordination. The convergence of afferent paths to form common paths occurs with great frequency in the central nervous system. A question whether any reflexes are in the intact organism wholly neutral one to another.

WE have hitherto dealt with reflex reactions under the guise of a convenient but artificial abstraction—the simple reflex. That is to say, we have fixed our attention on the reaction of a reflex-arc as if it were that of an isolable and isolated mechanism, for whose function the presence of other parts of the nervous system and of other arcs might be negligible and wholly indifferent. This is improbable. The nervous system functions as a whole. Physiological and histological analysis finds it connected throughout its whole extent. Donaldson opens his description of it with the remark: "A group of nerve-cells disconnected from the other nerve-tissues of the body, as muscles and glands are disconnected from each other, would be without physiological significance." A reflex reaction, even in a 'spinal animal'

Principle of the Common Path

where the solidarity of the nervous system has been so trenchantly mutilated, is always in fact a reaction conditioned not by one reflex-arc but by many. A reflex detached from the general nervous condition is hardly realizable.

The compounding together of reflexes is therefore a main problem in nervous co-ordination. For this problem it is important to recognize a feature in the architecture of the grey-centred (synaptic) nervous system which may be termed *the principle of the common path*.300 If we regard the nervous system of any higher organism from the broad point of view, a salient feature in its scheme of construction is the following.

At the commencement of every reflex-arc is a receptive neurone extending from the receptive surface to the central nervous organ. This neurone forms the sole avenue which impulses generated at its receptive point can use whithersoever be their destination. This neurone is therefore a path exclusive to the impulses generated at its own receptive point, and other receptive points than its own cannot employ it. A single receptive point may play reflexly upon quite a number of different effector organs. It may be connected through its reflex path with many muscles and glands in many different regions. Yet all its reflex-arcs spring from the one single shank or stem, i.e. from the one afferent neurone which conducts from the receptive point at the periphery into the central nervous organ.

But at the termination of every reflex-arc we find a final neurone, the ultimate conductive link to an effector organ (muscle or gland). This last link in the chain, e.g. the motor neurone, differs obviously in one important respect from the first link of the chain. It does not subserve exclusively impulses generated at one single receptive source, but receives impulses from many receptive sources situate in many and various regions of the body. It is the *sole* path which all impulses, no matter whence they come, must travel if they are to act on the muscle-fibres to which it leads.

Therefore, while the receptive neurone forms a private path exclusively serving impulses of one source only, the final or efferent neurone is, so to say, a public path, *common* to impulses arising at any of many sources of reception. A receptive field, e.g. an area of skin,

Interaction between Reflexes

is analysable into receptive points. One and the same effector organ stands in reflex connexion not only with many individual receptive points but even with many various receptive *fields*. Reflexes generated in manifold sense-organs can pour their influence into one and the same muscle. Thus a limb-muscle is the *terminus ad quem* of many reflex-arcs arising in many various parts of the body. Its motor-nerve is a path common to all the reflex-arcs which reach that muscle (cf. infra, Fig. 44, p. 150).

Reflex-arcs show, therefore, the general features that the initial neurone of each is a *private* path exclusively belonging to a single receptive point (or small group of points); and that finally the arcs embouch into a path leading to an effector organ; and that their final path is common to all receptive points wheresoever they may lie in the body, so long as they have connexion with the effector organ in question. Before finally converging upon the motor neurone the arcs converge to some degree. Their private paths embouch upon *internuncial* paths common in various degree to groups of private paths. The terminal path may, to distinguish it from internuncial common paths, be called *the final common path*. The motor-nerve to a muscle is a collection of final common paths.

Certain consequences result from this arrangement. One of these seems the preclusion of essential qualitative difference between nerve-impulses arising in different afferent nerves. If two conductors have a tract in common, there can hardly be essential qualitative difference between their modes of conduction; and the final common paths must be capable of responding with different rhythms which different conductors impress upon it. It must be to a certain degree aperiodic. If its discharge be a rhythmic process, as from many considerations it appears to be, the frequency of its own rhythm must be capable of being at least as high as that of the highest frequency of any of the afferent arcs that play upon it; and it must be able also to reproduce the characters of the slowest.*

A second consequence is that each receptor being dependent for final communication with its effector organ upon a path not exclusively its own but common to it with certain other receptors,

---

* Baglioni's results[285] support this inference.

Principle of the Common Path

such nexus necessitates successive and not simultaneous use of the common path by various receptors using it to *different or opposed* effect. When two receptors are stimulated simultaneously, each of the receptors tending to evoke reflex action that for its end-effect employs the same final common path but employs it in a different way from the other, one reflex appears without the other. The result is *this* reflex or *that* reflex, but not the two together.[183] Excitation of the central end of the afferent root of the eighth or seventh cervical nerve of the monkey evokes reflexly in the same individual animal sometimes flexion at elbow, sometimes extension. If the excitation be preceded by excitation of the first thoracic root the result is usually extension: if preceded by excitation of the sixth cervical root it is usually flexion. Yet though the same root may thus be made to evoke reflex contraction of the flexors or of the extensors, it does not, in my experience, evoke contraction in both flexors and extensors in the same reflex-response. Of the two reflexes on extensors and flexors respectively, either the one or the other results, but not the two together. Thus, in my experience, excitation of the seventh or eighth root never causes simultaneously with reflex contraction of the flexors of elbow a contraction of that part of the triceps which extends the elbow. The flexor-reflex when it occurs seems therefore to exclude the extensor-reflex, and vice versa. If there resulted a compromise between the two reflexes, so that each reflex had a share in the resultant, the compound would be an action which was neither the appropriate flexion nor the appropriate extension. Were there to occur at the final common path algebraical summation of the influence exerted on it by two opposed receptive arcs, there would result in the effector organ an action adapted to neither and useless for the purposes of either.

In the Coelenterate, *Carmarina*, a mechanical stimulus applied to the sub-umbrella causes, as in another Geryonid, *Tiaropsis indicans*,[72] a reflex movement that brings the free end of the manubrium to the spot touched. Bethe reports[263] that if two stimuli are applied simultaneously to opposite points of the discoid sub-umbrella, the points chosen being such that the manubrium is midway between them, the manubrium is moved toward the point at which the stimulus applied was the stronger. He adds that if both stimuli are of exactly equal strength the manubrium remains unmoved and uncontracted. To obtain such a result as this last with antagonistic spinal reflexes in the vertebrate would obviously be more difficult, because the more complex the preparation and the nervous system involved, the more difficult it will be at any moment to exactly balance the two reflexes. But, apart from that, the observation on *Carmarina* is an analogue of that in the monkey's arm.

This dilemma between reflexes would seem to be a problem of frequent recurrence in reflex co-ordination. We note an orderly sequence of actions in the movement of animals, even in cases where every observer admits that the co-ordination is merely reflex. We see one act succeed another without confusion. Yet, tracing this sequence to its external causes, we recognize that the usual thing in nature is not for one exciting stimulus to begin immediately after another ceases, but for an array of environmental agents acting concurrently on the animal at any moment to exhibit correlative change in regard to it, so that one or other group of them becomes—generally by increase in intensity—temporarily prepotent. Thus there dominates now this group, now that group in turn. It may happen that one stimulus ceases coincidently as another begins, but as a rule one stimulus *overlaps* another in regard to time. Thus each reflex breaks in upon a condition of relative equilibrium, which latter is itself reflex. In the simultaneous correlation of reflexes some reflexes combine harmoniously, being reactions that mutually reinforce. These may be termed *allied reflexes*, and the neural arcs which they employ *allied arcs*. On the other hand, some reflexes, as mentioned above, are antagonistic one to another and incompatible. These do not mutually reinforce, but stand to each other in inhibitory relation. One of them inhibits the other, or a whole group of others. These reflexes may in regard to one another be termed *antagonistic*; and the reflex or group of reflexes which succeeds in inhibiting its opponents may be termed 'prepotent' for the time being.

Allied Reflexes

ALLIED REFLEXES

The action of the principle of the final common path may be instanced in regard to 'allied arcs' in the scratch-reflex as follows. If, while the scratch-reflex is being elicited from a skin point at the shoulder, a second point distant, e.g. 10 cm. from the other point but also in the receptive field of skin, be stimulated, the stimulation at this second point favours the reaction from the first point. This is well seen when the stimulus at each point is of subminimal intensity. The two stimuli, though each unable separately to invoke the reflex, yet do so when applied both at the same time (Fig. 38). This is not due to overlapping spread of the feeble currents about the stigmatic poles of the two circuits used. Weak cocainization of either of the two skin points annuls it. Moreover, it occurs when localized mechanical stimuli are used. It therefore seems that the arcs from the two points, e.g. $R\alpha$ and $R\beta$ (Fig. 39, B) have such a mutual relation that reaction of one of them reinforces reaction of the other, as judged by the effect on the final common path.

It is obvious that such reinforcement—*immediate spinal induction*—may occur in either of two ways. The diagram (Fig. 39, B) treats the final common path as if it consisted of a single individual neurone. The single neurone of the diagram stands for several thousands. It may be (1) that when the reflex is excited from $R\alpha$, only a particular group of the motor neurones composing the final common path is thrown into action, and similarly another particular group when the reflex is excited from $R\beta$. If the two groups in the final common path are separate groups, the explanation of the reinforcement shown in the muscular response may be by mechanical summation of contraction occurring in two separate fields of muscular tissue, the contraction of each too slight to cause perceptible movement by itself without the other. In other words, the reinforcement would be due not to the response in the set of neurones comprising the final common path (*FC* Fig. 39, B), being neurone for neurone more intense under the combined stimulation of $R\alpha$ and $R\beta$ than under stimulation of either singly, but the result would arise from the number of neurones in action in *FC* being simply greater under the

Interaction between Reflexes

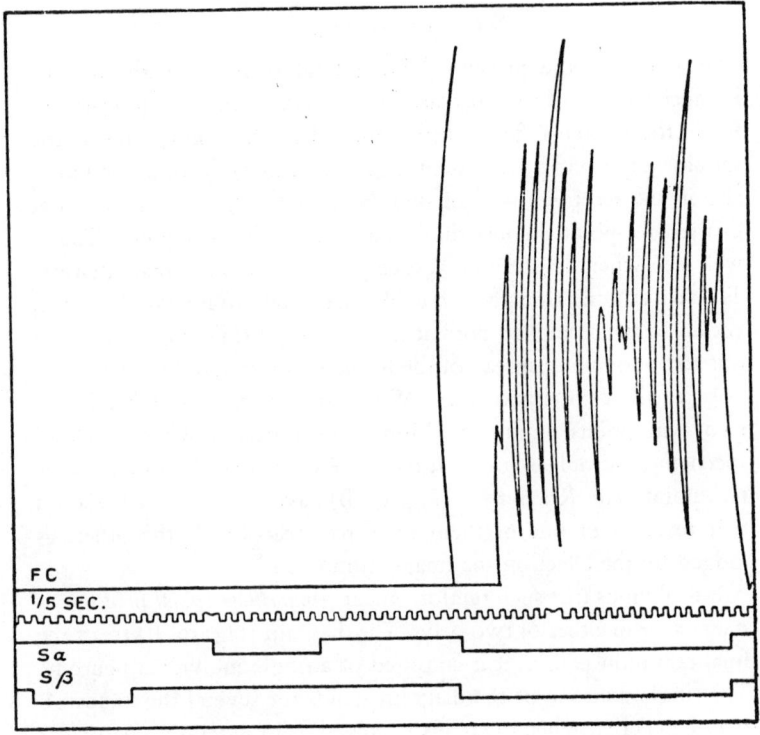

Fig. 38. Reflex summation (immediate spinal induction)

Records from above downwards (read from left to right):

FC, myograph curve of flexor muscle of hip (scratch-reflex). The vertical arc (preceding the response) coincides with the descent of the signal lines ($S\alpha$, $S\beta$).

Time in $\frac{1}{5}$ sec.

Signal line $S\alpha$: each descent of the line marks the period of stimulation of the skin belonging to arc $R\alpha$ (Fig. 39, B) of the shoulder skin. The strength of stimulus is arranged to be subminimal, so that a reflex-response in *FC* is not obtained.

Signal line $S\beta$: each descent of the line marks the period of stimulation, also subminimal of a point of shoulder skin 8 cm. from $R\alpha$.

Though the two stimuli applied separately are each unable to evoke the reflex, when applied contemporaneously they quickly evoke the reflex. The two arcs $R\alpha$ and $R\beta$, therefore, reinforce each other in their action on the final common path *FC* (summation effect, *immediate spinal induction*).

Allied Reflexes

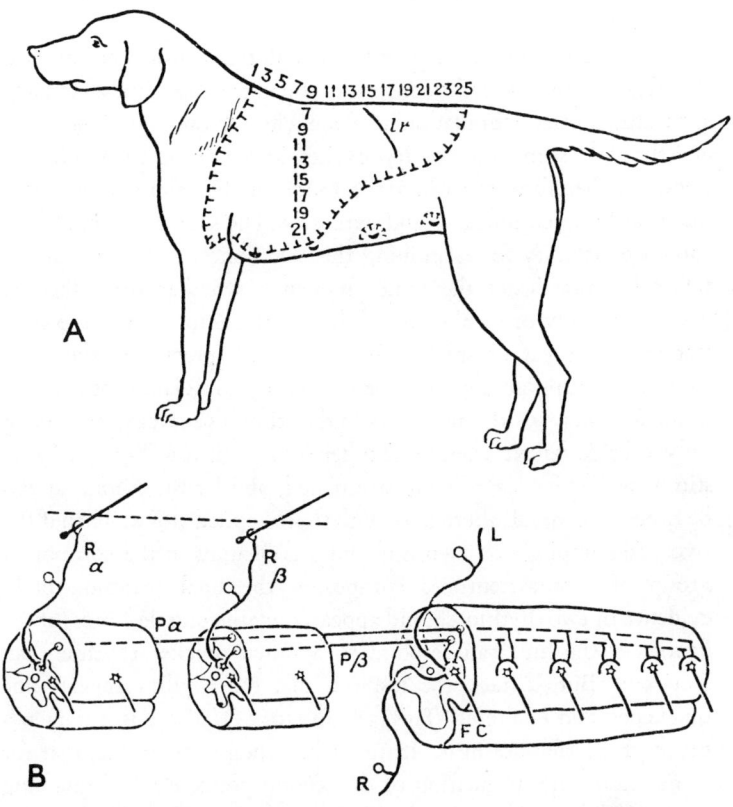

Fig. 39

A. The 'receptive field', as revealed after low cervical transection, a saddle-shaped area of dorsal skin, whence the scratch-reflex of the left hindlimb can be evoked. *lr* marks the position of the last rib.

B. Diagram of the spinal arcs involved. *L*, receptive or afferent nerve-path from the left foot; *R*, receptive nerve-path from the opposite foot; $R\alpha$, $R\beta$, receptive nerve-paths from hairs in the dorsal skin of the left side; *FC*, the final common path, in this case the motor neurone to a flexor muscle of the hip; $P\alpha$, $P\beta$, proprio-spinal neurones.

Interaction between Reflexes

stimulation of the two skin points than under stimulation of one of them only.

On the other hand, it may be (2) that all the neurones composing the final common path constitute together one almost unitary apparatus, so that stimulation at $R\alpha$ excites or can excite them all, and similarly stimulation at $R\beta$ excites or can excite them all. The question, therefore, regarding the mode of the reinforcement is a question between intensity and extensity. The scratch-reflex affords some opportunity for examining this question. The rhythm of the reflex has practically the same frequency whether the reflex be excited strongly or feebly: thus, whether the amplitude of the contractions be great or small, they recur with practically the same frequence. Suppose the reflex be excited by stimulation of the skin point $R\alpha$ (Fig. 39, B), and suppose the stimulus is weak, producing only a feeble reflex. Then let another skin point $R\beta$ (Fig. 39, B) be stimulated while $R\alpha$ is being stimulated, and let the stimuli at $R\beta$ be timed so as to fall alternately with those applied at $R\alpha$. Then if the two paths impinge on two different sets of units in the compound group of motor neurones composing the final common path, evidence of two rhythms should appear, since the muscle-fibres (of the flexors of the hip) can respond to a much quicker rhythm than 4 per sec. But, in fact, the result is that the rhythm appears unquickened and unaltered (Figs. 18, 19, 20, 21). There is not even a break or interference in it. It might be thought, therefore, that for some reason the stimulation of the second point, $R\beta$, is remaining ineffective altogether. But that is not so, because the stimulation at $R\beta$ has often the effect of increasing the amplitude (Fig. 18) of the individual beats of the rhythmic reflex, though it does not alter the rhythm. This change in amplitude proves that the reflex is also in action from the second skin point as well as from the first. But there is no interference of the rhythms of the two reflexes. Evidently the central mechanism on which $R\beta$ acts is subjected by $R\alpha$ to a refractory state which the stimulation at $R\beta$ does not break through. That is, the refractory state obtaining in the central mechanism under action from $R\alpha$ obtains at the same moment for excitation reaching it from $R\beta$. The central mechanism acted on by $R\beta$ must

Immediate Spinal Induction

therefore belong in common to the reflexes from $R\alpha$ and $R\beta$ respectively. And since the experiment can be repeated with a great number of different pairs of points in the receptive field, practically the whole of the neurones of FC are common to all the receptive points in the receptive field. Similarly it was shown by Zwaardemaker[272] that the refractory phase demonstrated by him in reflex deglutition spreads to the whole of the reflex centre, both right and left.

Again, it was shown above, under the heading of summation, that although a single-induction shock, even though strong, does not in my experience ever evoke a scratch-reflex, a series of even feeble shocks does so by summation. But in order to act by summation the individual shocks must follow each other at not too long an interval of time, the interval being *ceteris paribus* shorter the less intense the shocks. Suppose an induction shock be applied to $R\alpha$ at such a frequence, e.g. once a second, that at the intensity chosen they fail to evoke the reflex. Suppose that a series of induction shocks be applied to $R\beta$ similarly unable to evoke the reflex. Then suppose that while the stimuli are being applied to $R\alpha$ and fail to evoke the reflex, the other series of stimuli are applied to $R\beta$, and are so applied that each stimulus at $R\beta$ falls at a moment of time midway between the moments of application of the stimuli at $R\alpha$. The stimuli thus conjoined suffice to evoke the reflex. Evidently the internal excitatory change is not confined to the arcs to whose receptive ends the external stimulus is actually applied. It spreads to other arcs belonging to the same 'type-reflex', especially to those arising near to those actually stimulated in the receptive field. A subminimal stimulus at one point in the field favours response to a subsequent stimulus at a second point in the field even 8 cm. distant—so long as the second stimulus follows within summation time; but the summation time is shorter than when stimuli follow each other at one and the same spot, and is especially so when the points stimulated lie distant from one another. Hence we may draw some sort of picture of the extent of the excitatory internal change induced in this reflex mechanism by a single momentary stimulus: as to distribution in time the change fades off gradually from an early maximum to a trace just detectable

Interaction between Reflexes

after 1400σ, if the stimulus be strong: as to distribution in space it spreads from the peripherally stimulated arcs AA themselves as centre to the intraspinal parts of other arcs of the same type-reflex, but among these it affects those starting in the skin as neighbours to AA more than ones more distant in origin, and it endures less long in these than in its own arcs; hence the shorter summation time. Exner early insisted on the close connexion between 'facilitation' (bahnung) and summation. The above immediate spinal induction illustrates it well.

The mutual reinforcement of action exercised by the two scratch-reflexes one upon another appears therefore to be an affair of intensity. This does not, however, exclude the existence of extensity as a factor also in some degree. There is evidence, adverted to above (p. 78, Lect. III), that makes it likely that in very weak reflexes not all the individual neurones composing the final common path are in action, although in stronger reflex reactions all may be in action.

In the scratch-reflex the mutual reinforcing power between the reflexes falls as the distance between the receptors of the arcs increases. The nearer the skin points of $R\alpha$ and $R\beta$ lie together the greater the mutual reinforcement between the action of their arcs on FC. This suggests an explanation by physical diffusion of the stimulating currents applied to $R\alpha$ and $R\beta$; but for the reasons above mentioned this overlap of stimulus can, I consider, be excluded. Light is, however, thrown on this proportion between the degree of reinforcement and the degree of nearness of the receptive points by another feature of the reflex. The scratch-reflex in the spinal dog carries the foot approximately toward the place of stimulation. In the spinal dog the reflex does not succeed in bringing the foot actually to the irritated skin point, yet when the irritation lies far forward the foot is carried farther forward, and when the irritation is far back the foot is carried farther back. A scratch-reflex evoked by a stimulus applied far back and high up in the dorsal skin is therefore not wholly like a scratch-reflex evoked from far forward and low down. These differences are easily registered in graphic tracings of the movement at hip (Fig. 40). It is found that the greater the likeness between the two scratch-reflexes which two separate skin points initiate, the stronger the mutual reinforcement between the action of those two

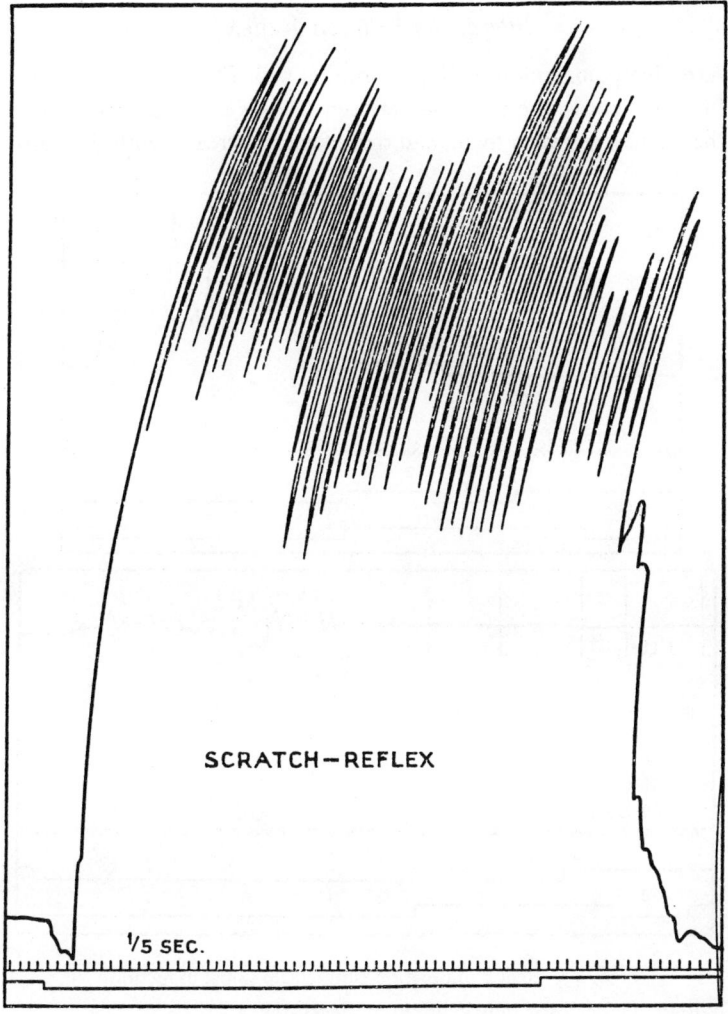

Fig. 40. Scratch-reflex

Records from above downwards:
Myograph curve: tracing of the hip flexion in the 'scratch-reflex'. The reflex was elicited by unipolar faradization of a point of skin rather far back and near the dorsum in the receptive field. Considerable tonic flexion is seen to accompany the clonic scratching movements.
Time in $\frac{1}{5}$ sec.
Signal line: descent indicates period of stimulation. Compare Figs. 14, 18, 19, in which the skin points excited lay farther forward and more ventral in the field and the substratum of steady flexion is much less.

Interaction between Reflexes

receptive points upon the final common path FC (Figs. 38 and 41). In other words, the coalition between reflexes is greater the greater the likeness between them, and that likeness increases with the near-

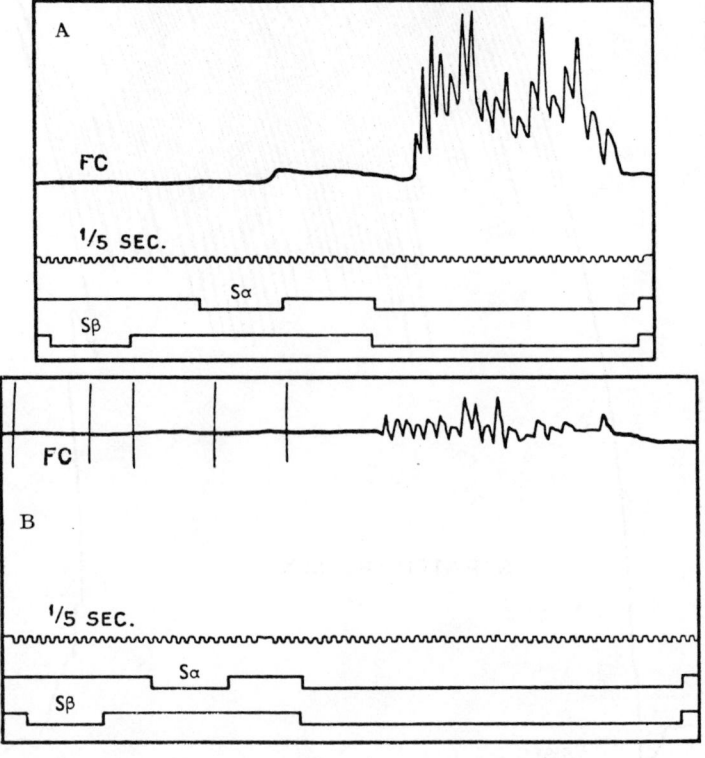

Fig. 41. Reflex summation (immediate spinal induction)

Response of flexor muscle of hip in scratch-reflex (FC).

Records as in Fig. 38, but with greater separation of the two skin points stimulated: in A the separation of the two points was 15 cm., in B it was 20 cm.

The vertical arcs on myograph curve (FC) in B indicate successively onset and cessation of stimulation of $S\beta$, onset and cessation of stimulation of $S\alpha$, onset and cessation of combined stimulation of $S\alpha$ and $S\beta$.

ness of their receptive points to one another in the skin surface. I have seen the mutual reinforcement demonstrable with skin points 20 cm. apart in the receptive field of the scratch-reflex, but I have

Type-Reflexes and Allied Reflexes

failed to find this mutual reinforcement between the most distant areas of the receptive field. Whether coalition fades into mere indifference or passes over into antagonism I have not at present the evidence to judge.

The whole collection of points of skin surface from which the scratch-reflex can be elicited may conveniently be termed the *receptive field* of that reflex. And the receptive field of a reflex is analysable into points from each of which the reflex can be evoked. But the reflex as elicited from various points in its receptive field is not in the case of all the points exactly the same reflex; e.g. the foot is directed to somewhat different places according as the scratch-reflex is elicited from this or that point. A similar feature is seen in the 'wisch-reflex' of the spinal frog's hind-leg. That is to say, when we speak of the 'scratch-reflex' in general, what we mean strictly speaking is a *group* of reflexes all more or less alike, all using approximately the same motor apparatus in approximately the same way, and all more or less conforming to the same type. And this group of individual reflexes forms a physiological group not only on account of their similarity, but also because they act harmoniously upon the same final common path, and in many cases reinforcement occurs between them in their action on that common path. Their intraspinal mechanisms are more or less knit together into an harmonious whole. A reflex, e.g. the scratch-reflex, when referred to in general, may be conveniently termed a *type-reflex*. The kind of harmonious relationship which holds between the individual reflexes comprised under one and the same type-reflex may be indicated by recognizing them as 'allied reflexes' and their arcs as 'allied arcs'.

Similarly with the various other reflexes. The flexion-reflex of the hind-limb, the pinna-reflex, the extensor-thrust, the crossed extension-reflex of the hind-limb, the torticollis reflex, etc.; these are each of them type-reflexes. Each is a group of reflexes. The individual reflexes comprised in each of these type-reflexes have such mutual relationship between themselves that they act harmoniously together on the same final common path, and are therefore 'allied reflexes' and employ 'allied arcs'.

The extent of the receptive field of each type-reflex is usually wide.

Interaction between Reflexes

It is much wider in some type-reflexes than in others; thus, that of the direct flexion-reflex of the hind-limb of the dog is more extensive than that of the extensor-thrust of the limb. Within the receptive field of any given type-reflex not all the receptive points equally potently excite the reflex. From certain areas of points the reflex can be most easily evoked, from certain others least easily, and from the rest of the field with intermediate degrees of facility. The area whence the reflex can be evoked with most difficulty is usually the circumferential zone of the field, the width of the zone varying along different radii. The area where the threshold stimulus is lowest lies usually fairly remote, though not equally remote, from all the borders of the field. The reflex effect of a weak stimulus in this central focal area seems to resemble the effect of a stronger stimulus applied in the border zone of the field. Reflexes of an intensity unobtainable from the border zone of the field can be easily provoked by stimulation of the focal area of the field. In the flexion-reflex of the dog's hind-limb the toe-pads and plantar cushion are in the focal area of the receptive field. In the scratch-reflex of the dog the focal area is along that part of the field that lies next to the mid-dorsal line of the trunk, and especially (as seen after low cervical transection) near the posterior end of the scapular region; e.g. in Fig. 39, A, from 5 to 15 in the horizontal figures and dorsal to 9 in the vertical row. The difference between the threshold value of the stimulus for the reflex at different points in the field is very considerable indeed. Although the absolute value of the threshold may vary considerably in one and the same animal at different times, even from day to day, the relative values as between separate areas in the same field is usually about the same. But this relative value may be upset by 'local fatigue', etc. The coalescence of allied reflexes excited from one receptive field tends to make weak stimuli applied to an extensive area equivalent to intenser stimuli applied to a smaller area. G. H. Parker[253] shows that in the positive phototropism of the frog to light falling on its skin the strength of the reaction varies in proportion with the extent of skin exposed to the light.

Receptive Field of a Reflex

REFLEX COMPLICATION

One and the same field of receptive surface may, and usually does, contain receptive points of more than a single species. Thus, a skin-field may contain receptors some of which are adapted for mechanical stimuli, some for chemical, some for thermal, and so on. In this case receptors of two different species may not both of them initiate reflexes which belong to the same type-reflex, i.e. which have the relation to one another of 'allied reflexes'. For instance, in the planta of the dog's foot receptors coexist[252] of which one set are excited by mechanical stimuli of harmless (tactual) kind, the other set by stimuli of nocuous kind. The reflexes elicited from the limb through these two kinds of receptors respectively do not reinforce each other but oppose each other. On the other hand, in the tentacles of the Actinian, *Aiptasis saxicola*, there coexist at the surface receptors of two species,[146] one receptive for tactual stimuli the other for certain chemical stimuli (Nagel). The reflexes elicited through these by combination of mechanical with certain chemical stimuli seem to combine harmoniously and mutually reinforce each other (Nagel). And a similar occurrence seems evidenced by observations on the barblets of Siluroid fishes, e.g. *Ameiurus*[250] (C. J. Herrick). The combining of such reflexes is comparable with the associative combination of disparate sensations for which Herbart[12b] introduced the term 'complication'.

Analogy exists here, as it should, between the compatibility of reflex movements from two receptors of different species and the compatibility of sensations which, judging by inference from our own introspection, might be initiated from such receptors. Skin-pain is sensually incompatible with pure touch, the dolorous suppressing the tactual, just as the noci-ceptive reflex in the 'spinal' dog's hind-leg suppresses the merely tango-ceptive. But gustatory and tactual sensations excited from the same receptive surface, e.g. the tongue, habitually blend harmoniously.

Interaction between Reflexes

PROPRIO-CEPTIVE REFLEXES

There exists a further important class of cases in which reflexes have 'allied' relation. Throughout a vast range of animal types the bulk formed by the organism presents to the environment a surface sheet of cells, and, beneath that, a mass of cells more or less screened from the environment by the surface sheet. Many of the agencies by which the environment acts on the organism do not penetrate it far enough to reach the cells of the deep mass inside. Bedded in the surface layer of the organism are numbers of receptor cells constituted in adaptation to the stimuli delivered by environmental agencies. But the organism itself, like the world surrounding it, is a field of ceaseless change, where internal energy is continually being liberated, whence chemical, thermal, mechanical, and electrical effects appear. It is a microcosm in which forces which can act as stimuli are at work as in the macrocosm around. The deep tissues underlying the surface sheet are not provided with receptors of the same kinds as those of the surface, yet they are not devoid of receptors. They have receptors specific to themselves. The receptors which lie in the depth of the organism are adapted for excitation consonantly with changes going on in the organism itself, particularly in its muscles and their accessory organs (tendons, joints, blood-vessels, etc.). Since in this field the stimuli to the receptors are given by the organism itself, their field may be called the *proprio-ceptive* field.

There exist, therefore, two primary distributions of the receptor organs, each a field in certain respects fundamentally different from the other. The surface field lies freely open to the numberless vicissitudes of the environment. It has felt for countless ages the full stream of the varied agencies for ever pouring upon it from the outside world. This field, *extero-ceptive* as it may be called, is rich in the number and variety of receptors which adaptation has evolved in it.

The excitation of the receptors of the *proprio-ceptive* field in contradistinction from those of the *extero-ceptive* is related only secondarily to the agencies of the environment. The proprio-ceptive receive their stimulation by some action, e.g. a muscular contraction,

Proprio-ceptive and Extero-ceptive Reflexes

which was itself a primary reaction to excitation of a surface receptor by the environment. The primary reaction is excited in the majority of cases by a receptor of the extero-ceptive field, that field so rich in the number and the variety of its receptors. Reflexes arising from proprio-ceptive organs come therefore to be habitually attached and appended to certain reflexes excited by extero-ceptive organs. The reaction of the animal to stimulation of one of its extero-ceptors excites certain tissues, and the activity thus produced in these latter tissues excites in them their receptors, which are *proprio-ceptors*. Thus, in a muscular movement induced by a stimulus to the skin of the spinal dog, the change in form and tension of the muscles, the movements of the joints, etc., excite the receptors in these structures, and these in turn initiate a reflex in their own arcs and their reaction often has an 'allied' relation to the reflex reaction excited from the skin.

ALLIANCE OF PROPRIO-CEPTIVE WITH EXTERO-CEPTIVE REFLEXES

In one of the type-reflexes previously described, namely the scratch-reflex, the reflex-arcs which provoke the reflex arise in a large continuous area of skin, and all excite the same motor neurones, that is, are mutually related as allied arcs. The area of skin whence these arcs arise we termed the *receptive field* of the reflex. The afferent nerves of the muscles which execute the scratching movement do not, when themselves excited, evoke the scratch-reflex; nor does the severance of the afferent nerves of the muscles obviously impair or alter the scratch-reflex. With the flexion-reflex of the limb it is different. The reflex, like the scratch-reflex, has a cutaneous field of origin. It is provocable from arcs arising in a large area of the skin covering the hind-limb. But the flexion-reflex can in addition be excited from various of the afferent nerves of the muscles of the limb. Thus stimulation of the central end of the nerve of the flexor muscles themselves excites the reflex. It is similarly elicitable from the afferent nerve of the extensor muscle (vasto-crureus) of the knee. And the reflex excited from the muscles of the limb allies itself with the reflex excited from the skin of the limb. A subliminal stimulation

Interaction between Reflexes

of the afferent nerve of the hamstring muscles applied simultaneously with a subliminal stimulation of the skin of the foot results in a marked flexion-reflex.

In the case of the flexion-reflex, therefore, the receptive field includes not only reflex-arcs arising in the surface field, but reflex-arcs arising in the depth of the limb. Combined therefore with an *extero-ceptive* area, this reflex has, included in its receptive field, a *proprio-ceptive* field. The reflex-arcs belonging to its extero-ceptive and proprio-ceptive components co-operate harmoniously together, and mutually reinforce each other's action. In this class of cases the reflex from the muscle-joint apparatus seems to *reinforce* the reflex initiated from the skin.

Reflex flexion of the leg is induced by stimulation of the central end of the nerve of a hamstring muscle. Since mechanical stimulation of these flexor muscles, e.g. kneading or squeezing them, excites a reflex inhibition of the contraction of their antagonists, which as we have seen is part of the flexion-reflex itself, it would seem likely that their own contraction will excite a flexion-reflex. A flexion-reflex excited from the skin would thus in its progress tend to induce a secondary flexion-reflex which would reinforce the primary one, for when excited apart the reflexes excited from an afferent nerve of the foot and from the hamstring nerve are closely similar (Fig. 37). The case therefore resembles that of the reflexes from two adjacent spots in the receptive field of the scratch-reflex. The reflex elicited from the skin of the foot and that elicited from the hamstring muscle are 'allied' reflexes. There is here alliance and 'bahnung' between a reflex of the proprio-ceptive field and a reflex of the extero-ceptive field.

Similarly, if the knee-jerk is accepted as a sign of a tonic reflex originated by the afferent nerve-endings in the knee-jerk muscles themselves, many reflexes elicitable from the extero-ceptive surface are well known to reinforce it. A comprehensive account of these was furnished in Sternberg's monograph[142] (1893). Here again the reflexes which are 'allied', exhibiting reinforcement and 'bahnung', belong not in the ordinary sense to the same category, but have reflex-arcs commencing in receptive organs of different species. Yet

Wider Combinations of Reflexes

the arcs are 'allied arcs', for they act harmoniously on the same final common path.

That the prolongation of the reflex contractions characteristic of strychnine is due to excitation of muscular (proprio-ceptive) reflexes (Baglioni[212, 245, 285]) secondary to a reflex elicited from other receptors is again a further illustration of the secondary relation of proprio-ceptive reflexes to extero-ceptive pointed out above.

WIDER COMBINATIONS OF REFLEXES

And reflexes whose arcs commence in receptive fields even *wider* apart than those mentioned above may also have 'allied' relation. In the bulbo-spinal dog stimulation of the outer digit of the hind-foot will evoke reflex flexion of the leg, and stimulation of each of the other digits evokes practically the same reflex; and if stimulation of several of these points be simultaneously combined the same reflex as a result is obtained more readily than if one only of these points is stimulated. And to these stimulations may be added simultaneously stimulation of points in the crossed fore-foot; stimulation there yields by itself flexion of the hind-leg; and under the simultaneous stimulation of fore- and hind-foot the flexion of the leg goes on as before, though perhaps more readily; that is, the several individual reflexes harmonize in their effect on the hind-limb. Further, to these may be added simultaneous stimulation of the tail, and of the crossed pinna; and the reflexes of these stimulations all coalesce in the same way in flexion of the hind-leg. Exner[99] has shown that in exciting different points of the central nervous system itself, points widely apart exert 'bahnung' for one another's reactions, and for various reflex reactions induced from the skin. Thus reflexes originated at different distant points, and passing through paths widely separate in the brain, converge to the same motor mechanism (final common path) and act harmoniously upon it. Reflex-arcs from widely different parts conjoin and pour their influence harmoniously into the same muscle. The motor neurones of a muscle of the knee are the *terminus ad quem* of reflex-arcs arising in receptors not only of its own foot, but from the crossed fore-foot and pinna, and tail, also un-

Interaction between Reflexes

doubtedly from the otic labyrinth, olfactory organs, and eyes. Thus, if we take as a standpoint any motor-nerve to a muscle it consists of a number of motor neurones which are more or less bound into a unit mechanism; among the reflex-actions of the organism a number can all be brought together as a *group*, because they all in their course converge together upon this motor mechanism, this *final common path*, activate it, and are in harmonious mutual relation with regard to it. They are in regard to it what were termed above 'allied' reflexes.

ALLIED INHIBITORY REFLEXES

The examples of allied reflexes cited so far have had for their result on the final common path an increase of its activity; that is to say, of its activity as a discharger of nervous impulses. But the same final common path can be shown to be connected also with certain reflexes initiable from other receptive points which depress its activity as a discharger of nervous impulses. The reflexes exerting this influence are 'inhibitory', whereas the reflexes mentioned before may be termed 'excitatory'. Inhibitory reflexes are accessible to study chiefly through the kind of refractory state which they impress upon the commencement of the efferent part of their arc, as tested by concurrent excitations of reflexes which should excite it.

Just as in regard to one and the same final common path certain excitatory reflexes act harmoniously together and reinforce one another, so also do certain inhibitory reflexes. Thus, reflex inhibition of the flexors of the knee (spinal dog) is regularly excitable by stimulation of the skin of a digit of the crossed hind-foot; and the concurrent stimulation of two or more digits and of the *dorsum pedis* of the crossed foot mutually combine and reinforce in their reflex inhibition of the knee-flexor: and to these may be added stimulation of the homonymous fore-foot: all these reflexes combine harmoniously together in exerting a conjoint inhibitory influence on the knee-flexors. The alliance between reflexes in regard to any one final common path may be as wide and strong when the end-result of those reflexes is in the form of inhibition as when it is in the form of excitation. In addition, therefore, to the category of 'allied

Antagonistic Reflexes

excitatory' reflexes above mentioned there is a category of 'allied inhibitory' reflexes. Under this latter category come subgroups analogous to the four already mentioned under allied excitatory reflexes. Thus: the reflex from the proprio-ceptive nerves of the hamstring muscles combines with and reinforces the flexion-reflex from the skin of the foot of the same leg in a resultant reflex inhibition of the extensors of the homonymous knee.

But there are, as we have seen, reflexes which are neither purely excitatory nor purely inhibitory. For instance, the flexion-reflex of the hind-leg (cat and dog) is, as we have seen, at one and the same time excitatory of the flexor neurones (knee) and inhibitory of the extensor neurones (knee).

These reflexes of simultaneous double-sign may have 'allied' relation with one another, e.g. the individual reflexes of the flexion type-reflex.

Also there are other reflexes neither purely excitatory nor purely inhibitory, namely, the reflexes which during the continuance or repetition of the exciting stimulus exhibit refractory period. Several rhythmic reflexes seem of this character, e.g. the swallowing reflex, the scratch-reflex. If we regard refractory phase as a kind of inhibition, then these reflexes are, as we have seen, reflexes of successive double-sign. And these also can be 'allied' in their relation one to another.

ANTAGONISTIC REFLEXES

But not all reflexes connected with one and the same final common path stand to one another in the relation of 'allied reflexes'. Suppose during the scratch-reflex a stimulus be applied to the foot not of the scratching side but of the opposite side (Fig. 39, B, R). The left leg, which is executing the scratch-reflex in response to stimulation of the *left* shoulder skin is cut short in its movement by the stimulation of the *right* foot, although the stimulus at the shoulder to provoke the scratch movement is maintained unaltered all the time. The stimulus to the right foot will temporarily interrupt a scratch-reflex, or will cut it short or will delay its onset; which it does of these depends on the time-relations of the stimuli (Fig. 42). The inhibition of the

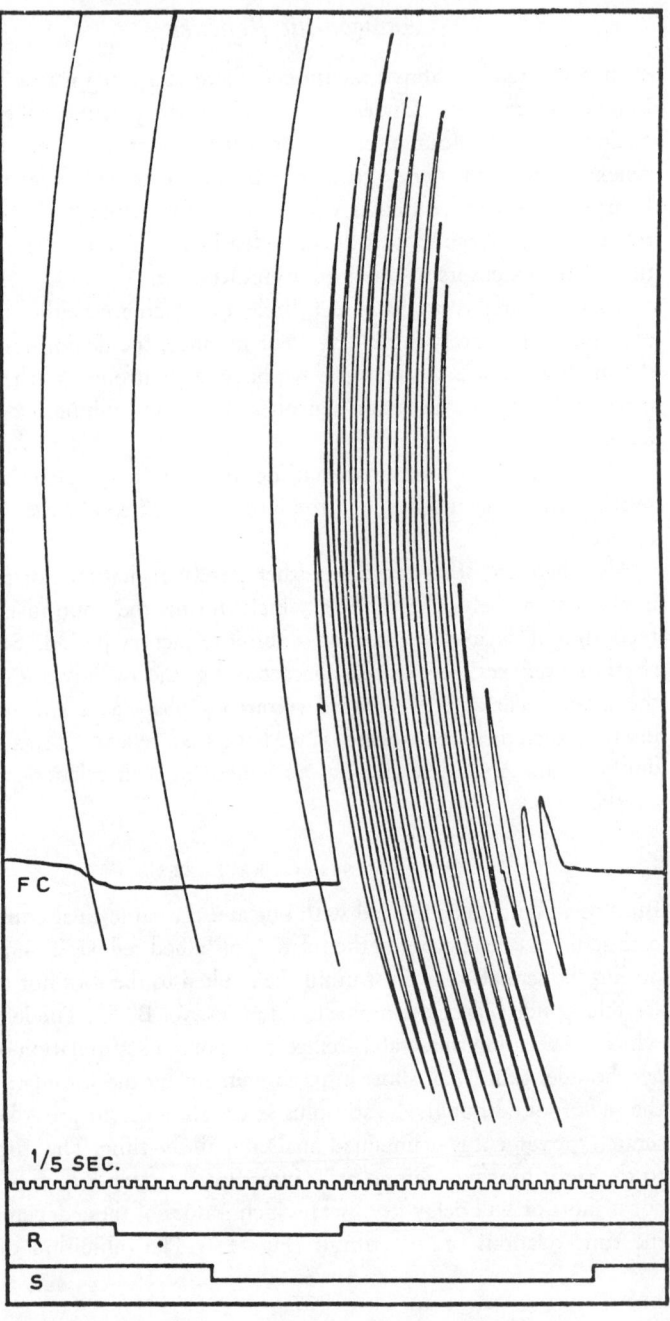

Fig. 42

Antagonistic Reflexes

scratch-reflex occurs sometimes when the contraction of the muscles innervated by the reflex conflicting with it is very slight. There is interference between the two reflexes and the one is inhibited by the other. The final common path used by the left scratch-reflex is also common to the reflex elicitable from the right foot. This latter reflex evokes extension at the opposite (left) knee; in doing this it causes steady excitation of extensor neurones of that knee and steadily inhibits the flexor neurones.300 But the scratch-reflex causes rhythmic excitation of the flexor neurones. Therefore these flexor neurones in this conflict lie as a final common path under the influence of two antagonistic reflexes, one of which would excite them to rhythmical discharge four times a second, while the other would continuously repress all discharge in them. There is here an antagonistic relation between reflexes embouching on one and the same final common path.

In all these forms of interference there is a competition, as it were, between the excitatory stimulus used for the one reflex and the excitatory stimulus for the other. Both stimuli are in progress together, and the one in taking effect precludes the other's taking effect as far as the final common path is concerned; and the precise form in which that occurs depends greatly on the time-relations of application of the two stimuli competing against each other.

Fig. 42. Antagonism of reflexes

Interference of the reflex from the skin of the opposite foot with the scratch-reflex.

Records from above downwards. Read from left to right:

FC: myograph curve of the flexor muscle of the left hip (Fig. 39, B, FC) recording scratch-reflex.

The vertical arcs mark respectively onset of stimulus R, onset of stimulus S, cessation of stimulus R.

Time in $\frac{1}{5}$ sec.

Signal line R: the notch marks the beginning, continuance, and conclusion of a skin stimulation of the right foot (Fig. 39, B, R).

Signal line S: similarly marks the period of stimulation of the skin of the left shoulder (Fig. 39, B, $R\alpha$).

The ability of stimulus S to produce the scratch-reflex takes effect only on concluding stimulus R; that is, S obtains connexion with the final common path (the motor neurone of the flexor muscle) only on R's relinquishing it. Stimulus R, while excluding S from FC causes slight contraction of FC's antagonist, and coincident slight relaxation of FC itself.

Interaction between Reflexes

Again, if, while stimulation of the skin of the shoulder is evoking the scratch-reflex, the skin of the hind-foot of the *same* side is stimulated, the scratching may be arrested 300 (Fig. 43). Stimulation of the skin of the hind-foot by any of various stimuli that have the character of threatening the part with damage causes the leg to be flexed, drawing the foot up by steady maintained contraction of the flexors of the ankle, knee, and hip. In this reaction the reflex-arc is (under schematic provisions similar to those mentioned in regard to the scratch-reflex schema) (i) the receptive neurone (Fig. 39, B, L), noci-ceptive, from the foot to the spinal segment, (ii) the motor neurone (Fig. 39, B, FC) to the flexor muscle, e.g. of hip; (a short intra-spinal neurone, a Schalt-zelle (v. Monakow) is probably existent between (i) and (ii) but omitted for simplicity). Here, therefore, there is an arc which embouches into the same final common path FC as do $R\alpha$ and $R\beta$, Fig. 39, B. The motor neurone FC is a path common to it and to the scratch-reflex arc; both these arcs employ the same effector organ, namely, the knee-flexor, and employ it by the common medium of the final path FC. But though the channels for both reflexes embouch upon the same final common path, the excitatory flexor effect specific to each differs strikingly in the two cases. In the scratch-reflex the flexor effect is an intermittent

---

Fig. 43. Antagonism of reflexes

Interference between the reflex action of the left hip flexor, FC, caused by the nervous arc from the left foot (L, Fig. 39, B) and the scratch-reflex.

Records from above downwards. The tracing reads from left to right:
 Time in $\frac{1}{5}$ sec.
 FC: myograph curve of left hip flexor.
 The vertical arcs indicate respectively onset of stimulus S, cessation of stimulus L, and cessation of stimulus S.
 Signal line L: stimulation of foot.
 Signal line S: stimulus for scratch-reflex.

The stimulation of the dorsal skin (Fig. 39, A) inducing the scratch-reflex began at the beginning of the notch in the signal line S, and continued throughout the period of that notch. Later, for the period marked by the notch in signal line L, the stimulation of the foot was made. This latter stimulation interrupts the clonic scratch-reflex in the manner shown. It is noteworthy that the interruption of the scratch-reflex by the foot-reflex is not established directly the foot-stimulus begins, and that it outlasts for a short time the application of the foot-stimulus.

Antagonistic Reflexes

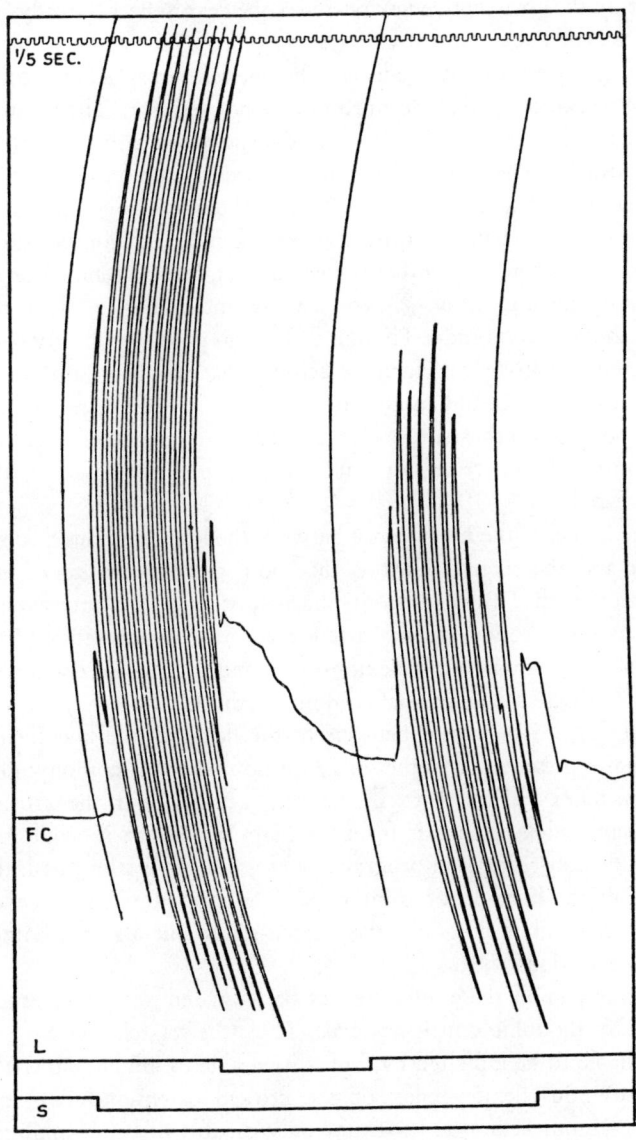

Fig. 43

Interaction between Reflexes

effect; in the noci-ceptive flexion-reflex the flexor effect is steady and maintained. The accompanying tracing (Fig. 43) shows the result of conflict between the two reflexes. The one reflex displaces the other at the common path. Compromise is not evident. The scratch-reflex is set aside by that of the noci-ceptive arc from the homonymous foot. The stimulation which previously sufficed to provoke the scratch-reflex is no longer effective, though it is continued all the time. But when the stimulation of the foot is discontinued the scratch-reflex returns. In that respect, although there is no enforced inactivity there is an *interference* which is tantamount to, if not the same thing as, inhibition. Though there is no cessation of activity in the motor neurone, one form of activity that was being impressed upon it is cut short and another takes its place. A stimulation of the foot too weak to cause more than a minimal reflex will often suffice to completely interrupt, or cut short, or prevent onset of, the scratch-reflex.

The kernel of the interference between the homonymous flexion-reflex and the scratch-reflex is that both employ the same final common path *FC* to different effect—just as in the interference between the crossed extension-reflex and the scratch-reflex. Evidently, the homonymous flexion-reflex and the crossed extension-reflex both use the same final common path *FC*. And they *use it to different effect*. The motor neurone to the flexor of the knee being taken as representative of the final common path, the homonymous flexion-reflex excites it to discharging activity, but the crossed extension-reflex inhibits it from discharging. Hence if, while the direct flexion-reflex is in progress the crossed foot is stimulated, the reflex of the knee-flexor is inhibited. The crossed extension-reflex therefore inhibits not only the scratch-reflex but also the homonymous flexion-reflex.

Further, in all these interferences between reflexes the direction taken by the inhibition is *reversible*. Thus, the scratch-reflex is not only liable to be inhibited by, but is itself able to inhibit, either the homonymous flexion-reflex or the crossed extension-reflex; the homonymous flexion-reflex is not only capable of being inhibited by the crossed extension-reflex (Fig. 32, p. 99), but conversely in its

Summation and Interference

turn can inhibit the crossed extension-reflex (Figs. 33, 35, pp. 102, 105). These interferences are therefore reversible in direction. Certain conditions determine which reflex among two or more competing ones shall obtain mastery over the final common path and thus obtain expression.

Therefore, in regard to the final common path FC the reflexes that express themselves in it can be grouped into sets, namely those which excite it in one way, those which excite it in another way, and those which inhibit it. The reflexes composing each of these sets stand in such relation to reflexes of the same set that they are with them 'allied reflexes'. But a reflex belonging to any one of these sets stands in such relation to a reflex belonging to one of the other sets that it is in regard to the latter an 'antagonistic' reflex. This correlation of reflexes about the flexor neurone in the leg, so that some reflexes are mutually allied and some are mutually antagonistic in regard to that neurone, may serve as a paradigm of the correlation of reflexes about every final common path, e.g. about every motor-neurone to skeletal muscle.[300]

As to the intimate nature of the mechanism which thus, by summation or by interference, gives co-ordination where neurones converge upon a common path it is difficult to surmise. In the central nervous system of vertebrates, afferent neurones A and B in their convergence toward and impingement upon another neurone Z, towards which they conduct, do not make any lateral connexion directly one with the other—at least there seems no clear evidence that they do. It seems then that the only structural link between A and B is neurone Z itself. Z itself should therefore be the field of coalition of A and B if they transmit 'allied' reflexes.

It was argued above (Lect. III), from the morphology of the perikaryon, that it must form, in numerous cases, a nodal point in the conductive lines provided by the neurone. The work of Ramon-y-Cajal, van Gehuchten, v. Lenhossék, and others with the methods of Golgi and Ehrlich, establishes as a concept of the neurone in general that it is a conductive unit wherein a number of branches (dendrites) converge toward, meet at, and coalesce in a single outgoing stem (axone). Through this tree-shaped structure the nervous

impulses flow, like the water in a tree, from roots to stem. The
conduction does not normally run in the reverse direction. The place
of junction of the dendrites with one another and with the axone is
commonly the perikaryon. This last is therefore a nodal point in the
conductive system. But it is a nodal point of particular quality. It is
not a nodal point where lines meet to cross one another, nor one
where one line splits into many. It is a nodal point where conductive
lines run together into one which is the continuation of them all. It is
a reduction point in the system of lines. The perikaryon with its
convergent dendrites is therefore just such a structure as spatial
summation and immediate induction would demand. The neurone
Z may well, therefore, be the field of coalition, and the organ where
the summational and inductive processes occur. And the morphology of the neurone as a whole is seen to be just such as we should
expect, arguing from the principle of the common path.

With the phenomenon of 'interference' the question is more
difficult. There it is not clear that the field of antagonism is within the
neurone Z itself. The field may be synaptic. We have the demonstration by Verworn[207] that the interference produced by A at Z for
impulses from B is not accompanied by any obvious change in
excitability of the axone of Z. Z, if itself the seat of inhibition, might
have been expected to exhibit that inhibition throughout its extent.
This, as tested by its axone, it does not do. There exist, it is true, older
experiments by Von Bezold & Uspensky,[42] Belmondo & Oddi,[122]
etc., according to which the threshold of direct excitability of the
motor root is lowered by stimulation of the afferent root. This points
to an extension of the facilitation effect through the whole motor
neurone, conversely to Verworn's demonstration for central inhibition. Verworn's experiment and its result is very clear. It leads us to
search for some other mechanism common to A and B to which
might be attributable their mutual influence on each other's reactions.
But if we admit the conception, argued above (Lect. I), that at the
nexus between A and Z, i.e. at synapse AZ, and similarly between B
and Z, i.e. at synapse BZ, there exists a surface of separation, a
membrane in the physical sense, a further consequence seems in-
ferable. Suppose a number of different neurones A, B, C, etc., each

Partial Interference

conducting through its own synapse upon a neurone Z. The synapses AZ, BZ, CZ, etc., are all surfaces or membranes into which Z enters as a factor common to them all. A change of state induced in neurone Z might be expected to affect the surface condition or membrane at all of the synapses, since the condition of Z is a factor common to all those membranes. Therefore a change of state (excitatory or inhibitory) induced in Z by any of the neurones A, B, C, etc., playing upon it would enter as a condition into the nervous transmission at the other synapses from the other collateral neurones. In harmony with this is the spread of refractory state in the neurones as mentioned above (p. 124). A change in neurone Z induced by neurone A playing upon it, in that case seems to affect its point of nexus with the other neurones B, C, etc., also. It is conceivable that the phenomena of interference may be based in part at least on such a condition. The neurone threshold of Z for stimulation through B will be to some extent a function of events at synapses AZ.

PARTIAL INTERFERENCE

It has to be remembered, however, that the total final common path, although a functional unity, is often, especially in compound reflexes, a complex one. It frequently happens that the set of final paths of one complex reflex is *partly* coextensive with the set of final common paths of another reflex. With two complex reflexes it can happen that the reflexes are 'allied reflexes' in regard to one part of their multiple final common path and are antagonistic reflexes in regard to another part of it. We may illustrate this from the scratch-reflex again. The scratch-reflex was mentioned above as being unilateral. That is not strictly the case. It is true that if the right scapular region be stimulated, the right hind-leg scratches; and if the left scapular region be stimulated the left hind-leg scratches. But if both shoulders be stimulated at the same time, one or the other leg scratches, but not the two together. This shows that the scratch-reflex, though at first sight it appears unilateral, is not strictly so. Suppose the left shoulder stimulated, the left leg then scratches; but if the right leg is examined it is found to present slight steady extension with some abduction.

Interaction between Reflexes

This extension of the crossed hind-leg which accompanies the scratching movement of the homonymous hind-leg contributes to support the animal on three legs while it scratches with the fourth. Suppose that stimulation at the left shoulder is evoking the scratching movement of the left leg, and the skin of the right shoulder is then appropriately and strongly stimulated. This latter stimulus often inhibits the scratching movement in the opposite leg and starts it in its own.[300] That is, the stimulus at the right shoulder not only sets the flexor muscles of the leg of its own side into scratching action, but it inhibits the flexor muscles of the opposite leg, because with excitation of the extensors of the latter leg goes inhibition of their antagonists, the flexors. The motor neurones of the flexor muscles of the left leg are part of the final common path not only of the scratch-reflex of the left shoulder, but also of the scratch-reflex of the right shoulder; but in the former case the final common path is thrown into rhythmic discharging activity, in the latter case it is steadily inhibited from discharging activity.

Again, the homonymous flexion-reflex of the hind-leg (spinal dog) is only the main part of a larger complex reflex which is bilateral (Fig. 37), and consists of flexion of the same side leg and extension of the crossed leg (the crossed extension-reflex). This being so, the mutual relation between the complete scratch-reflex, e.g. of left foot, and the complete noci-ceptive reflex of the same foot, is that the homonymous uncrossed parts of each reflex interfere and are related mutually as antagonistic reflexes; but the crossed parts of each reflex coalesce in excitation of the extensor neurones and inhibition of the flexor neurones of the right leg, and are related mutually as allied reflexes.

It is the transference of the final common path from the group of one set of reflexes to another which constitutes the change which occurs at each step of the orderly sequence of reaction that we see normally succeed each other in animal behaviour—leaving aside all question of consciousness in relation to the sequence. This transference is most obvious when the sets of reflexes between which the final common path is exchanged are antagonistic reflexes. Two classes of this kind of case of specially common occurrence are 'alternating reflexes' and 'compensatory reflexes' (Lect. VI).

Internuncial Common Paths

NUMBER OF COMMON PATHS

The interaction of reflexes has been here so far spoken of chiefly in regard to the final common path, as if the arcs of reflexes met at the *final* common path *only*. But, as stated above, reflex-arcs, especially the longer ones and those commencing in receptors far apart, converge and meet to some extent before they reach their *final* common path. The receptive neurones, i.e. private paths of the receptors, usually—perhaps always—reach internuncial paths (J. Hunter, 1770), which in turn conduct and converge to final paths or to further internuncial paths. The internuncial paths are thus themselves in various degrees common to groups of receptive neurones impinging upon them. They are therefore themselves, to some extent, *common paths*.300 There can be little doubt that in the scratch-reflex the long descending proprio-spinal neurone (Fig. 39, B, $P\alpha$ or $P\beta$) is connected not with one but with a whole group of afferent neurones (private paths) from the scalptor receptors in that part of the skinfield of the scratch-reflex which corresponds with its own spinal segment. Its internuncial path is therefore common to impulses transmitted to the central organ by many receptive paths. Again, the structure of the retina (Cajal), olfactory bulb (Cajal), etc., gives evidence that the conducting fibres of whole groups of receptors impinge together upon individual neurones of the next relay. Thalamic neurones form a path upon which the dorsal-column-fillet *and* spino-cerebellar-peduncular paths converge. Each internuncial path is therefore usually, to some extent, a common path,186 just as usually the receptive neurone, i.e. the private path, itself is common to a small number of receptors. The ultimate path, therefore, differs from the intermediate paths only in that it exhibits communism in the *highest* degree; it is to distinguish it from *internuncial* common paths that it was termed above the *final* common path.

Since each instance of convergence of two or more afferent neurones upon a third, which in regard to them is efferent, affords, as shown above, an opportunity for coalition or interference of their actions, each structure at which it occurs is a *mechanism for co-ordination*.300

Interaction between Reflexes

Whatever may be the intimate nature of this mechanism which gives co-ordination by the formation of a common path from tributary paths, such common paths exist in extraordinary profusion in the architecture of the grey-centred nervous system of Vertebrates. Two features of that system indicate this clearly. Enumerations by Donaldson and his co-workers[209] show that the afferent fibres (private paths) entering the human spinal cord three times outnumber the efferent (final common paths) which leave it. Add the cranial nerves and the so-called optic nerves (in the latter, of course, formation of common paths having already begun in the retina, the afferent paths are reduced in proportion), and the afferent fibres may be taken to be five times more numerous than the efferent. The receptor system bears, therefore, to the efferent paths the relation of the wide ingress of a funnel to the narrow egress. Further, each receptor stands in connexion not with one efferent only but with many—perhaps with all, though as to some of these only through synapses of high resistance. The simile to a funnel will therefore be bettered by supposing that within the general systematic funnel, of which the base is five times wider than the egress, the conducting paths from each receptor may be represented as a funnel inverted so that its wider end is more or less coextensive with the whole plane of emergence of the final common paths.[300] This gives some idea of the enormous formation of common paths from tributary paths which must take place.

Again, there is the accredited fact that under poisoning by strychnine a muscle can be excited from practically any afferent nerve in the body; in other words, that each final common path is in connexion with practically each one of all the receptors of the body. It is not necessary to accept this literally; even if approximately true, it shows the profusion in which common paths exist.

MUTUAL INDIFFERENCE BETWEEN REFLEXES

In view of such considerations the question arises, Are there in the body no reflexes absolutely neutral and indifferent one to another? That is, in regard to any one reflex using a given common path cannot another reflex be found which is wholly separate from it, and

Mutual Indifference between Reflexes

neither allied with it nor antagonistic to it? It was pointed out above that the coalition between scratch-reflexes gradually decreases as the interval between the receptive points at the skin surface becomes wider. Whether coalition fades into mere indifference or passes over into antagonism my own observations do not answer. But there are reflexes that do in the spinal dog appear neutral and indifferent to the scratch-reflex. For instance, a weak reflex of the tail may be obtained without any obvious interference between it and the scratch-reflex. The stronger two reflexes are, the less do they remain neutral one to another. Thus, a weak reflex may be excited from the tail of the spinal dog without interference with the stepping-reflex of the hind-limb; but a strong reflex (strong stimulus) in the tail inhibits (Goltz) the stepping-reflex. The spatial field of response of a reflex increases with its intensity. Two reflexes may be neutral to each other when both are weak, but may interfere when either or both are strong; when weak they remain 'local'.

But to show that reflexes may be neutral to each other in a spinal dog is not evidence that they will be neutral in the animal with its whole nervous system intact and unmutilated. It is a cardinal feature of the construction of the higher vertebrate nervous system that longer indirect reflex-arcs, attached as extra circuits to the shorter direct ones, all pass through the brain. With those former intact the number of reflexes neutral one to another might be fewer. In presence of the arcs of the great *projicient receptors* (Lect. IX) and the *brain* there can be few receptive points in the body whose activities are totally indifferent one to another. Correlation of the reflexes from points widely apart is the crowning contribution of the brain towards the nervous integration of the individual.

Our conception comes therefore to this. About any final common path a great number of, or all, the receptive arcs of the nervous system are arranged and are divisible into sets that do not act alike upon it. It might at first be thought that there would be simply two such sets, namely, those that excite it and those that inhibit it. But it must be remembered that we are only at the beginning of knowledge of differences of time-relations between different type-

Interaction between Reflexes

reflexes. Thus (Lect. II, III) at the knee of the spinal dog the time-relations of the extensor-thrust are vastly different from those of the crossed extension-reflex, and these again from the extensor tonus that supports the knee-jerk, and these again from the scratch-reflex, and so on. Of the reflexes that excite a final common path some

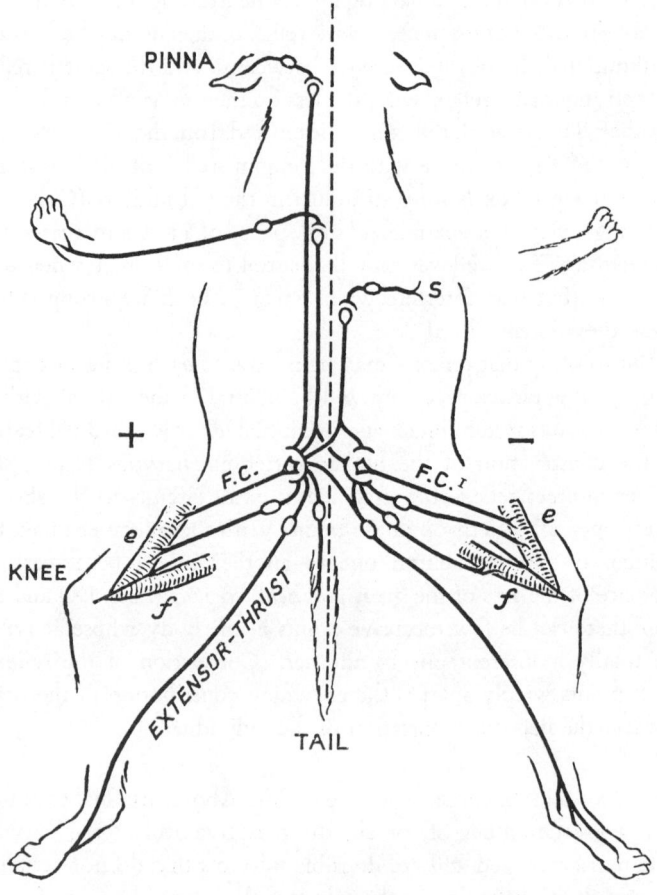

Fig. 44. Explanation mainly in text

s stands for scratch-receptor, *e* and *f* are extensor and flexor muscles of knee respectively.

Convergence on Final Common Path

evidently excite it in a manner very different from that in which some others excite it; their excitations if concurrent *interfere*. We must therefore allow that the sets may be more than two, if the criterion for distinguishing the sets be interference, i.e. interruption, displacement, or extinction at the final common path of one reflex by another.

The final common path is therefore an instrument passive in the hands of certain groups of reflex-paths. I have attempted to depict this very simply in Fig. 44. There certain type-reflexes are indicated by lines representing their paths. The final common path (FC) selected is the motor neurone of the vasto-crureus of the dog or cat. Reflexes that act as 'allied reflexes' on FC are represented as having their terminals joined together next to the final common path. Reflexes with excitatory effect (+sign) are brought together on the left, those with inhibitory (−sign) on the right. Of the reflex pairs formed by the two reflexes which two symmetrical receptive points, one right and one left, yield in regard to the final common path, one of the pair only is represented, in order to simplify the diagram. To have a further indication of the reflexes playing upon FC, all that is required is to add to the reflexes indicated in the diagram for FC, a set of reflexes similar to those given in the diagram for FC^1, for they *must* be added if the remaining members of the right and left reflex pairs from various parts of the body be taken into account. It is noteworthy that in many instances the end-effect of a spinal reflex initiated from a surface point on one side is bilateral and takes effect at symmetrical parts, but is opposite in kind at those two parts, e.g. is inhibition at one of them, excitation at the other. Hence reflexes initiated from points corresponding one with the other in the two halves of the body are commonly antagonistic.

Lecture V

COMPOUND REFLEXES: SIMULTANEOUS COMBINATION

ARGUMENT: Combination of reflexes simultaneously proceeding. Spread of reflex-response about a focus. Grey matter and lines of reflex resistance. 'Short' reflexes and 'long' reflexes. Rules decipherable in the spread of reflex reaction. Pflüger's 'laws' of spinal irradiation. The 'reflex figure'. Variability of reflex result. Irradiation of a reflex attaches itself to the problem of the simultaneous combination of reflexes. Co-ordination of reflex result obtains even when large mixed afferent nerve-trunks are stimulated. The movement excited by stimulation of the motor spinal nerve-root does not really resemble a movement evoked reflexly or by the will. Extent of simultaneous combinations of reflexes. Simultaneous stimuli arrange themselves naturally in constellations in which some component is usually of pre-eminent intensity. The resulting compound reaction has both positive and negative sides.

A LARGE part of co-ordination consists in the orderly combining of reflexes. In studying this co-ordination we have to deal with and discriminate between simultaneous combinations and successive combinations of reflexes. We may proceed to attempt the former problem.

IRRADIATION

If by appropriate stimulation of the skin of the foot, say by unipolar faradization of a spot of the plantar skin of a digit, the ordinary flexion-reflex of the hind-limb of the dog be evoked, the extent of the reflex increases with increase in the intensity of the stimulus. The reflex-effect spreads over a larger and larger field, irradiating as it were in various directions from a focus of reflex-discharge which takes effect on the limb itself.

The centrifugal discharge elicited by any reflex seems as regards its spatial distribution to be focused about a centre round which its irradiation varies according to circumstance. In the scratch-reflex the pretibial muscles that dorsi-flex the ankle seem to lie at the focus of

Irradiation

the motor discharge. In the 'flexion-reflex', if the reaction evoked is very weak a band of the deep inner hamstring muscle has often in my experience seemed the only part of the musculature thrown into action. On the other hand, when the reflex is evoked with medium strength it can often be seen that after the reflex (the exciting stimulation being continued unaltered) has been in progress for a few seconds, flexion at hip adds itself to the flexion at the knee (see Fig. 45, B). And by strong stimulation, strong flexion at hip occurs together with that at knee and practically from the very outset. In my experience the condition of 'spinal shock' is very favourable for noting the seat of the focus of the motor discharge in a reflex, because in that condition it happens often that the piece of musculature which is at focus of the discharge is the only one which can be got to give the reflex-response. It seems possible in this way to determine what reflex in, for instance, a 'spinal' monkey corresponds with this or that reflex in a 'spinal' dog. In the monkey the severity and long duration of spinal shock allows merely the focal reply in the musculature. Thus a feeble tightening of a part of a hamstring muscle, in response to a stimulus of the foot in the 'spinal' monkey, affords fair evidence that the flexor-reflex—for the full extent of which one must turn to the 'spinal dog'—is evoked. In man spinal shock seems still more severe and lasting than in the monkey. The situation of the weak brief contractions evoked can still reveal which they correspond with among reflexes better open to study in the lower mammals.

The more intense the spinal reflex—apart from strychnine and similar convulsant poisoning—the wider, as a general rule, the extent to which the motor discharge spreads around its focal area. Thus, as stimulation of the planta causing the flexion-reflex is increased there is added[182,275] to the flexion of the homonymous hind-limb extension of the crossed hind-limb, then in the homonymous fore-limb extension at elbow and retraction at shoulder, then at the crossed fore-limb flexion at elbow, extension at wrist, and some protraction at shoulder; also turning of the head toward the homonymous side, and often opening of the mouth, also lateral deviation of the tail.

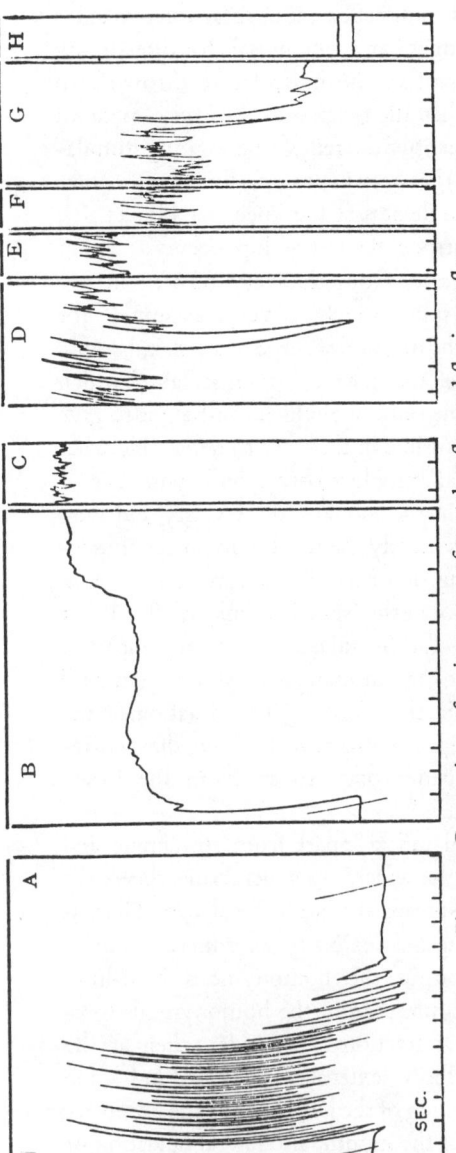

Fig. 45. Comparison of maintenance of scratch-reflex and flexion-reflex

Records from above downwards: Myograph curve. Time in seconds. Maintenance of the scratch-reflex (A) and the flexion-reflex (B, C, D, E, F, G, H) respectively under unipolar faradic stimulation of comparable intensity. The diffuse electrode (anode) was on the fore-limb in each case; the primary circuit and its rate of interruption was the same, and the secondary coil of the inductorium remained at the same distance from the primary. For the scratch-reflex the needle (stimulating) electrode was set in the skin of the loin, for the flexion-reflex in the plantar skin of the outermost digit. In A, after giving 28 beats the scratch-reflex died out, having lasted about 7 sec. Further continuation of the stimulation was cut short as useless after four more seconds. The flexion-reflex, B, on the other hand, is in full intensity at the end of the 13th sec. of continued application of the stimulus, and its amplitude is perfectly maintained at the end of the 20th (C), although the reflex is rather tremulant. At the 44th sec. (D), when it has become more tremulant still, it suddenly shows a brief, complete relaxation, lasting somewhat less than a second. This is accompanied by contraction of the extensor muscle of the knee (successive spinal induction, Lect. VI). After this the reflex is well maintained, although tremulant, to the 54th sec. (E); thence onward it shows gradual decline, reducing it by about a third of its original amplitude, when the stimulus is stopped at the 95th sec. (F). Relaxation then sets in promptly (G) and the tremor diminishes, but the original base line is hardly reached even 15 sec. later (H). At the 10th sec. (B) the flexion-reflex shows an increase due to sudden spread of the reflex to the flexors of the hip. The break shocks used in stimulation were at the rate of 33 per sec.

Irradiation

According to circumstance, especially according to intensity of stimulation, the field of end-effect of the flexion-reflex may vary from a minute field occupying part of a flexor muscle of the knee to a field including musculature in all four limbs and neck and head and tail.

That the reaction should spread in its spatial extent is not surprising. The afferent neurone on entering the central organ, the spinal cord, enters a vast network of conduction paths interlacing in all directions. A glance at any Weigert preparation of the spinal cord shows a tangle of branching nerve-fibres, the richness and intricacy of which seems practically infinite. Into this forest the receptive neurone conducts the impulses, and can itself be traced, breaking up into many divisions that pass in many directions and to various distances. And this web of conductive channels into which the centripetal impulses of the reflex are thus launched is known to be practically a continuum in the sense that no part of the nervous system is isolated from the rest. "A group of nerve-cells disconnected from the other nerve-tissues of the body, as the muscles or glands are disconnected from each other, would be without physiological significance. To understand the physiology of the nervous system it is important to keep in mind the fact that by histology it is found to be continuous throughout its entire extent."[209] And there is the generally accredited statement that on exhibition of strychnine centripetal impulses poured in via any afferent nerve, excite reflex-discharge over the efferent channels of the whole nerve-system. This, even if not strictly true, is sufficiently approximate to the truth to show the enormous interconnexions between any afferent channel and the congeries of arcs of the whole central nervous system. It is therefore not surprising that the reflex reaction should spread. On the other hand, the data leave unexplained certain features of the spread. How is it that the spread, as the reflex is intensified, does not extend everywhere, as it is said to do in strychnine poisoning? How is it that in the flexion-reflex, of the cat for instance, the spread does not extend to the muscles of the pinna of the ear? It is easy from certain parts to obtain the brisk reflex retraction of the pinna. Yet in my experience the stimulation of the foot that causes the flexion-

Compound Reflexes

reflex and all its various irradiations may be pushed without evoking retraction or other movement of the pinna. In other words, the irradiations of the reflex occur along certain lines only and not along others, and the line to the pinna is of these latter.

Evidently the irradiation from each entrant path tends to run in certain directions and not in all. This fact is sometimes stated in the form that grey matter offers to the entrant path lines of conduction possessing different degrees of resistance. To say this merely of course restates the fact in terms suggesting analogy between nerve-paths and electric circuits. Before the Golgi and methylene-blue methods had thrown doubt on the intricate forest of nerve-fibres in the grey matter being a network structurally continuous in all directions, as supposed from the Gerlach preparations and the universal irradiation under strychnine, the differences in conductive resistance were attributed mainly to differences in the length of the network to be traversed by some reflexes as compared with others. The longer that path in the grey matter the higher was thought to be the resistance. Evidence indicating slow travel of impulses in grey matter was taken as evidence of resistance in grey matter. In certain reactions the impulses were supposed to have very long paths of travel in grey matter. Thus, impulses of pain were supposed to ascend along the spinal grey matter to the brain. The path of impulses connected with pain does plunge into the grey matter very soon after entering the spinal cord; it then, probably after a short course, emerges into the lateral white columns, preponderantly of the side crossed from that on which it entered. This short in-and-out traverse of the spinal grey matter seems typical of all paths in the grey matter; they are probably all quite short.[205] If all synapses lie in the grey matter, each path where it involves a passage from one link to another of the neural chain must enter the grey matter to establish its linkage; it probably soon emerges thence again.

NEURONE-THRESHOLD

But one finds still very generally expressed the view that the differences of resistance to irradiation in different directions are referable to different conductive resistance offered by different fibres

Neurone-threshold

in the grey matter. The different resistance seems more probably referable to differences in the facility of conduction at different synapses. At each synapse there is a neurone-threshold.[187] At each synapse a small quantity of energy, freed in transmission, acts as a releasing force to a fresh store of energy not along a homogeneous train of conducting material as in a nerve-fibre pure and simple, but across a barrier which whether lower or higher is always to some extent a barrier. There is abundant evidence that different synapses differ from one another. That neurones should differ in the threshold value of the stimulus necessary to excite them seems only natural. The arguments adduced by Goldscheider point in this same direction. Many of the phenomena considered in the first three lectures are easiest explicable by such differences. The distinctions between different synapses in regard to ease of alteration by strychnine and by tetanus toxin emphasize this probability further. On this view the fact that irradiation of a reflex reaction spreads along certain conductive arcs more readily than along others, can be schematically figured as in the diagram (Fig. 46). A receptive neurone A enters the cord and forms synaptic connexions with three neurones; the neurone-threshold at the synapse with one of the neurones is higher than that at the synapses with the others. The threshold heights (resistances) are represented by whole numbers, two and one respectively. Each of the intraspinal neurones in its turn forms two synaptic connexions with two neurones, and in these cases also the thresholds at the synapses are of different heights, numerically, two and one respectively. On the view that the action of one neurone upon the next is that of a releasing force liberating a potential system across a barrier whose resistance we do not exactly know, it is impossible to predict how the resistance will sum along the whole conductive chain. It is clear that although the total resistance of the reflex-arc AB may be numerically represented by 1, the resistance along AD need not, on the numerical values assigned to the synapses in the diagram (Fig. 46), sum to the value 4. Yet it is also clear that the threshold for any whole arc cannot be lower than the highest individual threshold in it. Further, the individual thresholds will tend to sum, for an excitation of neurone A just sufficient to excite

Compound Reflexes

neurone *a* is hardly likely to excite *a* sufficiently to overcome the threshold of synapse *aD*. Thus, with even small grades of difference of threshold at different synapses, large differences in the conductive facility of different reflex-arcs can be established.

Similarly, an additive influence of the threshold will make a reflex-chain consisting of several neurones offer *ceteris paribus* higher resistance than a chain of fewer neurones. The diagram is

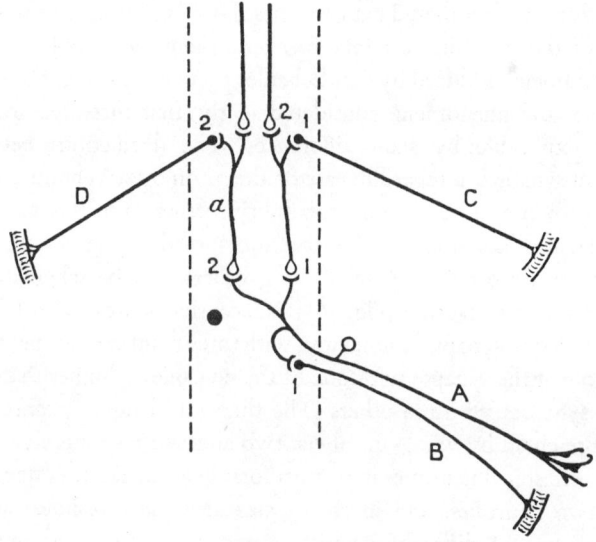

Fig. 46. Explanation in text

therefore in accord with the rule that the reflex-chains which conduct to parts segmentally distant require generally intenser stimulation to excite them than do merely local arcs.

SHORT AND LONG REFLEXES

For many purposes of description it is convenient to divide reflexes into 'short' and 'long'.205

The cord may, in its relation to the receptive surface and skeletal musculature, be considered divisible into right and left lateral halves,

Short and Long Reflexes

each subdivisible into regions of neck (cervical, including pinna), fore-limb (brachial), trunk (thoracic), hind-limb (crural), and tail (caudal). A reflex action in which the stimulus applied to a receptive area in one of the above regions evokes a reaction in the musculature of another of the regions is conveniently called a *long spinal* reflex. A reflex reaction in which the muscular reply occurs in the same region as the application of the stimulus is conveniently called a *short spinal* reflex. Short spinal reflexes are, as a rule, more easily and regularly elicitable than are long spinal reflexes. It might further be convenient to allocate hard-and-fast boundaries to these regions, but such limits would of necessity be artificial and arbitrary. The scope of the delimitation is indicated and its purpose better served by comparison with one retina, say of the bird, the one lateral half of the skin corresponding with one retina; one optic nerve would correspond with the lateral half of the spinal cord and bulb. Between these comparable surfaces a difference exists, in that the receptive field of the skin, unlike the retinal, has instead of one (or two, cf. Kalischer[310]) focal region of concentrated responsiveness, several such foci, e.g. the relatively highly responsive skin at the apex of each limb. As the retina has muscles at call, so also the skin. The closeness of nexus between a retinal point and the visual musculature is graduate in degree, e.g. most close for the muscles of its own bulbus, next for those of the contralateral, then for the neck muscles, etc. Similarly there are degrees of nexal closeness between a point of skin and the related musculature: its connexion is most close with muscles of its own limb, next with those of another limb or other region. The main interest of direction of nervous irradiation *per se*—apart from light it may incidentally cast upon the integrative work of the nervous system—lies in its elucidation of the machinery for working sentient surfaces. That the skin is a region which morphologically considered is composed of a segmental series seems to have been allowed greater weight in the estimation of its receptive functions than is fully justified, at least in the higher vertebrata. That its segmental innervation demonstrably limits existing reflex spinal functions in the mammal has not been shown.[136]

Compound Reflexes

RULES OBSERVED IN THE SPREAD OF IMPULSES IN SPINAL REFLEXES

Regarding short spinal reflexes, and the directions taken by the examples of intraspinal irradiation which they furnish, it is possible to make certain general statements.[136]

I. Broadly speaking, *the degree of reflex spinal intimacy between afferent and efferent spinal roots varies directly as their segmental proximity.* Thus excitation of the central side of a severed thoracic root, e.g. seventh, evokes with especial ease contraction of muscles or parts of muscles innervated by the corresponding motor roots, and next easily muscles innervated by the next adjacent motor roots. The spread of short spinal reflexes in many instances seems to be rather easier tailward than headward. This may be related with the oblique correlation that so largely holds between the distribution of the afferent root in the skin and the distribution of the efferent root in the underlying muscles.

II. Taken generally, *for each afferent root there exists in immediate proximity to its own place of entrance in the cord (e.g. in its own segment) a reflex motor path of as low a threshold and of as high potency as any open to it anywhere.* Further, in response to excitation even approximately minimal in intensity, a single afferent root, or a single filament of a single root, evokes a spinal discharge of centrifugal impulses through more than one efferent root, i.e. the discharge is plurisegmental. And this holds especially in the limb regions. In the limb region the nerve root is therefore a morphological aggregate of nerve-fibres, rather than a functionally determined assortment of impulse-paths. The view that the efferent spinal root is a functional assemblage of nerve-fibres is certainly erroneous. The formation of functional collections of nerve-paths (peripheral nerve-trunks) out of morphological collections (nerve-roots) seems to be the meaning of the limb-plexuses.

III. Motor mechanisms for the skeletal musculature lying in the same region of the cord, and in the selfsame spinal segment, exhibit markedly *unequal accessibility to the local afferent channels as judged by pressor effects.* For example, if pressor effects only, and the primary

Reflex Accessibility of Motor-Neurones

phase only, of the reflex movement be considered, the flexors of the homonymous knee and the extensors of the contralateral are in many animals much more accessible than the extensors of the homonymous and the flexors of the contralateral. Inasmuch as at many joints the flexors and extensors are *both* innervated by motor-fibres contained in one and the same efferent root, it follows that the reflex movement obtained by excitation of an afferent root in many cases is quite dissimilar from the movement obtained by excitation of the corresponding efferent root, in spite of the rule of segmental proximity.

It is necessary to insert the qualification 'pressor' before 'effects' ('reciprocal innervation'). It is only in regard to pressor effect that the above statement holds for such contrasted neurones as those of 'extensors' and 'flexors'. I have stated the rule in this way because it is in conformity with the oft-quoted rule of spinal reflexes coming to us from Ludwig's laboratory, which insisted on the rarity or impossibility of obtaining hind-limb extension as a primary homonymous spinal reflex. But how easy and direct is really the reflex nexus between the receptive surface of the limb and its extensor muscles, e.g. at knee, is shown by nothing better than by giving a small dose of strychnine. That alkaloid has, as has been mentioned, the property of converting spinal reflex inhibition into excitation. The same stimulus which normally reflexly excites the knee-flexors to contraction is seen after the strychnine to excite the knee-extensors to contraction. The reflex inhibition of the extensors which was previously the reflex-effect is more difficult to observe, but by turning it into excitation the facility of the reflex nexus with the extensors is found to be as close as with the flexors. Therefore, in the rule before us, if inhibition and excitation are *both*—as they should be—counted as evidence of the reflex nexus, then the reflex nexus with the homonymous knee-extensors and with the crossed knee-flexors, is as close as with the homonymous knee-flexors and the crossed knee-extensors.

In the question, therefore, that was put above, How is it that the spread of a reflex reaction, when the reflex is intensified, does not extend to all parts, as it is said to do in strychnine poisoning? there

Compound Reflexes

are two different things involved. It does not spread to some parts because, as argued above, an additive synaptic resistance intervenes across the potentially conductive path. An instance of such a path was given. But the absence of apparent irradiation to certain others is for a different reason. Keeping to the flexion-reflex as elicited by unipolar faradization of the plantar skin of a digit as illustration, the instance of the knee-extensor may be taken. However intensely the stimulation may be pushed, although the reflex reaction is thereby more and more intensified, contraction of the knee-extensor does not result—but for a wholly different reason than that suggested for the absence of spread of the reflex from the leg to the pinna. The muscles of the pinna, in my experience, do not at all easily become involved in the reaction; but the extensor muscle of the knee is really involved in the reaction from the beginning, only it is involved in a way that escapes observation unless special means be taken to reveal it. The reflex-effect upon it takes the form of an inhibition of the efferent path just central to its motor neurone, an inhibitory block, which in proportion as the intensity of the exciting stimulus of the reflex is increased simply becomes itself the more intense. There is no evidence that this can be broken down and converted into excitation by merely increasing the intensity of the stimulus that is evoking it. On the other hand, as shown above, strychnine and tetanus toxin convert it into excitation, and that is one reason why strychnine seems to increase the spread of reflexes so greatly; but in this case the increase of spread which that drug appears to cause is really merely apparent. The reflex-effect was there already, but had another form of expression.

IV. *The groups of motor nerve-cells contemporaneously discharged by spinal reflex action innervate synergic and not antergic muscles.* This is the reverse of the view that since Winslow and Duchenne[49] has been common doctrine concerning muscular co-ordination. It controverts an argument adduced for the view that the limb movement evoked by excitation of an *efferent root* represents a highly co-ordinate functional synergism.[96, 97] The spinal reflex in its intraspinal irradiation develops a combined movement and synthesizes a muscular harmony.

Irradiation in Long Reflexes

V. It follows almost as a corollary from this, and from the *rule of spatial proximity* (p. 160), that *the spinal reflex movement elicitable in and from any one spinal region will exhibit much uniformity despite considerable variety of the locus of incidence of the exciting stimulus*. Approximately the same movement, e.g. in the hind-limb flexion of the three great joints, will result, whatever piece of the limb surface be irritated. The locus of incidence of the stimulus will only influence the character of the general movement executed by the limb musculature, in so far that the flexion will tend to predominantly occur at that joint the flexor muscles of which are innervated by motor cells segmentally near to the entrance of the afferent fibres from the particular piece of skin the seat of application of the stimulus. Another way of expressing this rule is to say that the receptive field of a 'type-reflex' is usually of plurisegmental cutaneous extent.

Part of the question of spatial distribution of the motor discharge of a spinal reflex has long been studied, and a fundamental contribution to knowledge of it was made by Pflüger.[24] His inductions were based chiefly upon observations on the frog and on the records of clinical cases of spinal lesion in man. They were drawn up in the form of four 'laws'.

It was regarding the course of irradiation in *long spinal* reflexes, namely *those spinal reflexes that initiated from one* of the above mentioned spinal regions *spread over into others* that Pflüger,[24] in 1853, formulated his four 'laws'. These 'laws' have for many years been widely accepted.[132] They are stated as follows:

1. The law of homonymous conduction for unilateral reflexes. If a stimulus applied to a sensory nerve provokes muscular movements solely on one side of the body, that movement occurs under all circumstances and without exception on the same side of the body as the seat of application of the stimulus.

If, as is clear from the context in the original paper, by movement on the same side is meant contraction of muscles on the same side, this statement does not in reality very completely express the facts.[183] It is in part an outcome of the rule of spatial proximity, but certain cases which conform to the latter yet offer striking exception to the

Compound Reflexes

former; for instance, when the skin of the tail is stimulated on one side the organ is very frequently moved towards the opposite, and this in a great number of classes, from fish to mammal inclusive.

2. The law of bilateral symmetry of the reflex action. When the change produced in the central organ by excitation of a sensory nerve has already evoked a unilateral reflex, if it spreads farther, it excites in the contralateral half of the cord only those motor mechanisms which are symmetrical with those already excited in the homonymous half of the cord. This statement, although true of a number of instances, fails to conform with fact in many, even perhaps the majority.

The important cross-reflex from the hind-limb of the bird and mammal does not conform to it; so similarly with the fore-limb. The asymmetry of the crossed reflexes of the limbs is important because probably connected with the fundamental co-ordination of muscles for progression. Again, the wag-reflex of the tail, and a reflex I have called the 'torticollis reflex'[183] (cervical region), afford important exceptions to the 'law'. And many other exceptions can be found. In the spinal rabbit, on the other hand, and less often in the dog, the crossed reflex from one hind-limb to the other is sometimes not an asymmetrical movement, but a symmetrical one: this seems to stand in obvious relation to the hopping mode of progression of the animal.

3. The law of unequal intensity of bilateral reflexes. When the excitation of a sensory nerve elicits reflex action involving both halves of the body, and the action is unequal on the two sides, the side of stronger contractions is always that homonymous with the seat of application of the stimulus.

This statement is in conformity with a number of instances. The following are examples. When bilateral retraction of the abdomen is excited from the skin of the chest, the contralateral retraction is much the less marked: in the bilateral protraction of the 'whiskers' (cat, rabbit, dog) on the excitation of the skin of the face, the crossed movement is the less ample. An interesting illustration,[183, 205] because it involves inhibitory as well as pressor influence, can be demonstrated in the spinal cat or dog thus: The animal resting

Pflüger's 'Laws of Reflexes'

comfortably on its back, if one hind-paw be pressed that leg will be flexed at hip, knee, and ankle, in accordance with the rules laid down on p. 160, and if the stimulus be strong, or the reflex excitability good, the fellow hind-limb will be extended. If instead of one hind-paw both hind-paws be pressed, both hind-limbs are simultaneously flexed, and there is no trace of extension (Fig. 66, Lect. VI, p. 226). The homonymous reflex is prepotent, therefore, and inhibits the crossed reflex.

But there are also a number of exceptions to this 'law', among others, the abduction of the tail from the side stimulated already referred to.

4. The fourth of Pflüger's classical 'laws' of spinal reflex action states that with associated spinal reflex centres the irradiation spreads more easily in the direction toward than in the direction away from the head.

My own experience in the mammal is far from completely accordant with this statement: in, I think, the majority of instances, irradiation has spread more easily down than up the cord.[183,205,251] It is easy to obtain reflex movements of the limbs and tail by excitation of the skin of the pinna, whereas the reverse is rare. To elicit by excitation of the hind-limb a movement of the fore-limb, is more difficult than by excitation of the fore-limb to elicit movement of the hind-limb. To elicit movement of the tail by excitation of the fore-limb is easier than to move the fore-limb by excitation of the tail. The irradiation has in my experience been easier across the cord from hind-limb to hind-limb than from hind-limb to fore-limb; but it is often easier down the cord from fore-limb to hind-limb than across from fore-limb to fore-limb. In such reflexes also as the 'shake' reflex (a reflex in which the trunk is shaken, as when a dog comes out of water), which implicate the trunk more than the limbs, the radiation is away from the head, for it is well obtained as a rump reflex when the skin of the shoulder is the part rubbed. In the 'scratch-reflex', too, the skin stimulus is applied far headward of the region of the muscular contraction evoked.

These so-called 'laws' of reflex irradiation were so generally accepted as to obtain a doctrinal eminence which they hardly merit.

Compound Reflexes

It seems here less profitable to attempt adapting them to better fit the observed facts than to briefly describe the salient features of the long spinal reflexes as exhibited in an ordinary experiment on the spinal mammal.

THE REFLEX FIGURE

When the animal is supported freely from above, with its spine horizontal and the limbs pendant, a point that early strikes the

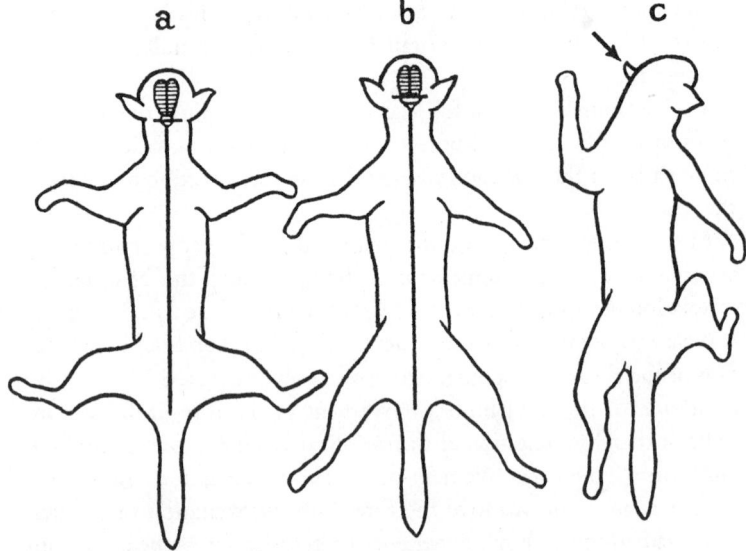

Fig. 47. *a.* Position of animal after transection at calamus scriptorius;
b. Position under decerebrate rigidity;
Change of attitude from *b* evoked by stimulation of left pinna.

observer is that there are ten areas whence bulbo-spinal reflexes employing skeletal musculature can be provoked with pre-eminent facility. These areas are the soles, the palms, the pinnae, the mouth, the snout, and the tail and cloacal region. It is significant that nine of these areas are those which possess the greatest range of motility if the axis of the animal be considered fixed. Stimulation at any one of these areas causes a particular attitude—a *reflex figure*—to be struck. From the pinna is excited movement of each limb, the neck, the

The Reflex Figure

tail, and the trunk (Fig. 47). The irradiation from this reflexigenous area usually presents the following order: (1) Neck and homonymous fore-limb, (2) homonymous hind-limb, (3) tail and trunk on both sides, (4) contralateral hind-limb, (5) contralateral fore-limb. From the fore-foot (Fig. 48) can be excited besides movements in the fore-limb itself, movements in the other limbs and tail. The facility of radiation is usually in the following descending series: (1) homonymous hind-limb and the tail, (2) crossed hind-limb, (3) crossed fore-

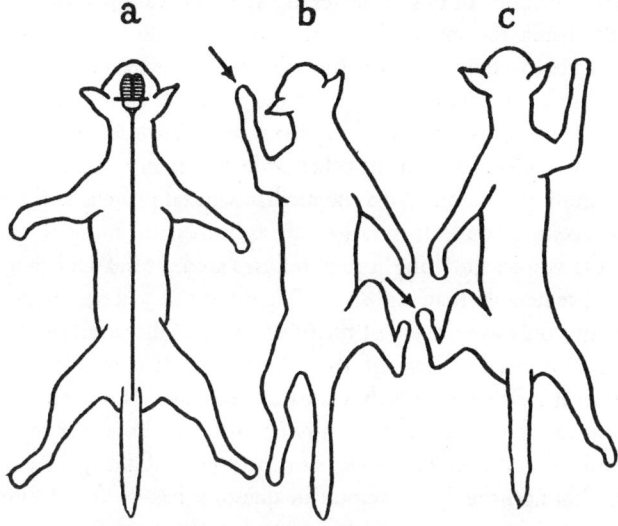

Fig. 48. *a*. Position under decerebrate rigidity;
  b. Change of attitude from *a* evoked by stimulation of left fore-foot;
  c. Change of attitude from *a* evoked by stimulation of left hind-foot.

limb. The relative facility of spread of the reaction to the crossed fore-limb seems subject to much variation. In the frog the path between the two fore-limbs is, especially in the breeding season, very open and facile. In the cat and monkey it seems to be much more open in the bulbo-spinal than in the spinal animal. From the hind-foot (Fig. 48) the frequency and ease of irradiation into other spinal regions usually appears to exist in the following order: (1) extension of crossed hind-limb and tail, (2) extension of homonymous fore-limb, (3) flexion of crossed fore-limb. The facility of

Compound Reflexes

'spread' from one lateral half of the cord to the other is very dissimilar at different levels of the cord. It is particularly easy in certain parts of the tail region. Motor mechanisms which are yoked together are for the most part, as with the flexion-extension mechanisms of the hip and knee, of an asymmetrical kind. In the hind-limb region the crossed irradiation is also fairly free, and largely connects asymmetrical muscle-groups; but one of the most facile and persistent of all bilateral reflexes resulting from unilateral stimulation is the adduction of both thighs, a bilaterally symmetrical movement.

In the trunk the spread across the median plane is most free for skin reflexes excited from near the midline; this is seen in the venter of the frog; the yoking is of bilaterally symmetrical muscles. To excite movement of one fore-limb from the other is less easy than to excite one hind-limb from the other, at least in many animals. In the neck region irradiation across the median sagittal plane is fairly easy, and the yoking connects in large part asymmetrical muscles.

On the whole, the 'long' spinal reflexes are more variable and less validly predictable than the short. They vary in a series of experiments, not only as to order of relative facility of direction of irradiation, but as to the sense of the movement elicited at the joint, whatever it may be, to which irradiation extends. Not unfrequently a region to which the reflex usually irradiates is altogether omitted, and omitted consistently throughout the whole of a lengthy experiment, although the spinal region in question has, so far as known, suffered no damage, nor indeed been directly implicated in any of the procedure. Thus, excitation of the skin of the neck or pinna will sometimes spread back along the cord and produce movement in the tail, or in the hind-limbs, and in doing so pass by the fore-limbs without evoking a twitch in either of them. The motor mechanisms of the fore-limb thus skipped over may show no sign when examined by the local reflexes of being less amenable than usual.

The inconstancy of the irradiation as to the kind of movement produced, e.g. whether it flex or extend a limb, is different in different reflexes. The irradiations from the 'drawing-up reflex' of the hind foot (i.e. the flexion-reflex) have great constancy; the irradiation is shown in Fig. 48; to the figure the turning of the head

Variability of Reflex Response

to the homonymous side may be added; the irradiation from the fore-foot reflex is less regular; sometimes flexion at crossed knee, sometimes extension. The variation is from experiment to experiment, not during a single experiment.

There is some evidence that the influence exerted on a common path by one and the same afferent arc may not always be of the same kind. It is true that the regularity with which the same end-result appears and reappears in observations dealing with certain reflexes is very great, and inclines the observer to regard the reaction of the reflex-arc as perfectly constant. But that is not equally clear of all the reflexes. Instances of inconstancy seem to occur in some reflex-arcs, and these suggest the possibility that in some cases one and the same afferent arc may exert on a final common path even reverse effects at different times; in other words, under different conditions. The effect of stimuli to the pinna of the 'bulbo-spinal' cat seems sometimes to be flexion of the hind-limb, sometimes extension of that limb. Stimulation of the afferent nerve of a part of the vasto-crureus muscle is often inhibition of the rest of that muscle, but sometimes not. In my experience these results, though variable from experiment to experiment, do not vary during the same experiment. Again, the afferent nerve, stimulation of which excites reflex rise of arterial pressure under curare, is known to yield reflex fall of pressure under chloral. It must be admitted that here other explanations are indeed possible, besides the supposition that the kind of influence excited by the afferent arc on the efferent path has changed.

Irradiation of a reflex attaches itself to the problem of the simultaneous combination of reflexes. It does so because it affords clear evidence that by irradiation a reflex assumes use of a number of final common paths which do not in the first instance belong to it, but belong in the first instance rather to reflexes arising in their own immediate segmental locality. From them a 'reflex figure' is formed. Thus, by irradiation, the flexion-reflex of the right *planta* causes reflex-discharge down the motor nerve of the cubital extensor (part of triceps) of the homonymous fore-limb. But this reflex motor discharge to the cubital extensor is more easily excited by stimulation of the left fore-paw. Again the flexion-reflex of the right planta, if

Compound Reflexes

strong, will irradiate as motor discharge into the flexors of the left elbow, but the reflex motor discharge into the flexors of the left elbow is much more easily obtained by stimulation of the left fore-paw; so that the irradiation welds into a single combined reflex-effect belonging primarily, as it were, to several reflexes. But the reflexes whose effects are thus combined are always reflexes of what was termed above 'allied' relation. Thus, if a stimulus exciting the flexion-reflex from the right planta be just subliminal for evoking the irradiation to the homonymous cubital extensor and a stimulus be applied to the left fore-paw of an intensity by itself just subliminal for provoking crossed elbow-extension, the two stimuli applied simultaneously mutually facilitate and the reflex of the right fore-limb results.

Moreover, it seems to me significant that the irradiation extends rather *per saltum* than *gradatim*. As the flexion-reflex is continued, flexion at hip (Fig. 45, p. 154) can be seen to add itself almost suddenly to flexion already in progress at knee.

Romanes[72] writes of irradiation in Medusa as follows: "It is not difficult to obtain a series of lithocysts connected in such a manner that the resistance offered to the passage of the waves by a certain width of the junction-tissue is such as just to allow the residuum of the contraction wave which emanates from one lithocyst to reach the adjacent lithocyst, thus causing it to originate another wave, which in turn is just able to pass to the next lithocyst in the series, and so on, each lithocyst acting in turn like a reinforcing battery to the passage of the contraction wave. Now this, I think, sufficiently explains the mechanism of ganglionic action in those cases where one or more lithocysts are prepotent over the others; that is to say, the prepotent lithocyst first originates a contraction wave which is then successively reinforced by all the other lithocysts during its passage round the swimming-bell." If we read for 'prepotent lithocyst' the 'exciting external stimulus' of the arc primarily stimulated and for the other lithocysts the other arcs to which the excitement of the one primarily stimulated extends, it seems to me we have in the above description of *Aurelia aurita* a description that applies well to the process of reflex irradiation in the central nervous organ of vertebrates.

Irradiation of Reflexes

It may be objected that in the case of Medusa the wave of contraction is reinforced by, on reaching the lithocyst, initiating through that a new reflex which reinforces the one already in progress; whereas in the spread of the flexion-reflex to the reflex-arcs of the fore-limb, the reaction does not initiate in these latter anything that can be called a new reflex because the reaction in them is not excited through their local receptors, the normal point of departure for their reflexes. That is a difference certainly, and a significant one. But it does not vitiate the analogy from the point of view under consideration now. In Medusa the irradiation of the reflex is in its propagation reinforced at the certain points mentioned by the reaction in its spread exciting a new neurone, attached to its path, across a definite threshold resistance. In Medusa the threshold lies in Romanes' view at the receptor organ. In the irradiation of the flexion-reflex the reaction also breaks at certain points into new arcs across a threshold resistance, and once over the threshold, propagates itself along those arcs, as evidenced by the movements produced. It is in accordance with that mode of propagation that the irradiation of the reflex appears to occur *per saltum* rather than *gradatim* (Fig. 45). Here again it is noteworthy that the places of reinforcement in the spread of the reaction which are peripheral in Medusa are central in the vertebrate; in other words, just as refractory state, inhibition, interference, etc., which are peripheral in Medusa are central in the vertebrate, so with this latter instance of 'reinforcement'. The reason which seemed obvious before, applies in the present instance also, and is the same as that which explains the centrality of the central nervous system itself (Lect. IX).

It is not only when the spot stimulated is a *receptor* that the reflex shows itself co-ordinate. The stimulation of the central end of any even large afferent nerve-trunk, or even the central end of a whole spinal afferent root, evokes reflexly a movement that is co-ordinate. This result is familiar and commonplace, but it is also remarkable.

For stimulation of the central ends of that vast medley of afferents, from different sources and of various species, collected together in one afferent spinal root (e.g. eighth cervical), to evoke no inharmonious confusion of various reflexes, such as the component fibres

Compound Reflexes

in it must, taken individually, represent but one allied group of harmonious reflexes, is a result that, though regularly obtainable, is surely not what the observer might have expected would occur. Stimulation of the central end of the tibial nerve behind the ankle causes flexion at knee, hip, and ankle, in which the normal inhibitions of extensor muscles accompany the contractions of the flexor muscles. Yet in that nerve are included the afferent fibres from the *planta* which evolve the powerful extension-reflex, the extensor-thrust. How is it that this reflex does not appear conjoined with the flexion-reflex produced by the other afferent fibres in the posterior root or tibial nerve? The principle of interference of antagonistic reflexes central to the mouth of the common path on which both embouch precludes such confusion of reflexes. Such simultaneous combination of flexion and extension reflexes would be inco-ordination. The formation of a common path from tributary paths is a mechanism ensuring co-ordination against that. The stimulation of the nerve containing admixed receptive paths of different and antagonistic reflexes excites reflexly through the central organ an effect in the skeletal musculature which is co-ordinate and synergic. It is as though a solvent were simultaneously supersaturated with two crystalloids, and as though when a pair of these crystals was simultaneously dropped into the solution the crystallization out took place of one salt or of the other, but not of both together. What happens resembles what occurs when there is presented to the eye one of the plane figures suggesting visual perspective, but equivocally in either of the two ways; the *whole* of the beaker or of the flight of steps appears set in one way or in the other, never partly in one way, partly in the other. And this is a really germane analogy.

The mode of preclusion of the antagonistic reflexes seems so closely akin to the process which occurs when one reflex in its supervention on another dispossesses an antagonistic reflex from the common path that its discussion may be deferred until treating of the co-ordination of successive reflexes. But it is obvious that in the irradiation of a reflex so as to produce a combined movement of remote parts we have really a synthesis of simultaneous reflexes. The parts of the reflex finding simultaneous expression in the efferent

Reflex Figure not given by Motor Root

paths of other reflexes are combined by a process which tends to exclude the antagonistic reflex for each component part. It is obvious that while 'allied' reflexes can be compounded together both in simultaneous and successive combination, antagonistic reflexes can be combined only in successive combination.

THE COLLECTION OF FIBRES IN A MOTOR SPINAL ROOT DOES NOT REPRESENT A 'REFLEX FIGURE'

The supporters of the view that the motor-fibres gathered together in a motor spinal root form a collection assorted so as to represent the fibres that normally are excited together in willed and other actions adduce the fact that antagonistic muscles are together thrown into contraction on exciting this or that spinal motor nerve root supplying a limb—e.g. the arm. This fact, as I pointed out some years[136] ago, is in reality one of the clearest evidences that their view is erroneous, because most commonly in normal movements the antagonistic muscles, far from being thrown into contraction together, are reciprocally innervated, one antagonist being made to contract and the other to relax. Further, far from a normal action ever throwing into activity all the motor-fibres of a single motor root, still less using that one root thus solely without other roots, in reality the evidence is that in all normal actions, reflex or voluntary, especially in the limb regions, the centrifugal discharge to the muscles takes place through scattered motor-fibres contained in several roots, even when the action provoked and the movement effected are weak. Outside the limb region, those who argue that the aggregation of motor-fibres in each efferent spinal root represents some definite synergic contraction of muscles for a co-ordinate movement must disregard the observation of Newell Martin and Hartwell[79] that in the normal breathing of the dog the action that goes forward in the internal and external intercostal muscles is alternating in them. One relaxes as the other contracts; yet both the external and the internal intercostal muscles of the space receive their motor supply from one and the same motor spinal root.

Those who hold the view that the assortment of the fibres of the motor root is functional, state that the movements which result

Compound Reflexes

from stimulation of these individual roots in the brachial region are not mere contractions more or less strong of various muscles, but are a highly co-ordinated functional synergy in each case. To this one may reply that the mere superficial resemblance of the position assumed by the limb, to one of the manifold positions assumed by it in the normal activity, is a slender analogy. The hind-limbs of a frog, when it tries to climb the side of the bell-jar which confines it, assume an attitude of extreme extension, in outward semblance like that of a strychnine cramp, or that due to excitation of the eighth root; but is it permissible from that resemblance to argue that excitation of the eighth root produces a co-ordinate movement of the limb? The same analogy would argue that the strychnic cramp is also a co-ordinate movement of the limb, whereas it is definitely known to be inco-ordinate.

Myself I have not been struck by resemblance between the movement produced by excitation of the motor spinal root of a limb-plexus and the co-ordinate normal movements of the limb. It may be urged that in order to obtain the resemblance the excitation employed must be strong, so as to bring into full action every component of the complex entity of the root. When I have done this the resulting movement has seemed to me, e.g. in the case of the sixth subthoracic root of the monkey, like a strychnine cramp rather than a movement of co-ordinate adjustment. If, on the other hand, it be urged that minimal excitation must be used, I have not been able to obtain in that way any more obvious relation to a co-ordinate movement. For instance, in the lumbo-spinal region of the monkey, excitation when just effective induces through the ninth subthoracic motor root abduction of the tail and flexion of the toes without any movement elsewhere. Similar excitation of the eighth motor root induces flexion of minimus and hallux without the intervening digits, not infrequently accompanied by pursing of the anus. Such combinations strike the observer as bizarre and give little suggestion of the bringing into play of a highly co-ordinate functional synergy.

On the view that the compound muscular contraction obtained by excitation of one whole motor root is highly co-ordinated and due to a group of contractions combined in accordance with some plan for

Motor Root not a Functional Unit

a functional result, it might be expected that the severance of one such motor root in a limb region would result in loss of some particular co-ordinate movement, and that the disappearance of that movement might be fairly clearly detectible. I was unable to detect such a result and saw no evidence in support of its existence. The severance of a single motor root seemed to produce not the complete loss of any one particular movement, but a weakened condition of many movements. Even when two of the motor spinal roots were cut the effect on the movements of the limb was rather weakness of movement than inco-ordination of movement. When the number of consecutive nerves cut was more than two there appeared limitation of the range of movement by loss in some particular direction. I inferred from my experiments that the mechanism for specific movement of each part of a limb (e.g. a digit) is so placed in the cord that the efferent fibres debouching from it into the motor roots pass via many root filaments and via at least two, usually more, spinal roots. Thus there is not in any one motor root filament, nor even in any one motor root, a perfect representation of any one movement, but only an imperfect representation of several adjacent local movements, though not for each equally imperfect.

Against the view that the aggregation of efferent fibres in a motor spinal root represents a functionally co-operative collection is the fact that between them there may intervene a high resistance; that is to say, afferent impulses that easily throw some of them into action have great difficulty in throwing others of them into action. Thus, the ninth subthoracic motor root of the monkey sometimes contains efferent fibres to the urinary bladder and to the muscles of the leg. It is easy to obtain a reflex on the latter through the afferent root of the ninth, but relatively difficult to obtain a reflex upon the bladder. The synergic view of the character of the collection of fibres in the spinal motor root presupposes or infers that mere spatial juxtaposition possesses curiously high value for spinal co-ordination; but are the separate spinal and bulbar elements of the respiratory centre less perfectly associated in function because in the neural axis they are placed apart? Likeness of quality rather than proximity in space insures the harmony of their reactions. I conclude, therefore, that

Compound Reflexes

the collection of fibres in a spinal motor root is not a functional collection in the sense that it is representative of any co-ordination.[136]

THE RECEPTIVE FIELD OF A REFLEX DOES NOT CONFORM WITH THE FIELD OF DISTRIBUTION OF AN AFFERENT SPINAL ROOT

Similarly with the afferent root. The distribution in the skin of any afferent root does not correspond with the receptive field of any cutaneous reflex. The skin-field of the scratch-reflex is made up of parts of the skin-fields of many adjacent spinal roots (compare Fig. 49 with Fig. 39, p. 123). The skin-field of the flexion-reflex of the hind-limb similarly; that of the fore-limb similarly. Even the relatively limited receptive field[251] of the extensor-thrust is a patch into which parts of the fields of at least two spinal roots enter. Nor do the *limits* of the receptive fields of cutaneous reflexes respect the limits of spinal root skin-fields. Again, the afferent nerve of the extensor cruris muscle evokes the same reflex as does that of the flexor muscle, yet the two belong to wholly different spinal nerves.

REINFORCEMENT

The overflow of reflex action into channels belonging primarily to other reflex-arcs than those under stimulation, leads to the production by the single stimulus of a wide, compound reflex which is tantamount in effect to a simultaneous combination of several allied reflexes.

When in the spinal animal the one fore-foot is stimulated, flexion of the hind-leg of the crossed side is often obtained. Stimulation of that hind-foot itself also causes a like reflex of that limb. When these two are concurrently stimulated, the flexion movement is obtained more easily than from either singly. These widely separate reflex-arcs therefore reinforce one another in their action on the final common paths they possess in common. Similarly with certain reflex-arcs arising from the skin of the pinna of the crossed ear. In them excitation reinforces that of the just mentioned arcs from the fore-foot and opposite hind-foot.

This reinforcement is significant of the solidarity of the whole spinal mechanism; but significant of more extensive solidarity still

Skin Fields of Spinal Afferent Roots

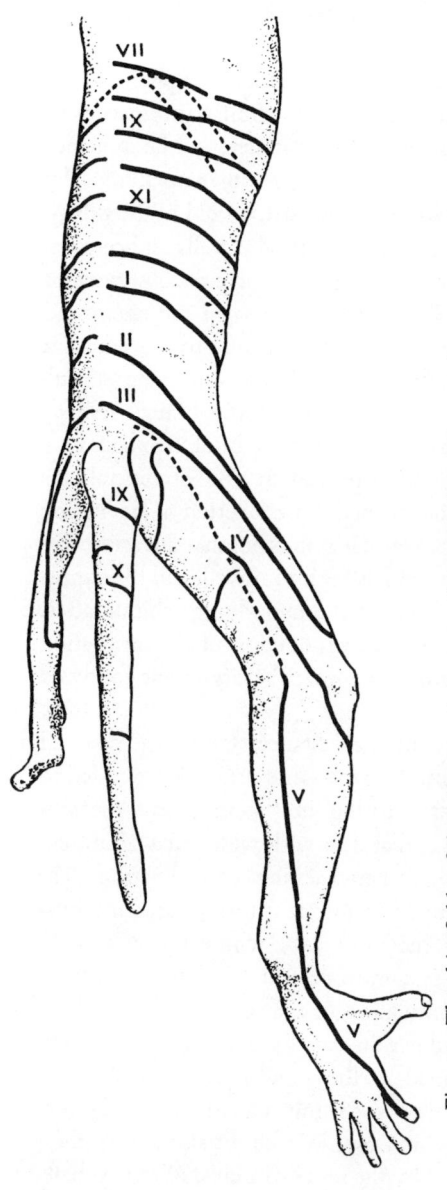

Fig. 49. The skin-fields of the afferent spinal roots of the monkey (*Macacus rhesus*), showing their general arrangement in the trunk and hind-limb

On the right side only the posterior limit, on the left side only the anterior limit. The fields were observed by the method of 'remaining aesthesia'. After determination of the limits of the field for a spinal root in a number of individuals the mean of the observations for that root was transferred to a plaster cast of *Macacus rhesus*, and the lines thus gradually built up on the model. The dotted line extending from the mid-dorsum outward along the dorsal aspect of the thigh is the 'dorsal line' of the hind-limb, and to it the fields of the sensory roots distributed to the skin of the limb behave as do those of the skin-fields of the trunk to the mid-dorsal line of the body. It will be noticed that the boundaries of the spinal root-fields neither in the limb nor in the trunk conform with the limits of the 'receptive-fields' of cutaneous reflexes. The cutaneous fields of the 'scratch-reflex', the 'flexion-reflex', the 'extensor-thrust', are areas which in nowise fit in with the pattern of the cutaneous fields of the afferent spinal roots. Compare this figure with Fig. 13, A, p. 46.

Compound Reflexes

are results observed by Exner.99, 149 A sound conveyed to the ear of a chloralized rabbit, he found, increased the amplitude of a reflex movement of the foot, induced by the stimulus applied to the foot a moment later. Sternberg has studied similar summation of reflexes.130 The same significance probably attaches to the influence of various precurrent stimuli on the knee-jerk in man, studied by Jendrassik, 105 Mitchell and Lewis, 107 Lombard, 119 and by Bowditch and Warren.123 In these cases of course cerebral as well as subcerebral arcs were in action. And in regard to these, we have the observations by Bubnoff and Heidenhain, 92 and by Exner, 99 in the narcotized dog and rabbit. In their experiments gentle stimuli to the skin of a limb exerted a reinforcing influence on closely following stimuli applied to the limb region of the cortex of the brain. Exner's observations proved that minimal electrical stimuli applied near together in point of time to the fore-limb region of the rabbit's cortex and to the skin of the crossed foot, exerted a facilitating influence, 'bahnung', on each other. He points out that this reinforcement occurs when the cortex itself has been removed, and the stimulation of the brain is applied direct to the underlying white matter. He argues, therefore, that the seat of production of the facilitation lies in the spinal centres. With that view, the argument followed here is in complete accord.

The co-ordination, in some of the instances taken, has covered but one limb or a pair of limbs. But the same principle extended to the reactions of the great arcs arising in the projicient receptor organs of the head, e.g. the eye, that deal with wide tracts of musculature as a whole, involves further-reaching co-ordination. The singleness of action from moment to moment thus assured is a keystone in the construction of the individual whose unity it is the specific office of the nervous system to perfect. And in the instance taken, namely, concurrent stimulation of the one fore-foot and the crossed hind-foot, the co-ordination can be easily traced further; the crossed fore-foot is extended at elbow and retracted at shoulder under the combination of the two stimuli, and the homonymous hind-limb is extended at knee and hip. We might also add to these movements others, also caused by the same stimulus, of the eyeballs,

Simultaneous Combination of Reflexes

the lips, the larynx, and the arterial wall of the splanchnic area. But these would not for the present purpose emphasize the main point further.

As remarked above, it is not usual for the organism to be exposed to the action of only one stimulus at a time. It is more usual for the organism to be acted on by many stimuli concurrently, and to be driven reflexly by some group of stimuli which is at any particular moment prepotent in action on it. Such a group often consists of some one pre-eminent stimulus with others of harmonious relation reinforcing it, forming with it a constellation of stimuli, that, in succession of time, will give way to another constellation which will in its turn become prepotent.

The concurrent stimuli keep a number of arcs in active touch with their final paths, and a number of other arcs out of active touch with the final paths belonging to them. In the particular instance taken, they keep arcs of one fore-limb and one hind-limb in action upon final common paths of flexion of those limbs, upon final common paths of extension in the diagonal pair of limbs, and upon final common paths of flexion of the neck. And the concurrent stimuli simultaneously check other arcs from getting into active touch with the final common paths of extension of one fore-limb and hind-limb, namely, those of the seat of stimulation, and of flexion in the opposite fore-limb and hind-limb, and of retraction of the neck. Further, these reactions certainly receive reinforcement through the arcs of receptors in the muscles and through arcs arising in the receptors of the otic labyrinth. An instance of reinforcement of this very kind from muscular receptors we have already given (Lect. IV, p. 133).

Thus at any single phase of the creature's reaction, a simultaneous combination of reflexes is in existence. In this combination the positive element, namely, the final common paths (motor neurone groups) in active discharge, exhibits a harmonious discharge directed by the dominant reflex-arc, and reinforced by a number of arcs in alliance with it. The dominant reflex-arc in the instance taken is that from the noci-ceptors of the right hind-foot. The reinforcing arcs are at this phase of the reaction certain direct extension arcs, certain

Compound Reflexes

proprio-ceptive arcs, and certain labyrinthine arcs. But there is also a negative element in this simultaneous combination of reflexes. The reflex not only takes possession of certain final common paths and discharges nervous impulses down them, but it takes possession of the final common path whose muscles would oppose those into which it is discharging impulses, and checks their nervous discharge. This negative part of the field of influence of the reflex is more difficult to see, but it is as important as the positive, to which it is indeed complemental. Therefore it is that the reflex initiated by one group of receptors while in progress excludes in various directions the reflexes of other receptors, although these latter may be being stimulated. In this way the motor paths at any moment accord in a united pattern for harmonious synergy, co-operating for one effect.

The notion, therefore, that we arrive at of such a motor reflex reaction is that it is referable to a constellation of congruous stimuli of which one is prepotent, and that the reaction taken in its totality gives the nervous intercommunications of the central organ a certain pattern, which pattern may ramify through a great extent of the central organ. This reaction has its positive side traceable as active discharge from a number of end-points of the nervous network, and its negative side symmetrically opposed to its positive, and traceable conversely by check, depression, or absence of nervous discharge. Even in extensive reflexes of the bulbo-spinal animal it is probable that though great fields of the nervous centres are involved in the reaction at any one time, large parts are still left outside the reaction. This part of the neural network would therefore be indifferent to that particular reaction. That amounts to saying that it is open during the reaction to be thrown into activity by some concurrent and distinct other reaction. But this possible neutrality and discreteness of reflex reaction and its fields is probably far less in the intact higher vertebrate than in the lower or in the mutilated higher vertebrate.300 In the presence of the brain the knitting together of the whole nervous network is probably much greater than in its absence.

A question arises concerning the simultaneous combination of

Mode of Simultaneous Combination of Reflexes

reflexes which is closely related to that regarding the grading of intensity of a reflex.

Some reflexes exhibit many grades of intensity under grading of intensity of stimulus. The flexion-reflex is an instance. There as the skin stimulus is increased the height to which the foot is flexed is increased. But it seems obvious that such an effect is not to be expected in all reflexes. Where, as, for instance, in the scratch-reflex, the foot has, in response to irritation at a certain spot, to be moved to that spot, it would defeat the use of the reflex for a strong stimulus to flex the limb further, so as to carry it beyond the spot required. And we see that as the scratch-reflex is increased in intensity the increase does not appreciably increase the amount of tonic flexion exhibited by the reflex, but spends itself in increasing the clonic beat of the reflex, which still oscillates about the same median position. When the scratch-reflex is elicited by simultaneous combination of two reflexes initiated from spots near together in the receptive field the tonic flexion underlying either reflex does not in my experience appear to sum with that of the other; the summation that appears seems confined to the more vigorous clonic beating of the combined reflex.

It seems therefore likely that in the simultaneous combination of reflexes the reinforcement that goes on, although it is sometimes expressed as greater amplitude of contraction, is not necessarily so expressed in all cases. Just as various type-reflexes exhibit extreme individuality of time-relations, intensity grading, etc., so also they exhibit in their mode of simultaneous combination individual differences of high degree.

Lecture VI

COMPOUND REFLEXES:
SUCCESSIVE COMBINATION

ARGUMENT: Co-ordination of reflex sequences. Chain-reflexes (Loeb). Overlapping of successive stimuli in time. The sequence of allied reflexes. Spread of *bahnung*, 'immediate induction'. Sequence of antagonistic reflexes. The role of inhibition in this transition. Views of the nature of inhibition: Rosenthal, Wundt, E. Hering, Gaskell, Verworn, J. S. Macdonald. The 'interference' of reflexes. 'Alternating reflexes.' W. Macdougall's view of 'drainage of energy'. 'Compensatory reflexes.' Factors determining the issue of the competition between antagonistic reflexes. 'Successive induction.' Rebound-effects in spinal reactions; tend to restore reflex equilibrium. Fatigue in reflexes. Relative high resistance to fatigue possessed by the final common path, i.e. motor neurone. Intensity of reaction a decisive factor in the competition of afferent arcs for possession of the final common path. Noci-ceptive nerves. Prepotency of reflexes generated by receptors that considered as sense organs initiate sensations with strong affective tone. Resistance of tonic reflexes to fatigue. All these factors render the conductive pattern of the central nervous system mutable between certain limits.

WE considered last the co-ordination of reflexes in simultaneous combination. We now turn to sequence of reflexes. Reflexes are seen to follow one another in consecutive combination. And in this chaining together of successive reflexes in different instances different kinds of processes seem traceable. Of these, one consists in the reaction to one external stimulus bringing about an application of an external stimulus for a second reflex. The dart-reflex of the frog's tongue provoked by the seen fly provides, if successful, the stimulus (contact with the mucosa of the mouth) which provokes closure of the mouth, and this probably insures the stimulus for the ensuing deglutition, and so on. Exner has dealt with this kind of chaining together of reflexes by one stimulus leading to another in his *Entwurf einer physiologischen Erklärung psychischer Erscheinungen*. Loeb has illustrated it luminously in his *Physiology of the Brain*. He calls sequence of reflexes proceeding by this process from one segmental reflex to another 'chain-reflexes' (*Ketten-reflexe*). Mosso,[66]

Reflex Sequence

Kronecker and Meltzer,[89,90,101] Chauveau,[218] and Zwaardemaker,[235,272] have traced such reflexes analytically in deglutition.

Mosso[66] showed that in the oesophageal stage of deglutition each reflex in a part of the tube above is immediately succeeded by a reflex ensuing in the adjoining part below, and yet in this sequence the distant bulbar centre is itself concerned, since the sequence ceases if the branches of the vagus containing the nerve paths to and from that centre be severed. Biedermann has recently demonstrated a very similar procession of reflexes in the crawling of the earthworm, and there again the sequence involves reflexes conducted through the central nervous system. It appears that the action of each preceding segment provides a stimulus for the reflex act of the next succeeding segment.

Orderly sequence of movement characterizes the outward behaviour of animals. Not least so where, as in the earthworm crawling,[273] or the insect in flight, or the fish swimming, every observer admits the coadjustment is essentially reflex. One act succeeds another without confusion. Yet, tracing this sequence to its external causes, we recognize that the usual thing in nature is not for one exciting stimulus to begin immediately after another ceases, but for an array of environmental agents acting concurrently on the animal at any moment to exhibit correlative change in regard to it, so that one or other group of them becomes—generally by increase in intensity—temporarily prepotent. Thus there dominates now this group, now that group, in turn. It may happen that one stimulus ceases coincidently as another begins, but as a rule the stimuli overlap one another in regard to time. Thus each reflex in the unmutilated animal breaks in upon a condition of relative equilibrium; and this latter is itself reflex.

It was shown that reflex movements can be grouped as regards their mutual relation into those which have allied relation and mutually facilitate and reinforce, and those which are mutually antagonistic. Antagonistic reflexes do not enter into simultaneous combination. Simultaneous combination unites 'allied' reflexes only. But into reflex combinations of *successive* kind, reflexes both allied and antagonistic enter as components.

Reflex Sequence

If the scratch-reflex be excited from a spot in its receptive skin-field and then, while the reflex is in progress, another scratch-reflex is excited from a receptive point not far removed from the first one, the scratch-reflex under the double excitation may differ very little in appearance from that first excited, and on the first stimulation being discontinued the reflex persists, maintained by the second stimulation, and hardly or not perceptibly altered in character from its outset. In this case the second reflex which succeeded the first resembles the first; that is, it is to outward appearance and for practical purposes merely a prolongation of it.

But if the point of application of the second stimulus be, although still in the receptive field of the scratch-reflex, widely distant from that of the first stimulus, the reflex becomes obviously modified when the second stimulus is thrown in. Thus, if the stimulus be so located in the receptive field that the first excites the low form of the reflex and the second the high form, the reflex, though initiated in the low form, assumes the high form when the second stimulus—if that is of appropriate strength—is thrown in. Or, conversely, it assumes the low form if the second stimulus be appropriately located for producing that form.

And between the component scratch-reflexes there are grades of likeness corresponding with degrees of proximity of the points of application of the stimuli in the receptive field. When, therefore, a reflex occurs in immediate sequence to a reflex to which it is allied, it smoothly maintains the reaction that is already in progress, and if its own character differs in some respect from the foregoing reflex, impresses that character on the reflex without, however, any hitch or hindrance of the reflex.

For a reflex to be immediately succeeded by a reflex of allied relation to it is of common occurrence. Any stimulus that moves over a receptive field is likely to excite such a sequence—a morsel of food moving over the surface of the tongue, a stimulus moving in the field of vision, an object moving along the skin, and, as an instance of the last, a parasite travelling across the receptive field of the scratch-reflex.252

In such successive combinations the reflexes are, in the scratch-

Sequence of Allied Reflexes

reflex at least, linked together by more than the mere external circumstance of the incidence of the stimulus. In such a sequence the *threshold of each succeeding reflex is lowered by the excitation just preceding its own.*

A subliminal stimulus applied at a point A will render a subliminal stimulus applied at a point B near A supraliminal if the second stimulus follow within a short time, e.g. 500 σ. The space of receptive surface across which this can be demonstrated in the scratch-reflex amounts to 5–6 cm. It is best worked out by unipolar application of the induced current through a stigmatic electrode—a fine gilt entomological pin. In that way numerical values can be assigned to the results. But the phenomenon is characteristically and simply illustrated[287] by the difference between the potency as a stimulus of the edge of a card, say 6 in. long, pressed simultaneously over its whole length against the receptive skin-field, say for 5 sec., and on the other hand lightly drawing one corner of the card along the same line in the skin-field also for 5 sec. The former application simply evokes a reflex of a few beats, which then dies out. The latter evokes a vigorous reflex that continues and outlasts the application of the stimulus. A successive line is more effective as a stimulus than a simultaneous line of equal length and duration. Again, if a light disk 3 cm. in diameter and a fraction of a millimetre thick be freely pivoted in bearings at the end of a handle, so that it turns when pushed by its handle over the skin surface, such a wheel may not, when pushed against a spot of the receptive surface, excite the reflex, but it excites it when it is rolled along it. The same thing is seen with a spur wheel. Even when the points are 2 cm. apart, as the spur wheel is rolled over the surface successive summation occurs, and the reflex is evoked as the progress of the wheel proceeds. If a parasite in its travel produces excitation which is but close below the threshold, its progress is likely to so develop the excitability of the surface whither it passes that the scalptor-reflex will be evoked. In the skin and the parasite respectively we have, no doubt, two competing adaptations at work. It is perhaps to avoid the consequences of the spatial spread of the 'bahnung' that the hop of the flea has been developed.

Reflex Sequence

This *bahnung*, which spreads around a stimulated point, must be the same phenomenon which finds still more marked expression in the summation of stimuli individually subliminal applied successively at one and the same point. That it influences other points in the neighbourhood as well as its own seat of application, is another item of evidence of the central conjunction of the neighbouring reflex-arcs of any one type-reflex. It is an influence which, with barely supraliminal stimuli, is short-lived; but it is one of the factors in the card-experiment just mentioned. This spread of influence to adjacent points is important because, though short-lived, it can contribute effectively to maintain one and the same reflex. It favours the occurrence of sequences of closely allied reflexes. It is convenient to have a term for such a species of *bahnung*, and *immediate induction* seems the most suitable here.

Phenomena akin to these are met with in the physiology of vision. A moving point in the peripheral field is more visible than a line of similar length, direction, and duration. Again, a row of dots individually below the *minimum visibile* and too far apart for their retinal images to overlap by diffusion, becomes visible. Probably this same process is contributory toward the seeing of lines the diameter of which is narrower than the diameter of the circular *minimum visibile*. I have found osmic-stained nerve-fibres of 4μ diam. visible to the naked eye both for myself and other workers in the laboratory. Reinforcement by positive induction appears to be at work in these visual effects just as in the scratch-reflex.

In the sequence of reflexes the supervening reflex may differ imperceptibly or slightly, though distinctly, from the precedent, or may be in part quite different from that.

If the reflexes are closely similar, it is difficult to say at what moment the transition under overlapping stimuli occurs, since the initial reflex on discontinuance of the first stimulation is maintained unaltered by the second. But if the reflexes are recognizably dissimilar, e.g. a low scratch-reflex and a high scratch-reflex, the moment of transition is obvious, for the reflex then takes the form of the response which the second stimulation would excite, and, on discontinuing the first stimulation, is continued in that form (Fig. 50).

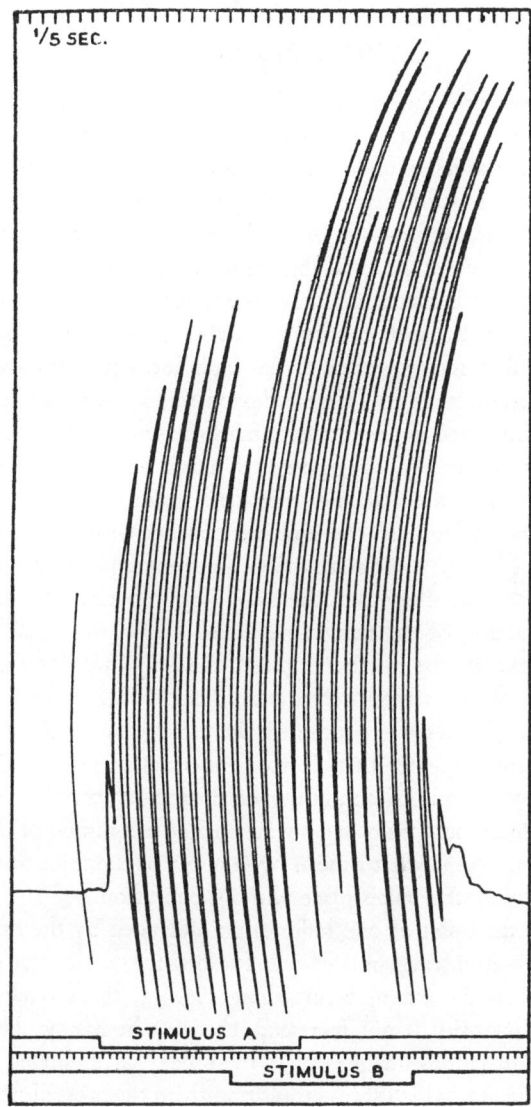

Fig. 50. Scratch-reflex

Records from above downwards:
  Time in ⅕ sec.
  Myograph curve of the scratch-reflex initiated from one receptive spot A in the form of a 'low' reflex and then concurrently from a receptive spot B, lying more dorsal than A, in the form of a 'high' reflex, the tonic flexion at hip supporting the clonic being greater.
  Signal line A: descent of line marks period of excitation of spot A.
  Rhythm of induction shocks delivered as stimuli.
  Signal line B: descent of line marks period of excitation of spot B.

Reflex Sequence

In my experience the transition does not, in the case of this reflex at least, include a period of summation of the two reflexes in the sense that the reflex under the two stimulations A and B consists of the response to stimulation A summed with that to stimulation B. So also in the transition from one reflex to another of even greater dissimilarity. There is the same absence of any period of fusion of the two reflexes. Such fusion might be appropriately termed confusion. The rule seems that such confusion is avoided in the transition. In the hind-limb a scratch-reflex of the high form presents a certain degree of resemblance to a simple flexion-reflex, inasmuch as there can be distinguished in the former a marked tonic flexion on which the clonic is, so to say, superposed. When a scratch-reflex of this form supervenes on the flexion-reflex the result is commonly that which is seen in Fig. 51. The transition occurs without confusion; even in regard to the tonic contraction, an element possibly common to the two reflexes, there is in the transition no period at which the tonic contraction of the flexion-reflex has added to it that of the scratch-reflex. In the instance figured, the amplitude of the tonic contraction of the scratch-reflex was about equal to that of the flexion-reflex; if these were summed, therefore, their joint amplitude would be much greater than that of either reflex singly. But the record shows a smooth continuity of flexion-reflex with scratch-reflex in which there is no stage of summated amplitude of the two contractions. This is what I mean by saying that the transition from one reflex to another takes place without confusion.

Not that the onset of one reflex is uninfluenced by the existence of the other—its interval of latency is, for instance, liable to be greatly influenced. In the example furnishing Fig. 51, the scratch-reflex, though its intensity is not increased, shows a hesitancy about the opening of its clonus not present in the reflex when elicited singly. Again, in Fig. 52, which shows transition from the crossed stepping-reflex to the scratch-reflex, though no period of confusion occurs in the transition from the former reflex to the latter, there is yet, on cessation of the latter, evidence of modification of the former. The crossed stepping-reflex returns, but considerably modified and after a longer latency than before. The amount of modification is greater

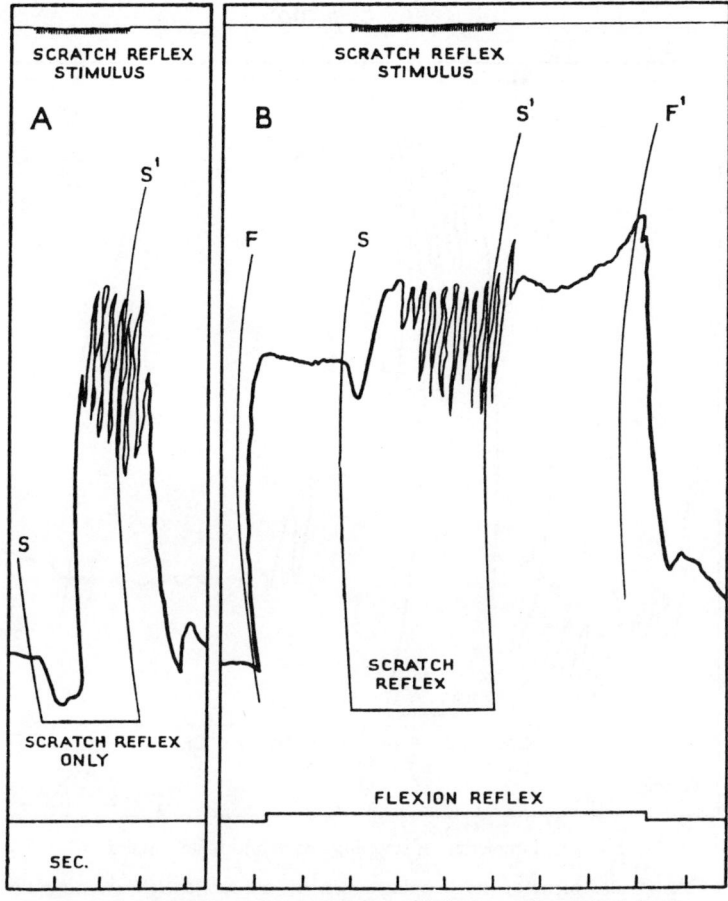

Fig. 51. Interaction of scratch-reflex and flexion-reflex (spinal dog)

Effect of overlapping in time of the stimuli for the flexion-reflex and the scratch-reflex.

Records from above downwards are:
  Signal line: stimulus for scratch-reflex (A and B).
  Myograph curve: in A the vertical arcs indicate onset (S) and cessation (S^1) of scratch-reflex stimulus only. In B, S and S^1 as in A; F and F^1 represent onset and cessation of stimulus for flexion-reflex.
  Signal line: in B, ascent of lever marks stimulus for flexion-reflex.
  Time in sec.

The scratch-reflex seems to displace the flexion-reflex; had it fused with it, the combined lift of the lever would have been much higher than it is. Compare the scratch-reflex in A and B.

Reflex Sequence

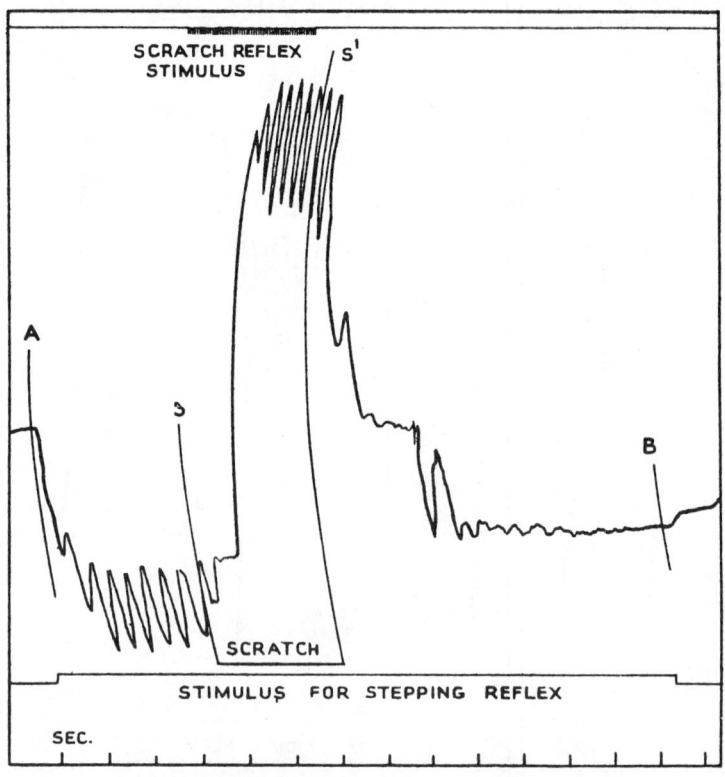

Fig. 52. Interaction of stepping-reflex and scratch-reflex

The displacement of the stepping-reflex by the scratch-reflex during the continuance of the stimulation appropriate for the former.

Records from above downwards:

    Signal line: stimulus for the scratch-reflex, namely, 75 break shocks delivered (unipolar faradization) at a rate of 30 per sec.

    Myograph curve: A, B, onset and cessation of stimulus for stepping reflex; S, S^I, onset and cessation of stimulus for scratch-reflex.

    Signal line: ascent marks onset of stimulus for the stepping-reflex, a crossed reflex, the stimulus (unipolar faradization) being delivered to the opposite foot.

    Time in sec.

The scratch-reflex, after a considerable latency, displaces the stepping-reflex. The crossed stepping-reflex reappears only in modified and imperfect form, though its stimulus is continued unaltered for some 7 sec. after the end of the stimulus for the scratch-reflex.

Transition from Reflex to Reflex

than would in my experience be ascribable with probability to the effect of mere fatigue for the period during which the stimulus was at work, although the movement itself was in abeyance; the rhythm is present but weakened.

If it is advantageous for the transition from one reflex to another of like type to occur without a period of confusion, it is still more advantageous that it should be so in the case of transitions from one reflex to another of converse type. Confusion in the literal sense above would in that case involve not merely inaccuracy at the outset of each new reflex, but would mean mutual destruction of the two reflex effects; an interval of impotent mutual self-hindrance would disadvantageously intervene between successive motor acts of opposite direction. In the transition from one reflex to another of antagonistic kind the avoidance of confusion of the two reflexes emphasizes at the same time the impossibility of co-ordinating them in a simultaneous combination.

Though the stimulus exciting the reflex that is displaced continues while the new reflex is introduced, the displacement of the former reflex occurs without confusion.

Taking the flexion-reflex and the scratch-reflex, the one may temporarily interrupt the other in mid career (Figs. 43, 53) or may cut it short or may defer its onset; in all these cases it does so without a phase of confusion in the transition, although the stimuli belonging to both reflexes continue in contemporary operation (Figs. 43, 51, 52, etc.) all the time. And the same holds between other antagonistic reflexes, e.g. flexion-reflex and crossed extension-reflex (Figs. 30, 32, 33), extension-reflex and scratch-reflex (Figs. 42, 54), etc.

And the direction of the interference is reversible. The flexion-reflex may be made to interrupt the scratch-reflex (Fig. 43) or the scratch-reflex to interrupt the flexion-reflex (Fig. 51). The scratch-reflex may be made to interrupt the crossed stepping-reflex (Fig. 52) or the crossed stepping-reflex to interrupt the scratch-reflex (Fig. 55); and similarly with other pairs of antagonistic reflexes.

Reflex Sequence

INHIBITION

The process in virtue of which this transition from one antagonistic reflex to another occurs is obviously one of active intervention. In many cases the form which the intervention takes is inhibition. For instance, where a crossed extension-reflex is interrupted by a brief

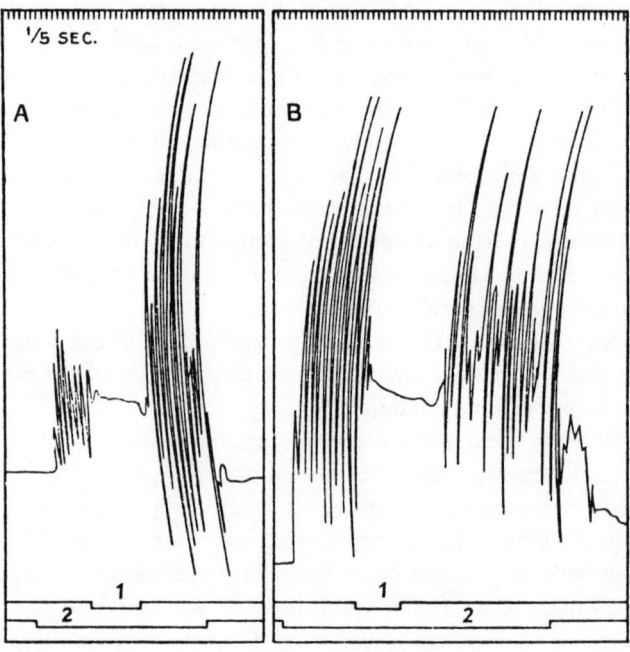

Fig. 53

A. Scratch-reflex interrupted by a brief flexion-reflex.
Records from above downwards:
    Time in ⅕ sec.
    Myograph curve.
    Signal 1: descent of signal indicates time of application of stimulus for flexion-reflex.
    Signal 2: descent of signal indicates time of application of stimulus evoking scratch-reflex.
The scratch-reflex returns with increased intensity after the interruption.
B. Similar to A, but the scratch-reflex is interrupted later and returns more slowly and with marked irregularity in its beat.

Reflex Inhibition

flexion-reflex, two transitions occur, the first at a moment α from the E-reflex to the F-reflex, the second at a moment β from the F-reflex back to the E-reflex (Fig. 33, p. 102). Although stimuli for the two reflexes are both in operation continuously from α to β, there is a clean transition from one reflex to the other. The tracing is taken from the extensor muscle of the knee. The flexion-reflex expresses itself by inhibition of the reflex contraction in progress in that muscle at that time under the combined influence of the crossed extension-reflex and of the tonic extensor rigidity due to the animal being decerebrate. It causes the contraction due to these conjoined reflexes to cease. In such a case the transition from the extension-reflex to the flexion-reflex evidently occurs by inhibition. So also in the transition from the flexion-reflex to the extension-reflex when the hamstring muscles are examined (Fig. 32, p. 99).

We do not yet understand the intimate nature of inhibition. In the cases before us now, its seat is certainly central, and in all probability is, as argued above, situated at points of synapsis. I have urged that a prominent physiological feature of the synapse is a synaptic membrane. It seems therefore to me that inhibition in such cases as those before us is probably

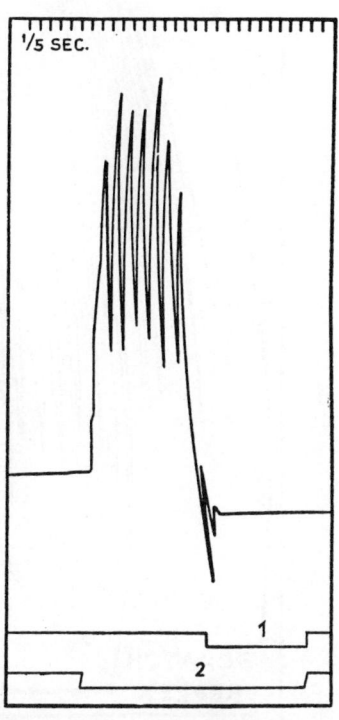

Fig. 54. The scratch-reflex cut short by excitation of the skin of a digit of the opposite hind-foot

Records from above downwards:
Time in $\frac{1}{5}$ sec.
Myograph curve: Scratch reflex.
Signal 1: descent of signal marks the period of application of the stimulus to the opposite hind-foot.
Signal 2: descent of signal marks the period of application of the stimulus exciting the scratch-reflex.

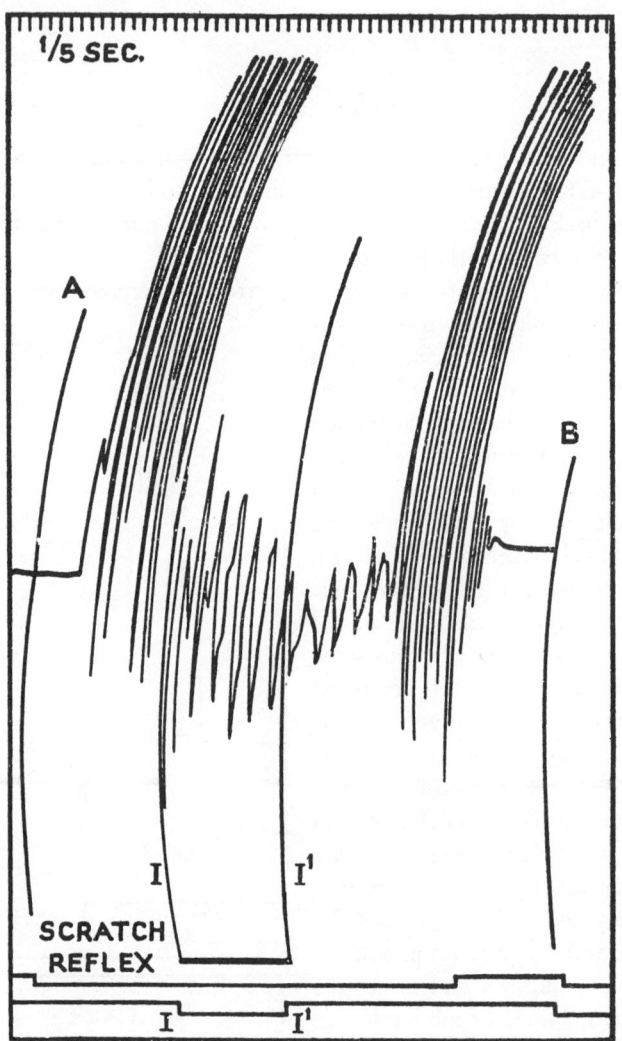

Fig. 55. The scratch-reflex interrupted by the crossed stepping-reflex

Records from above downwards:
    Time in $\frac{1}{5}$ sec.
    Myograph curve: The vertical arc A marks the onset of the stimulus for the scratch reflex; the vertical arcs I, I^1 mark respectively the onset and cessation of the contralateral stimulus evoking the crossed stepping reflex.
    Upper Signal: descent of signal represents onset of stimulus for the scratch-reflex (unipolar faradization of shoulder skin).
    Lower Signal: between I and I^1 a fairly strong stimulation of the crossed foot was applied.
The inhibition outlasts the application of the second stimulus by some 3 sec.; the scratch-reflex then returns, and only ceases on cessation of its own stimulus.

Nature of Inhibition

referable to a change in the condition of the synaptic membrane causing a block in conduction. But what the intimate nature of the inhibitory change may be we do not know.

The views of some of those who have authoritatively treated of the nature of inhibition may be cited here, both for their intrinsic interest and the suggestion of lines of investigation. One view has been that, as the process of conduction along nerve-fibres is an undulatory one in the sense that the nerve-impulse travels as a disturbance with wave-like configuration of intensity, inhibition is due to a mutual suppression of two wave-like disturbances impinging on the same point of the conductor but in opposite phases of disturbance.

In those cases where stimulation through one nerve inhibits the action of a tissue acted on by another nerve we can imagine a process which leaves the tissue unaffected but simply interferes with another stimulus, as in the physical interference of vibrations. Rosenthal's[30] resistance theory of the action of the afferent vagus-fibres upon the respiratory centre is a supposition of this kind. It recognizes during the inhibition no change of total output of energy in the particular function inhibited. The alteration of a hypothetical resistance only distributes the discharge of the nerve-centre over an altered time-rhythm—smaller and more frequent discharges representing the same liberation of energy as larger and less frequent. Such a view of the nature of inhibition is that which Gaskell[103] termed the *neutral* one; according to it the inhibition leaves the tissue in the same ultimate condition as that in which it found it, neither exhausted nor surcharged. "As far as the central nervous system is concerned, there exists a strong general tendency to look upon the inhibitory processes occurring there as *neutral* in their character."[103]

This view, originally put forward by v. Cyon,[39] has been abandoned by him, although it has since been supported by Lauder Brunton[107a] and others. It was expressly dissented from by Wundt.[83] And the grounds of Wundt's objection are valid, the kernel of them being that though in a certain sense of the word the nerve-impulse can be described as wave-like it is not an undulatory disturbance at all in the sense in which those reactions are which show

Reflex Sequence

physical interference. It is therefore to physical interference that in this view of inhibition the analogy is drawn, but the similarity between the process of nerve-conduction and conduction of light and electrical waves or sound, etc., is not real enough to strictly justify such analogy. Moreover, as we shall see presently, central inhibition is not a *neutral* process, for, at least in many cases, it leaves the reflex centre surcharged for subsequent response (vide infra, pp. 207-214, 'successive induction').

The most striking thing that we know of inhibition is that it is a phenomenon in which an agent such as in other cases excites or increases an action going on, in this case stops or diminishes an action going on. Now, the activity of a tissue can be lowered or abolished by production in it of deleterious changes such as exhaustion or, in the highest degree, death. But there is no evidence that inhibition of a tissue is ever accompanied by the slightest damage to the tissue; on the contrary, it seems to predispose the tissue to a greater functional activity thereafter.

We can imagine that a material continuously produced by a tissue, and yielding on decomposition the particular activity which is inhibited, may by an inhibition be checked in its decomposition, and accumulate, so that at the end of the period of inhibition the tissue contains more of the particular decomposable material than before. This molecular rearrangement would diminish activity for the time being, but lead to increase of activity afterwards. There would ensue a rebound effect. This is, as is well known since Gaskell's [99a] researches, what actually happens in the pure vagus action on the heart. A similar rebound-effect is perfectly obvious in many instances of inhibition in the central nervous system.[304] It constitutes a point of resemblance between central and peripheral inhibition.

Such an explanation as this second one may take the chemical structure of the living material, the *bioplasm*, of the cell as the field of operation for the decomposition and the synthetic process that it pictures. The living cell is constantly liberating energy in its function, and rebuilding its complex structure from nutrient material. Its life is therefore an equilibrium of balanced katabolism and anabolism; at any given moment the one process or the other may

Nature of Inhibition

predominate in the cell. At a moment when the cell is vigorously discharging some function which involves conversion of internal energy into external energy it is in a katabolic phase. In subsequent relative repose from the discharge of that function the replenishment of its store of potential energy by assimilation may predominate and the cell be in an anabolic phase. Katabolism and activity of external function, anabolism and rest from external function, come on this view to be almost synonymous terms. But Hering, Gaskell, Verworn, and others have taught us to attach important external functions to the assimilatory (anabolic) phase. The first mentioned has dealt with the visual sensations in assimilation-dissimilation pairs. Black-white sensation is thus traced to a pair of reactions affecting the trophism of the cell in exactly opposite directions. Gaskell relates vagus inhibition of the heart to the throwing of the cardiac muscle-cell into a phase predominantly anabolic. Verworn in his 'Biogen-hypothese' has developed this trophic theory with further elaboration still. These views all take the actual nutritive activity of the cell as the direct and immediate field in which inhibition has its seat. The tendency to rebound or after-effect in the opposite direction, is in this view a natural trophic result. Hence Gaskell expressively speaks of the vagus as the 'trophic nerve of the heart'. And Hering (1872)48a, 113 formulated his experience somewhat as follows: The action of a stimulus affects the cell's autonomic trophic equilibrium; it may increase or lessen either the cell's assimilation or the cell's dissimilation; in whichever of these ways the stimulus acts the excitation of the cell, owing to a self-regulation proper to it, dwindles for that stimulus and for all stimuli producing a similar change, while the excitability increases for stimuli that produce an opposite effect. On all these views inhibition is in its intimate and essential nature a trophic process.

An hypothesis not built immediately on views of the nutritive processes of the cell has recently been put forward by Macdonald.306 Dealing with nerve and muscle fibres, he does not take the purely chemical structure of the living framework of the cell as the field of operation for either excitation or inhibition. The explanation he offers of these two latter processes is as follows.

Reflex Sequence

From study of the part played by inorganic salts in the function of nerve, he sees in the attachment of these salts to the proteins present, and in their partial detachment from the proteins, normal occurrences underlying the conditions of rest and excitation respectively. He assumes the connexion between salt and protein involved in this matter to be of purely physical nature. The axis-cylinder, for example, is composed of a colloid solution in which there are present minute particles of colloid protein. These may increase in size—indeed, so much as finally to become visible—under the influence of factors determining a tendency towards coagulation. Upon the surface of these particles the major portion of the inorganic salts present is held restrained in a condition of condensed solution. An increase in the size of the particles is accompanied by a diminution in the total surface separating the particles from the solvent in which they lie. Such a diminution in surface is equivalent to a diminution in the forces restraining the motion of the inorganic salts. It occasions the liberation of salt molecules in a state of free motion into the surrounding aqueous solution. This release of hitherto restrained molecules is the cause of alterations in osmotic pressure, of new processes of diffusion, of resultant electrical phenomena, and thus of the phenomena of excitation.

Macdonald thus considers a stimulus as an agency determining an approach to the condition of coagulation. He regards as the important characteristic of the excited state the release of inorganic salts resulting from this change. According to him inhibition is a condition in which the inorganic salts are more securely packed away upon the surface of the 'colloid particles' than usual by reason of diminution in the individual size of the particles and an increase in the surface they present to the surrounding solution. He supposes the communication of a negative electrical charge to be a stimulus provoking a tendency to coagulation with all the just-mentioned dynamic consequences of the enlargement of the colloid particles. So he considers that conversely the communication of a positive charge produces a change of an exactly opposite kind in which inorganic salts hitherto in motion are brought to a static condition of rest.

It does not seem at once clear that the condition of greater sub-

Nature of Inhibition

division of particles should also be a condition of greater stability, although it is clear that such a conception might explain the greater store of potential energy possessed by an inhibited tissue. Macdonald, in fact, does not, I take it, assume this to be the case. To explain this separate fact he appeals to the evidence upon which the conception is based and points out a distinction between the amount of inorganic salt involved in changes above (inhibition) and changes below (excitation) the equilibrium line of the normal resting state. Thus there is quantitative evidence to show that the amount of salt remaining for withdrawal from the resting colloid solution is only a small fraction of the total amount of salt present; the major portion is already withdrawn, and is, so to speak, in reserve in this large quantity for such changes of excitation as occur below the base line of rest. Changes from the normal to the hypernormal, and from the hypernormal to the normal, cannot therefore involve a redistribution of salt comparable in quantity to those taking place down from, and up to, the normal. It is in this way conceivable that the application of a stimulus to an inhibited tissue—although productive of an effect akin to the phenomenon underlying the process of excitation—might yet lead only to such a subminimal change in the amount of inorganic salt in motion as to determine no externally appreciable manifestation of its occurrence. Imagine a tissue which has been placed in a condition of inhibition by the communication of a positive electrical charge. The application of a negative charge to such a tissue would produce no visible effect, although productive of an internal change. The application of a second negative charge would give rise to a characteristic excitation, its efficiency determined by 'summation'. Let us on the other hand suppose that the tissue has not only been inhibited, but is maintained in a continuous state of inhibition by the steady arrival of positive charges. In this case the application of a succession of stimuli would result in nothing more than a series of subminimal, and therefore unnoticed, changes.

In an excited tissue, summarizing this conception, an unusual quantity of inorganic salts is in motion. Excitation is ended by the reduction of this excessive motion. Inhibition is the condition in which the possibilities of free motion are most reduced.

Reflex Sequence

This view is fertile in suggestion for further experiment. Based on examination of the physical structure of nerve by electrical methods irreproachably employed, and on the revelation, under the microchemical test which we owe to Macallum,[307] of potassium appearing in quantity at injured points of nerve-fibres, and explaining naturally as it does the injury-current of nerve as similar in production to the current of a 'concentration' battery[234] the concentrations of which can be known from the current, it merits very careful consideration. The features and conditions of occurrence of inhibition harmonize strikingly with what on Macdonald's view we should expect them to be.

INTERFERENCE

Whatever the intimate nature of the inhibition, it is, however, only one part of the processes involved in transition from one antagonistic reflex to another. In the transition from the crossed extension-reflex to the flexion-reflex the inhibition of previous excitation in the extensor neurone is accompanied by excitation of the previously inhibited flexor neurone. And conversely in the transition from flexion-reflex to extension-reflex. Transition from one form of reciprocal innervation to another will obviously involve such changes wherever the transition is from one reflex of simultaneous double-sign to an antagonistic of simultaneous double-sign. There will be inhibition at one set of points and excitation at another. The process of transition, therefore, in many cases is one half of it inhibitory, one half excitatory. It seems advisable, therefore, to avoid employing the term 'inhibition' for the displacement in general of one reflex by another. To avoid confusion, some expression of broader scope, including excitation as well as inhibition proper, seems required. The term 'interference' already used by Wundt[83] and by A. Tschermak[186] in an almost similar way seems to me well suited for this purpose. In employing it Wundt expressly stipulated that it had in this use no reference to its technical employment by physicists for the mutual interaction of vibrations, as in light and sound. The term 'interference' as applied to reflexes would mean simply the interaction between antagonistic reflexes, that is,

Interference of Reflexes

reflexes which are incapable of simultaneous combination. These reflexes are capable of successive combination, and in that process the influence of one reflex replaces that of another upon a common path potentially belonging to each. The replacement may take place by inhibition succeeding excitation, or by excitation succeeding inhibition, or by excitation of one kind succeeding excitation of another kind, as when the steady tonic flexion of the flexion-reflex is succeeded by the rhythmic clonic flexion of the scratch-reflex. In all these cases the process of displacement of one reflex action by the other may be termed interference. We thus get a comprehensive convenient term for embracing the whole series of cases.

The frequency with which, in co-ordination of reflexes by successive combination, the reflex which succeeds to another is antagonistic to this latter is very great. Two important classes of such sequence are especially common. One is that which forms what are known as 'alternating reflexes'; the other is the class of 'compensatory reflexes'.

Alternating reflexes are seen very clearly in cyclic reversals of direction of movement; thus, when extension succeeds flexion in the stepping-reflex. Here antagonistic reflexes succeed one another alternately at two final common paths. In the motor neurones for the knee, in the stepping-reflex, excitation and inhibition alternately ensue in the flexor neurones, while synchronously with that, inhibition and excitation alternately ensue in the extensor neurones.

The essence of an alternating reflex is that excitation and inhibition ensue in succession at two (or more) final common paths, a sequence of antagonistic reflexes possessing them in turn. In an ordinary rhythmic reflex a periodic excitation (and a periodic refractory or inhibitory state) is recurrently produced in the reflex-arc at rhythmic intervals. Every alternating reflex, therefore, is a rhythmic reflex, but not every rhythmic reflex is an alternating reflex. The movements of the vertebrate limb in locomotion give instances of alternating reflexes; probably the movement of the tail of fishes in swimming is a similar instance, but has not yet been analysed as to its reflex composition. Alternating reflexes form an excellent field for examination of reciprocal innervation of antagonistic muscles.

Reflex Sequence

It is particularly by the case of 'alternating reflexes' that MacDougall illustrates his view of the central process in reciprocal innervation. His scheme also offers an explanation for the transition from one antagonistic reflex to another. Based more immediately on the behaviour of visual images, it is applied by MacDougall specifically to the case of the reciprocal innervation of antagonistic muscles. "Let us", he writes,262 "imagine each arc in a simple schematic form as a chain of three neurones afferent (a_1), central (a_2), efferent (a_3), and let us call them a_1, a_2, and a_3, and b_1, b_2, and b_3, in the two arcs respectively (Fig. 56). ...When a strong stimulus is applied to

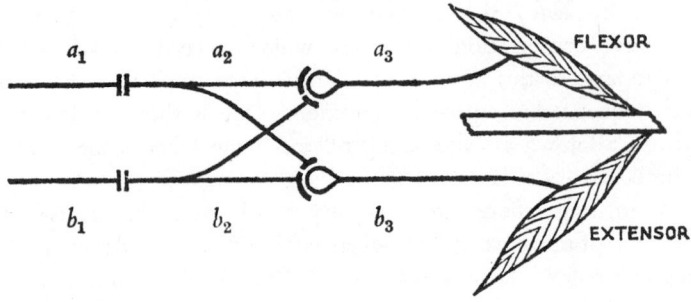

Fig. 56. Explanation in text

the afferent neurone of arc a it generates neurin rapidly, so that it becomes very rapidly charged, and the resistance of synapse a_1—a_2 is lowered until a series of discharges takes place from a_1 to a_2, and again from a_2 to a_3. The problem is, then, to imagine such a mode of connexion between arc a and arc b as will cause arc a during stimulation to drain off from the afferent and central neurones of b the smaller quantities of neurin generated in them. Several forms of such a connexion may be imagined, but I think that probably it takes the form of a collateral fibre coming from neurone b_2, and taking part with the axone of a_2 in forming a synapse with a_3.... Whatever the exact constitution of this synapse may be, we may assume that, when its resistance is lowered by the stimulation of a, and consequent charging of a_2, the collateral of b_2, making connexion with a_3, through this synapse, becomes the path of least resistance for

Alternating Reflexes

the escape of neurin from b_1 and b_2. These neurones are therefore drained by a_3, while b_3 ceases to receive any neurin from b_2, and the tone of the muscle-group supplied by it is abolished. ...In a similar way, if both a_1 and b_1 be stimulated, but one more strongly than the other, the more strongly stimulated arc will drain the afferent and central neurones of the less strongly stimulated arc, because the resistance of synapses of the former will be reduced to a lower level than that of the synapses of the latter."

This scheme fits a number of facts of reciprocal inhibition. Thus, in reciprocal innervation, as the term itself implies, the inhibition at one part always appears as the negative aspect of positive excitation at another. To 'alternating' reflexes, which are common as spinal reactions, MacDougall applies the scheme thus: "We must suppose the collateral connexion of the arc a (to which we may suppose the stimulus to be applied) with the neurone b_3 to be but little inferior in conducting capacity to its direct connexion with a_3. When, then, the neurone a is stimulated continuously, the arc will first discharge into a_3 and drain b_1 and b_2 (i.e. inhibit b_3) until after some little time fatigue causes the resistance of synapse a_2—a_3 to become slightly greater than that of synapse b_2—b_3, when a_2 will discharge with b_2 wholly into b_3, and a_3 will be in turn 'inhibited'. So the charges of the afferent neurones of both arcs will be discharged into b_3 until fatigue causes rise of resistance of the synapse on b_3." The high influence of intensity of reaction in determining whether the reaction shall or shall not replace another reaction is expressed by this scheme very lucidly. Also the occurrence under strychnine[304] and tetanus toxin of excitation at a synapse where inhibition is otherwise the rule seems a contingency which the view answers well. If these agents (strychnine presumably from the afferent side, tetanus toxin from the efferent) reduce the resistance at synapse a_2—b_3, there will, on stimulation of a_1, be conversion of the inhibition of b_3 in excitation, just as in the second phase of an alternating reflex, but the resistance at synapse a_2—a_3 not being raised, as it is in the second phase of the alternating reflex, a_3 will also be excited as usual, and both antagonistic muscles will contract, as I have shown they do in fact in strychnine reflexes and as they do in the convulsions of strychnine poisoning. The scheme

Reflex Sequence

makes it clear, too, that this double discharge, or leakage, will prove rapidly exhausting on the central arcs, and indeed the phasic character of the attacks in strychnine poisoning does seem due to rapid exhaustion following each convulsive discharge.

Again, in working with tetanus toxin, I have,304 in the gradual progress of the disease, several times found the afferent nerves produce a slight reflex inhibition of the extensor of the knee, if the initial posture at the knee were at the time extension (i.e. the extensor arc in high activity), and yet produce distinct excitation of the extensor if the initial posture at the time were flexion (i.e. the extensor arc in less activity). These effects of strychnine and tetanus toxin the view of MacDougall seems well fitted to meet, though they were not known at the time the view was formulated. The view seems also applicable to some of the results obtained in the interesting experiments by v. Uexküll on Invertebrata.

One difficulty, however, seems to me presented by MacDougall's view, and it is that the diversion of the influence of a_1 through a_2 away from a_3 which constitutes inhibition does not suggest a reason for the superactivity (successive induction) in a consequent on the inhibition. And a more serious difficulty, attaches, in my thinking, to the view—at least, as it at present stands—in that it seems to sever this central nervous inhibition—of which I regard reciprocal innervation of antagonistic muscles as but one widely spread case—from other forms of inhibition met peripherally in the heart, blood-vessels, and viscera, rather than to connect it with them. It appears to me unlikely that in their essential nature all forms of inhibition can be anything but one and the same process.

Another important class of sequence of antagonistic reflexes is that which gives the 'compensatory reflex'. A compensatory reflex occurs where the reflex is a return to a state of reflex equilibrium which had been disturbed by an intercurrent reflex to which the compensatory reflex is the diametrical antagonist. Some compensatory reflexes are excited by passive movements, others by active movements. It is the latter which come under consideration here. Many reflex movements are intercurrent reactions, breaking in

Compensatory Reflexes

on a condition of neural equilibrium itself reflex. Take the case of the flexion-reflex of the leg (spinal dog) induced by a brief stimulus during 'decerebrate rigidity', where the animal may be regarded as a bulbo-spinal machine. Suppose the animal suspended with spine horizontal and limbs pendent. The limbs are then in slight active extension, much as if the animal were standing. This slight extension is active, for it is reflex, and the peripheral source of the maintained reflex pose is traceable to arcs arising in the extensor muscles, in alliance probably with some from the otic labyrinth. The creature breathes quietly and regularly. Its skeletal musculature otherwise exhibits no movements, although its reflex activity is considerable and in progress all the time, as shown by the steady reflex extension of the limbs. If, then, the foot be excited by a brief stimulus and thus a flexion-reflex induced in the limb, the limb is drawn up at hip, knee, and ankle. The movement is brief; after being drawn up, the limb returns to its previous pendent posture. It is easy in many instances to perceive that the pose of extension, as resumed, is more marked than it was prior to the intercurrent reflex or flexion. It is also equally easy to perceive that in the replacement of the limb the extension is not a mere passive drop under gravity, but is a reversion to the previous posture by an active movement. In such a case the reflex effect of the intercurrent stimulus seems to cease with the cessation of the intercurrent reflex (flexion) which the stimulus immediately provoked. But closer examination shows that this is not really the case. There is an *active* reflex return to the pre-existing pose. Thus, the disturbing stimulus brought about not only the flexion-reflex, but, secondarily to that, a reflex antagonistic to that. This latter antagonistic (extension) reflex is 'allied' to that which originally held the field. When the flexion-reflex disturbed the neural equilibrium it dispossessed the opposed reflex of extension from certain final paths common to that and itself. In other words, its own reaction induces an after-coming reflex antagonistic to itself, and this brings resumption of the original reflex attitude that, under the condition (gravity, etc.) obtaining at the time, satisfies neural equilibrium. The whole intercurrent reflex disturbance is really ended by a 'compensatory reflex'. The compensatory reflex in this

Reflex Sequence

case seems traceable primarily to proprio-ceptive (muscular) afferents from the muscles, joints, etc., of the limb. But compensatory reflexes are particularly evident in reflex reactions started by labyrinthine afferents (Ewald, Lee, Loeb, Lyon, Muskens, Nagel, and others), and in the decerebrate animal this compensatory reflex of the limb is presumably due to muscular afferents of the limbs and to labyrinthine afferents acting in reflex alliance.

Among the afferent nerves of importance to this compensating reflex there seems particularly that of the vasto-crureus muscle itself, the extensor of the knee. Electrical stimulation of the central end of that nerve excites contraction of the flexors of hip and knee and inhibits the vasto-crureus itself. It therefore reinforces the flexion-reflex, but its stimulation is, on being discontinued, immediately succeeded by contraction of the extensor muscles. This rebound (successive induction) is particularly marked in the vasto-crureus itself. These instances exemplify further what was said as to the close connexion of secondary, not immediate, kind between reflexes initiated by receptors of the extero-ceptive (e.g. skin) surface and reflexes initiated by receptors of the deep, i.e. proprio-ceptive field. But in the instances given earlier the proprio-ceptive reflex which was initiated secondarily in consequence of the foregoing extero-ceptive (skin) reflex is antagonistic to the latter; the two reflexes are related as antagonistic reflexes. The secondary association which, as pointed our earlier, holds so generally between certain extero-ceptive and proprio-ceptive pairs of reflexes and connects them, forms some of its pairs from 'allied reflexes' and others from 'antagonistic reflexes'. In the former case the coupling is 'simultaneous', in the latter 'successive'. Proprio-ceptive reflexes may themselves be coupled in antagonistic pairs; of this, one example is the reflex contraction of the hamstring muscles, which sometimes undoubtedly ensues on stimulation of the central end of the nerve of the extensor of the knee (I was at first inclined to attribute this to escape of current, but am convinced it occurs truly reflexly 'sometimes); and another example is Mislawski and Baglioni's interesting expiratory reflex elicitable from the afferent fibres of the phrenic nerve.

Factors Determining the Sequence

FACTORS DETERMINING THE SEQUENCE

The formation of a common path from tributary converging afferent arcs is important because it gives a co-ordinating mechanism. There the dominant action of one afferent arc, or set of allied arcs in condominium, is subject to supersession by another afferent arc or set of allied arcs, and the supersession normally occurs without intercurrent confusion. Whatever be the nature of the physiological process occurring between the competing reflexes for dominance over the common path, the issue of their competition, namely, the determination of which one of the competing arcs shall for the time being reign over the common path, is largely conditioned by four factors. These are 'spinal induction',[304] relative intensity of stimulus, relative fatigue, and the functional species of the reflex.

I. SPINAL INDUCTION

The first of these occurs in two forms, one of which has been already considered, namely, 'immediate induction'. It is a form of 'bahnung'. The stimulus which excites a reflex tends by central spread to facilitate and lower the threshold for reflexes allied to that which it particularly excites. A constellation of reflexes thus tends to be formed which reinforce each other, so that the reflex is supported by allied accessory reflexes, or if the prepotent stimulus shifts, allied arcs are by the induction particularly prepared to be responsive to it or to a similar stimulus.

Immediate induction only occurs between allied reflexes. Its tendency in the competition between afferent arcs is to fortify the reflex just established, or, if transition occur, to favour transition to an allied reflex. Immediate induction seems to obtain with highest intensity at the outset of a reflex, or at least near its commencement. It does not appear to persist long.

The other form of spinal induction is what may be termed *successive induction*. It is in several ways the reverse of the preceding.[304]

In peripheral inhibition exemplified by the vagus action on the heart the inhibitory effect is followed by a rebound after-effect opposite to the inhibitory (Gaskell). The same thing is obvious in

Reflex Sequence

various instances of the reciprocal inhibition of the spinal centres. Thus, if the crossed-extension reflex of the limb of the spinal dog be elicited at regular intervals, say once a minute, by a carefully adjusted electrical stimulus of defined duration and intensity, the resulting reflex movements are repeated each time with much constancy of character, amplitude, and duration. If in one of the intervals a strong prolonged (e.g. 30 sec.) flexion-reflex is induced from the limb yielding the extensor-reflex movement, the latter reflex is found intensified after the intercurrent flexion-reflex.[304] The intercalated flexion-reflex lowers the threshold for the aftercoming extension-reflexes, and especially increases their after-discharge (Figs. 57, 58). This effect may endure, progressively diminishing, through 4 or 5 min., as tested by the extensor-reflexes at successive intervals. Now, as we have seen, *during* the flexion-reflex the extensor arcs were inhibited: *after* the flexion-reflex these arcs are in this case evidently in a phase of exalted excitability. The phenomenon presents obvious analogy to visual contrast. If visual brightness be regarded as analogous to the activity of spinal discharge, and visual darkness analogous to absence of spinal discharge, this reciprocal spinal action in the example mentioned has a close counterpart in the well-known experiment where a white disk used as a prolonged stimulus leaves as visual after-effect a grey image surrounded by a bright ring (Hering's 'Lichthof'). The bright ring has for its spinal equivalent the discharge from the adjacent reciprocally correlated spinal centre. The exaltation after-effect may ensue with such intensity that simple discontinuance of the stimulus maintaining one reflex is immediately followed by 'spontaneous' appearance of the antagonistic reflex. Thus the 'flexion-reflex' if intense and prolonged may, directly its own exciting stimulus is discontinued, be succeeded by a 'spontaneous' reflex of extension, and this even when the animal is lying on its side and the limb horizontal—a pose that does not favour the tonus of the extensor muscles. Such a 'spontaneous' reflex is the spinal counterpart of the visual 'Lichthof'. To this 'spinal induction', as it may be termed, seems attributable a phenomenon commonly met in a flexion-reflex of high intensity when maintained by very prolonged excitation. The reflex-flexion is then frequently broken at

Successive Spinal Induction

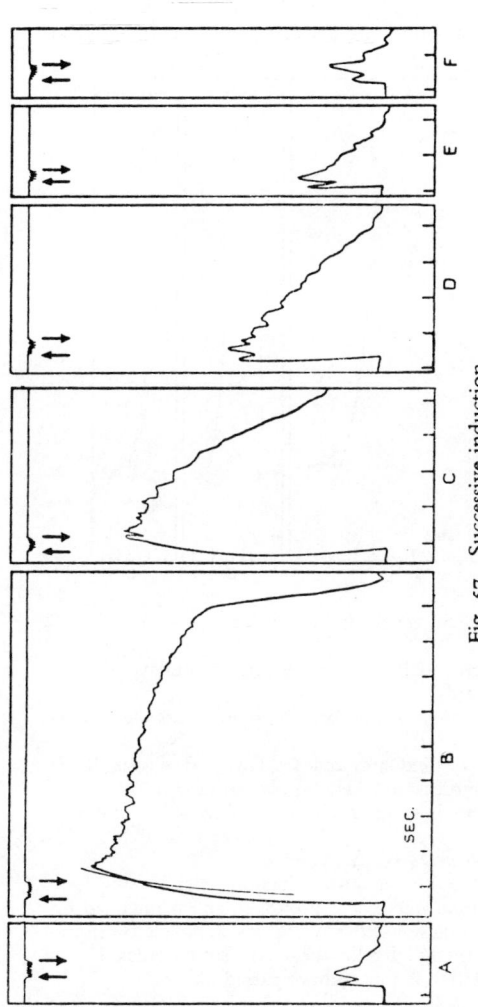

Fig. 57. Successive induction

The crossed extension-reflex of the hind-limb (dog) augmented by a precurrent flexion-reflex.
Records from above downwards:

Signal line: between arrows, short series of break shocks of each stimulation evoking the crossed extensor-reflex. The break shocks were applied (unipolar faradization) to the skin of a digit of the opposite foot. The reflex was of small intensity, the break shocks being weak.

Myograph curve of crossed extensor-reflex.

Time in sec.

Between A and B a strong flexion-reflex of the limb responding by contraction in the crossed extension-reflex was provoked and maintained for 55 sec. The next crossed extension-reflex, B, after the intercalated flexion-reflex, shows marked augmentation in amplitude and duration (after discharge). This augmentation subsides gradually, but is obvious in the three ensuing crossed reflexes C, D and E, elicited at 1 min. intervals. In reflex F, evoked in the 5th min. after the intercalated flexion-reflex, the augmentation has passed off.

Reflex Sequence

irregular intervals by sudden extension movements (Fig. 45). It would seem, therefore, that some process in the flexion-reflex leads to exaltation of the activity of the arcs of the opposed extension-reflex. And electrical stimulation of the proximal end of the severed

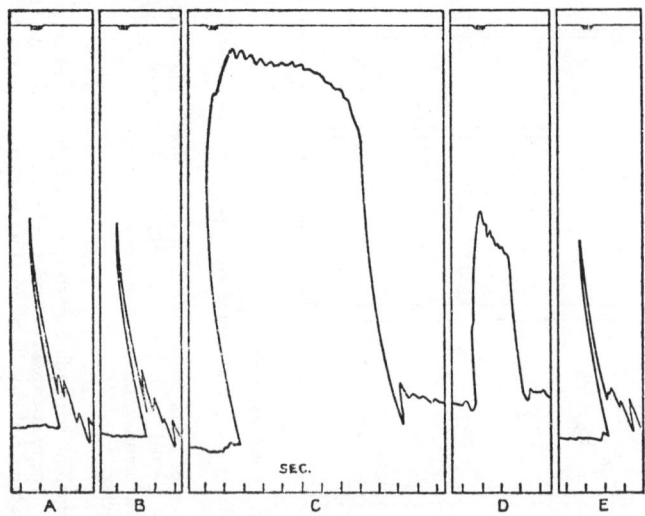

Fig. 58. Successive induction

Crossed extension-reflex augmented by precurrent flexion-reflex.
Records from above downwards:
    Signal line: break shocks of each stimulation evoking crossed extensor-reflex.
    Myograph curve: crossed extensor-reflex. This reflex was being elicited regularly by eleven break shocks (unipolar faradization to skin of opposite foot) at 1 min. intervals, stimulus and reflex being of low intensity.
    Time in sec.
    Intervals of 1 min. between A, B, C, D and E.
In the interval between B and C a strong flexion-reflex of the limb responding in the crossed extension-reflex was provoked and maintained for 45 sec. The next following extension-reflex C shows augmentation; this augmentation is also evident, though less in the next crossed-reflex D. In E, a minute later, the augmentation is seen to have passed off.

nerve of the extensor muscles of the knee (cat), though it does not in my experience directly excite contraction of the extensors of the knee, is on cessation often immediately followed by contraction of them.

Rebound in Mark-time Reflex

As examples of the rebound exaltation following on inhibition the following may also serve. 304 The so-called 'mark-time' reflex of the 'spinal' dog is an alternating stepping movement of the hind-limbs which occurs on holding the animal up so that its limbs hang pendent. It can be inhibited by stimulating the skin of the tail. On

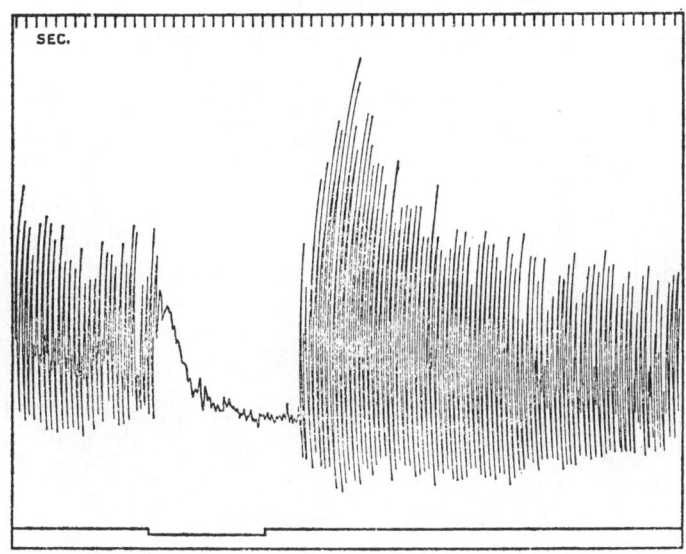

Fig. 59. 'Mark-time' reflex arrested by inhibition

Records from above downwards:
  Time in sec.
  Myograph curve: record of movement of limb (spinal dog). The upstrokes correspond with flexions.
  Signal line: descent of signal indicates period of stimulation of the tail which interrupts the 'mark-time' reflex. This arrest is followed, after discontinuance of the inhibitory stimulus, by increased amplitude and some quickening of the leg movement.

cessation of that stimulus the stepping movement sets in more vigorously and at quicker rate than before (Fig. 59). The increase is chiefly in the amplitude of the movement, but I have also seen the rhythm quickened even by 30 per cent of the frequence.

This after-increase might be explicable in either of two ways. It

Reflex Sequence

might be due to the mere repose of the reflex centre, the repose so recruiting the centre as to strengthen its subsequent action. But a similar period of repose obtained by simply supporting one limb—which causes cessation of the reflex in both limbs, the stimulus being stretch of the hip-flexors under gravity—is not followed by after-increase of the reflex (Fig. 60).

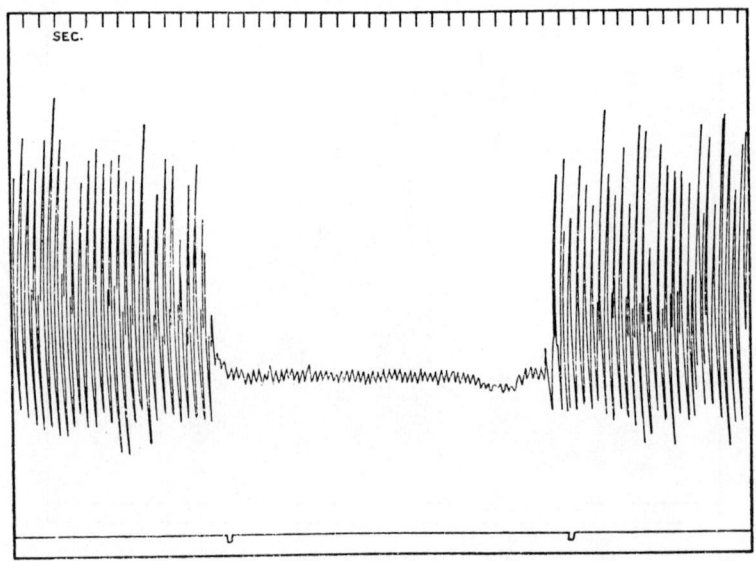

Fig. 60. 'Mark-time' reflex arrested by removing the exciting stimulus

Records from above downwards:
   Time in sec.
   Myograph curve: record of movement of limb (spinal dog). The upstrokes correspond with flexions.
   Signal line: during the period between the two marks on the signal line the reflex was interrupted by lifting the fellow-limb to that yielding the tracing. On letting the leg hang again, the reflex starts afresh, but without increase beyond its previous activity.

Or the after-increase might result from the inhibition being followed by a rebound to superactivity. This latter seems to be the case. The after-increase occurs even when both hind-limbs are passively lifted from below during the whole duration of the inhibitory stimulus applied to the tail. It is the depression of

Successive Spinal Induction

inhibition and not the mere freedom from an exciting stimulus that induces a later superactivity. And the reflex inhibition of the knee-extensor by stimulation of the central end of its own nerve is especially followed by marked rebound to superactivity of the extensor itself.

Again, the knee-jerk, after being inhibited by stimulation of the hamstring nerve, returns, and is then more brisk than before the inhibition (Fig. 29, p. 89).

By virtue of this spinal contrast, therefore, the extension-reflex predisposes to and may actually induce a flexion-reflex, and conversely the flexion-reflex predisposes to and may actually induce an extension-reflex. This process is qualified to play a part in linking reflexes together in a co-ordinate sequence of successive combination.[304] If a reflex-arc *A* during its own activity temporarily checks that of an opposed reflex-arc *B*, but as a subsequent result induces in arc *B* a phase of greater excitability and capacity for discharge, it predisposes the spinal organ for a second reflex opposite in character to its own in immediate succession to itself. I have elsewhere[183] pointed out the peculiar prominence of 'alternating reflexes' in prolonged spinal reactions. It is significant that they are usually cut short with ease by mere passive mechanical interruption of the alternating movement in progress. It seems that each step of the reflex movement tends to excite by spinal induction the step next succeeding itself.

Much of the reflex action of the limb that can be studied in the 'spinal' dog bears the character of adaptation to locomotion. This has been shown recently with particular clearness by the observations of Phillipson. In describing the extensor-thrust of the limb I drew attention at the time to its significance for locomotion. 'Spinal induction' obviously tends to connect flexion of the limb as an after-effect to this extensor-thrust. In the stepping of the limb the flexion that raises the foot and carries it clear of the ground prepares the antagonistic arcs of extension, and, so to say, sensitizes them to respond later in their turn by the supporting and propulsive extension of the limb necessary for progression. In such reflex sequences an antecedent reflex would thus not only be the means of

Reflex Sequence

bringing about an ensuing stimulus for the next reflex, but would predispose the arc of the next reflex to react to the stimulus when it arrives, or even induce the reflex without external stimulus The reflex 'stepping' of the 'spinal' dog does go on even without an *external skin* stimulus: it will continue when the dog is held in the air. The cat walks well when the soles of all four feet are anaesthetic.

Each reflex movement must of itself generate stimuli to afferent apparatus in many parts and organs—muscles, joints, tendons, etc. This probably reinforces the reflex in progress. The reflex obtainable by stimulation of the afferent nerve of the flexor muscles of the knee excites those muscles to contraction and inhibits their antagonists: the reflex obtainable from the afferent nerve of the extensor muscles of the knee excites the flexors and inhibits their antagonists.

Where a reflex by spinal induction tends eventually to bring about the opposed reflex, the process of spinal induction is therefore probably reinforced by the operation of any reflex generated in the movement. This would help to explain how it is that a reflex reaction, when once excited in a spinal animal, ceases on cessation of the stimulus as quickly as it generally does. Such a reaction must generate in its progress a number of further stimuli and throw up a shower of centripetal impulses from the moving muscles and joints into the spinal cord. Squeezing of muscles and stimulation of their afferent nerves and those of joints, etc., elicit reflexes. The primary reflex movement might be expected, therefore, of itself to initiate further reflex movement, and that secondarily to initiate further still, and so on. Yet on cessation of the external stimulus to the foot in the 'flexion-reflex' the whole reflex comes usually at once to an end. The 'scratch-reflex', even when violently provoked, ceases usually within 2 sec. of the discontinuance of the external stimulus that provoked it.

We have as yet no satisfactory explanation of this. But we remember that such reflexes are intercurrent reactions breaking in on a condition of neural equilibrium itself reflex. The successive induction will tend to induce a *compensatory* reflex, which brings the moving parts back again to the original position of equilibrium.

Reflex Fatigue

II. FATIGUE

Another condition influencing the issue of competition between reflexes of different source for possession of one and the same final common path is 'fatigue'.300 A spinal reflex under continuous excitation or frequent repetition becomes weaker, and may cease altogether. This decline is progressive, and takes place earlier in some kinds of reflexes than it does in others. In the spinal dog the scratch-reflex under ordinary circumstances tires much more rapidly (Fig. 45) than does the 'flexion-reflex'.

A reflex as it tires shows other changes besides decline in amplitude of contraction. Thus, in the 'flexion-reflex', the original steadiness of the contraction decreases (Figs. 45, 61); it becomes tremulous, and the tremor becomes progressively more marked and more irregular. The rhythm of the tremor in my observations has often been about 10 per sec. Then phases of greater tremor tend to alternate with phases of improved contraction as indicated by some regain of original extent of flexion of limb and diminished tremor. Apart from these partial evanescent recoveries the decline is progressive. Later, the stimulation being maintained all the time, brief periods of something like complete intermission of the reflex appear, and even of a replacement of flexion by extension. These lapses are recovered from, but tend to recur more and more. Finally, an irregular phasic tremor of the muscles is all that remains. It is not the flexor muscles themselves which tire out, for these, when they contract no longer during the flexion-reflex, still contract in response to the scratch-reflex which also employs them.

Similar results are furnished by the scratch-reflex with certain differences in accord with the peculiar character of its discharge.287 One of these latter is the feature that the individual beats of the scratch-reflex usually become slower and follow each other at slower frequency (Fig. 62). Also the beats, instead of remaining fairly regular in amplitude and frequency tend to succeed in somewhat regular groups. The beats may disappear altogether for a short time, and then for a short time reappear, the stimulus continuing all the while (Fig. 63). Here, again, the phenomena are not referable to

Reflex Sequence

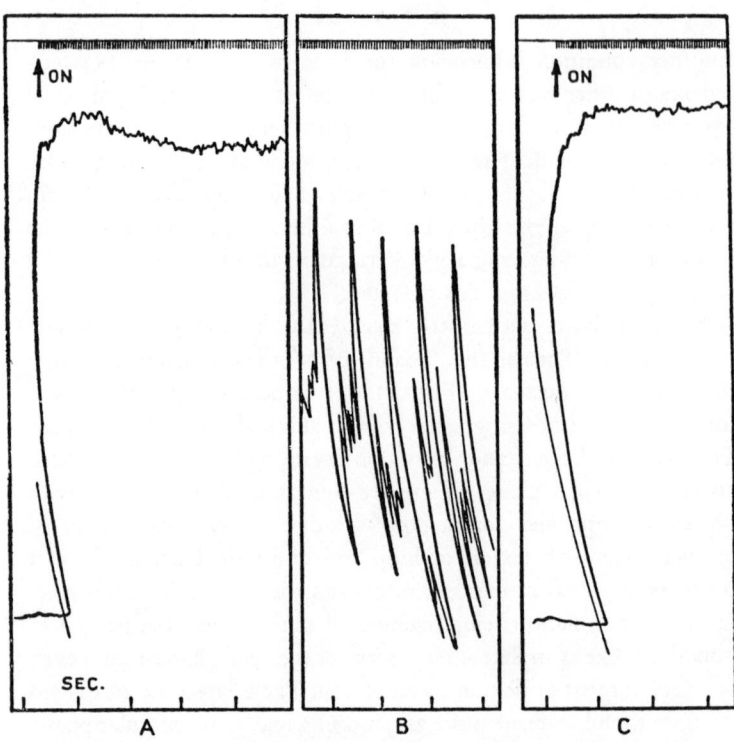

Fig. 61. Fatigue and recovery of flexion-reflex

The reflex was being elicited (by unipolar faradization applied to a point in the plantar skin of the outermost digit) with intervals of about 60 sec. between the end of one reaction and the commencement of the next.

Records from above downwards:
    Signal line: interruptions in primary circuit at rate of 40 per sec.
    Stimulation begins at ON.
    Myograph curve: flexion-reflex. The vertical arcs in A, C indicate onset of stimulation.
    Time in sec.

A shows the commencement of the third reaction in the series, and this reaction was continuously elicited for 50 sec.; B shows it in its latest stage. The stimulation was then stopped for 70 sec. and then recommenced: C shows the opening of the next reaction, the fourth of the series. In the 70 sec. interval the reflex has fully recovered from the 'fatigue' exhibited in B.

Fatigue of Scratch Reflex

the muscle, for when excited through other reflex channels, or through its motor-nerve directly, the muscle shows its contraction

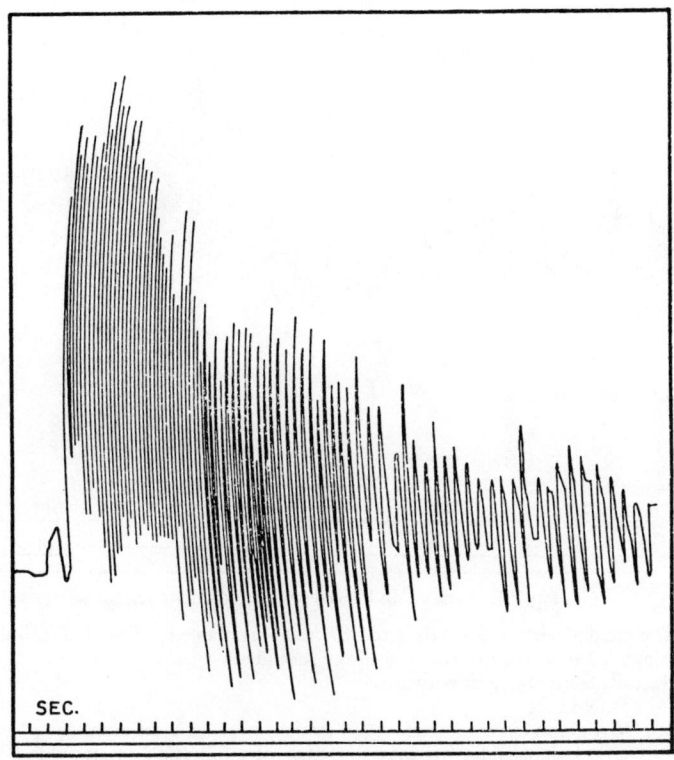

Fig. 62. Fatigue of scratch-reflex

The scratch-reflex evoked in spinal dog by mechanical stimulation at a spot in the skin of the shoulder. The reflex shows the rapid waning of the movement under continued application of stimuli to one spot of skin—this occurs with the same general features both under mechanical or electrical stimulation. The beats become of slower rhythm and more irregular and smaller amplitude and finally occur in groups. Time is marked below in seconds.

well. Part of the decline of these reflexes under electrical stimulation in the spinal dog may be due to reduction of the intensity of the stimulus itself by physical polarization. That does not account in the

Reflex Sequence

main for the above described effects. The graphic record of fatigue of the flexion of the scratch-reflex obtained by continued *mechanical*

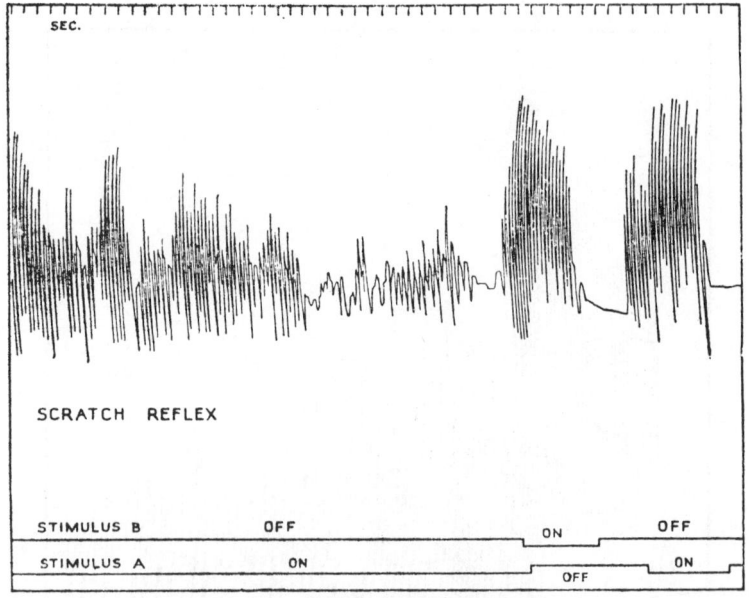

Fig. 63. Fatigue and recovery of scratch-reflex

The scratch-reflex toward the end of a long-maintained mechanical stimulation applied to a point of the skin of the shoulder.
Records from above downwards:
  Time in sec.
  Myograph curve: scratch-reflex evoked initially by stimulus A.
  Upper signal line: ON indicates time of application of stimulus B to second point.
  Lower signal line: ON indicates time of application of stimulus A for scratch-reflex.
  Time in sec.
Stimulus A was in operation at the beginning of the record. When the reflex was nearly tired out, stimulus A was remitted for about 10 sec. and then repeated. The reflex then returns showing considerable recovery. During the intermission of stimulus A, stimulus B was applied to a neighbouring point; the scratch-reflex response shows little evidence of fatigue.

stimulation does not appreciably differ from that yielded under electrical stimulation. The different speed of the decline due to fatigue proceeds characteristically in different kinds of reflex, and in

Seat of Reflex Fatigue

the same kind of reflex under different physiological conditions e.g. 'spinal shock': this indicates its determination by other factors than electrical polarization. Polarization has in a number of cases been deferred as far as possible by using equalized alternate shocks applied in opposite directions through the same gilt needle; this precaution has not yielded results differing appreciably from those given by ordinary double shocks or by series of make or break shocks of the same direction. The slowing of the beat in 'fatigue' is also against the explanation by polarization, since merely weakening the stimulus does not lead to a slower beat.

When the scratch-reflex elicited from a spot of skin is fatigued, the fatigue holds for that spot but does not implicate the reflex as obtained from the surrounding skin.[287, 300] The reflex when tired out to stimuli at that spot is easily obtainable by stimulation two or more cm. away (Fig. 63). This is seen with either mechanical or electrical stimuli. When the spot stimulated second is close to the one tired out, the reflex shows some degree of fatigue, but not that degree obtaining for the original spot. This fatigue may be a local fatigue of the nerve-endings in the spot of skin stimulated, to which in experiments making use of electric stimuli some polarization may be added. Yet its local character does not at all necessarily imply its reference to the skin. It may be the expression of a spatial arrangement in the central organ by which reflex-arcs arising in adjacent receptors are partially confluent in their approach toward the final common path, and are the more confluent the closer together lie their points of origin in the receptive field. The resemblance between the distribution of the incidence of this fatigue and that of the spatial summation previously described argues that the seat of the fatigue is intraspinal and central more than peripheral and cutaneous; and that it affects the afferent part of the arc inside the spinal cord, probably at the first synapse. Thus, its incidence at the synapse $R\alpha - P\alpha$ and at $R\beta - P\beta$ (Fig. 13, B, or Fig. 39, B) would explain its restrictions, as far as we know them, in the scratch-reflex.

The local fatigue of a spinal reflex seems to be recovered from with remarkable speed, to judge by observations on the reflexes of the limbs of the spinal dog. A few seconds' remission of the stimulus

Reflex Sequence

suffices for marked though incomplete restoration of the reaction (Fig. 63). In a few instances I have seen return of a reflex even during the stimulation under which the waning and disappearance of the reflex occurred. The exciting stimulus has usually in such cases been of rather weak intensity. In my experience, these spinal reflexes fade out sooner under a weak stimulus than under a strong one. This seeming paradox indicates that even under feeble intensities of stimulation the threshold of the reaction gradually rises, and that it rises above the threshold value of the weaker stimulus before it reaches that of a stronger stimulus. This is exemplified by Fig. 64, where the scratch-reflex which has ceased to be elicited by the stimulus A is immediately evoked—often without any sign of fatigue in its motor response—by increasing the intensity of the stimulus (applied at the same electrode) to $A+a$, $5\,\Omega$ having been short-circuited from the current in the primary circuit. But the occurrence of 'fatigue' earlier under the weaker stimulus than under the stronger also shows that the fatigue consequent under the weaker stimulus may often be greater relatively to the *production of the natural discharge* than when a stronger stimulus is employed. This, which has been of frequent occurrence in my observations on the leg of the spinal dog, if obtaining widely in reflex actions has evident practical importance.

It is easy to avoid in some degree the local fatigue associated with excitation of the scratch-reflex from one single spot in the skin by taking advantage of the spatial summation of stimuli applied at different points in the receptive field. Brief-lasting stimuli can be shifted from point to point in the field. When this is done, a curious result has met me. The provocation of the reflex has been made through ten separate points in the receptive field, the distance between each member of the series of points and the point next to it being about 4 cm. Each point is stimulated by a double-induction shock delivered twice a second. When this is done a series of scratch movements is elicited, and continues longer than when the stimuli are applied at the same interval, not to succeeding series of skin points but to one point. Thus three or four hundred beats can be elicited in unbroken series. But the series tends somewhat abruptly to cease.

Reflex Fatigue

If then, in spite of the cessation of the response, the stimulation be *continued* without alteration during three or four minutes or more, the scratching movement breaks out again from time to time and

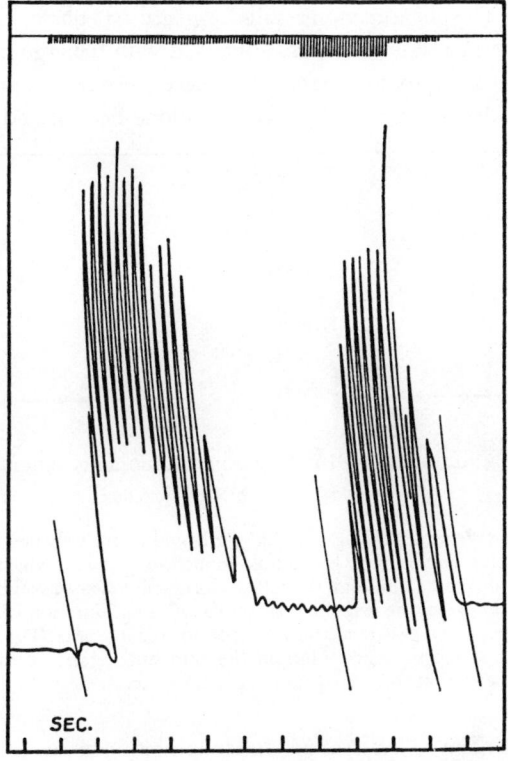

Fig. 64. Fatigue of scratch-reflex

Records from above downwards:
   Signal line marks the stimulation by an electromagnet in the primary: the armature is arranged so that the increase in intensity of the stimulation is shown by greater amplitude of excursion.
   Myograph curve: scratch-reflex.
   Time in sec.
The scratch-reflex evoked by a relatively feeble stimulation and disappearing under that stimulation. On increasing the intensity of the stimulus the reflex reappears, and does not reappear on reverting again to the original intensity of stimulation.

Reflex Sequence

gives another series of beats (Fig. 65), perhaps longer than the first. These experiments indicate that physical polarization at the stigmatic electrode is not answerable for the fading out of the scratch-reflex. It shows also the complexity of the central mechanisms involved in the reflex. The phenomenon recalls Lombard's[116] phases of briskness and fatigue in a series of records obtained with the ergograph.

It is interesting to note certain differences between the cessation of a reflex under 'fatigue' and under inhibition. Figs. 60 and 43 can be

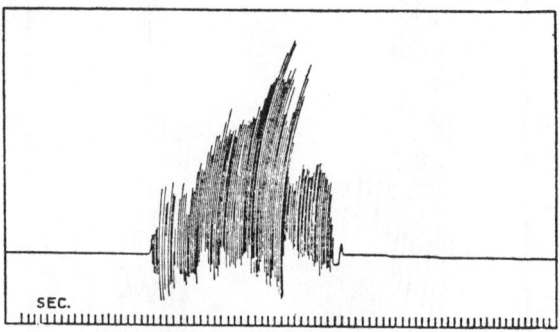

Fig. 65. Fatigue of scratch-reflex

A scratch-reflex reappearing after having lapsed completely under a stimulation (unipolar faradization by double-induction shocks) which has been maintained unaltered although the reflex it originally evoked had lapsed. The reappearances occur at irregular intervals of long duration, e.g. 50 sec., and the reflex on reappearance may last for 20 sec. at a time. The stimulation was applied at ten separate points in the skin surface and at each point by unipolar faradization from a separate secondary circuit.

compared. The reflex ceasing under inhibition is seen to fade off without obvious change in the frequency of repetition of the 'beats', or in the duration of the individual beats. The reflex ceasing under fatigue is seen to show a slower rhythm and a sluggish course for the latter beats, especially for the terminal ones.

Among the signs of fatigue of a reflex action are several suggesting that in it the command over the final common path exercised for the time being by the receptors and afferent path in action becomes less strong, less steady, and less accurately adjusted. Under prolonged excitation their hold upon the final common path becomes loosened.

Reflex Fatigue

This view is supported by the fact that its connexion with the final common path is then more easily cut short and ruptured by other rival arcs competing with it for the final common path in question. The scratch-reflex interrupts the flexion-reflex more readily when the latter is tired out than when it is fresh.

In the hind-limb of the spinal dog the extensor-thrust is inelicitable during the flexion-reflex. That is to say, when the flexion-reflex is evoked with fair or high intensity I have never succeeded in evoking the extensor-thrust, though the flexed posture of the limb is itself a favouring circumstance for the production of the thrust if the flexion be a passive one. But when the flexion-reflex is kept up by appropriate stimulation of a single point over a prolonged time, so that it shows fatigue, the 'extensor-thrust' becomes again elicitable. Its elicitability is, then, not regular nor facile, but it does become obtainable, usually in quite feeble degree at first, later more powerfully. In other words, it can dispossess the rival reflex from a common path when that rival is fatigued, though it cannot do so when the rival action is fresh and powerful.

Again, the crossed 'extension-reflex' cannot inhibit the flexion of the flexor-reflex under ordinary circumstances if the intensity of the stimulation of the competing arcs be approximately equal; but it can do so when the flexion-reflex is tired.

The waning of a reflex under long maintained excitation is one of the many phenomena that pass in physiology under the name of 'fatigue'. It may be that in this case the so-called fatigue is really nothing but a negative induction. Its place of incidence may lie at the synapse. It seems a process elaborated and preserved in the selective evolution of the neural machinery. One obvious use attaching to it is the prevention of the too prolonged continuous use of a 'common path' by any one receptor.[300] It precludes one receptor from occupying for long periods an effector organ to the exclusion of all other receptors. It prevents long continuous possession of a common path by any one reflex of considerable intensity. It favours the receptors taking turn about. It helps to insure serial variety of reaction. The organism, to be successful in a million-sided environment, must in its reactions be many-sided. Were it not for

Reflex Sequence

such so-called 'fatigue', an organism might, in regard to its receptivity, develop an eye, or an ear, or a mouth, or a hand or leg, but it would hardly develop the marvellous congeries of all those various sense-organs which it is actually found to possess.

The loosening of the hold upon the common path by so-called 'fatigue' occurs also in paths other than those leading to muscle and effector organs. If instead of motor effects sensual are examined, analogous phenomena are observed. A visual image is more readily inhibited by a competing image in the same visual field when it has acted for some time than when it is first perceived (W. McDougall).[223]

One point, on *a priori* grounds a natural corollary from the 'principle of the common path', is indicated by the experimental findings relative to the incidence of fatigue. The reflex-arcs, each a chain of neurones, converge in their course so as to impinge upon and conjoin in links (neurones) common to whole varied groups—in other words, they conjoin to *common paths*. This arrangement culminates in the convergence of many separately arising arcs in the final efferent-root neurone. This neurone thus forms the instrument for many different reflex arcs and acts. It is responsive to them in various rhythm and in various grades of intensity. In accordance with this, it seems from experimental evidence to be *relatively indefatigable*.[300] It thus satisfies a demand that the principle of the common path must make regarding it.

III. INTENSITY

In the transition from one reflex to another a final common path changes hands and passes from one master to another. A fresh set of afferent arcs becomes dominant on the supersession of one reflex by the next. Of all the conditions determining which one of competing reflexes shall for the time being reign over a final common path, the *intensity* of reaction of the afferent arc itself relatively to that of its rivals is probably the most powerful. An afferent arc strongly stimulated is *ceteris paribus* more likely to capture the common path than is one excited feebly. A stimulus can only establish its reflex and

Intensity of Stimulus

inhibit an opposed one if it have intensity. This explains why, in order to produce examples of spinal inhibition, recourse has so frequently been made in past times to *strong* stimuli. A strong stimulus will inhibit a reflex in progress, although a weak one will fail. Thus in Goltz's inhibition of micturition in the 'spinal' dog a *forcible* squeeze of the tail will do it, but not, in my experience, a weak squeeze. So likewise any condition which raises the excitability and responsiveness of a nervous arc will give it power to inhibit other reflexes just as it would if it were excited by a strong stimulus. This is much as in the heart of the Tunicate. There the prepotent spot whence starts the systole lies from time to time at one end and from time to time at the other. The prepotent region at one end which usually dominates the common path is from time to time displaced by local increase of excitability at the other under local distension of the blood-sinuses there.

In judging of intensity of stimulus the situation of the stimulus in the receptive field of the reflex has to be remembered. One and the same physical stimulus will be weak if applied near the edge of the field, though strong if applied to the focus of the field.

Crossed reflexes are usually less easy to provoke, less reliable of obtainment, and less intense than are direct reflexes. Consequently we find crossed reflexes usually more easily inhibited and replaced by direct reflexes than are these latter by those former. Thus the crossed stepping-reflex is easily replaced by the scratch-reflex (Fig. 52), though its stimulus be continued all the time, and though the scratch-reflex itself is not a very potent reflex. But the reverse can occur with suitably adjusted intensity of stimuli.

Again, the flexion-reflex of the dog's leg is, when fully developed, accompanied by extension in the opposite leg. This crossed extensor movement, though often very vigorous, may be considered as an accessory and weaker part of the whole reflex of which the prominent part is flexion of the homonymous limb. When the flexion-reflex is elicitable poorly, as, for instance, in spinal shock or under fatigue or weak excitation, the crossed extension does not accompany the homonymous flexion and does not appear. But, where the flexion-reflex is well developed, if not merely one but *both* feet be

Reflex Sequence

stimulated simultaneously with stimuli of fairly equal intensity, steady flexion at knee, hip, and ankle results in *both* limbs (Fig. 66) and extension occurs in neither limb.[205] The contralateral part of each reflex is inhibited by the homolateral flexion of each reflex. In other words, the more intense part of each reflex obtains possession

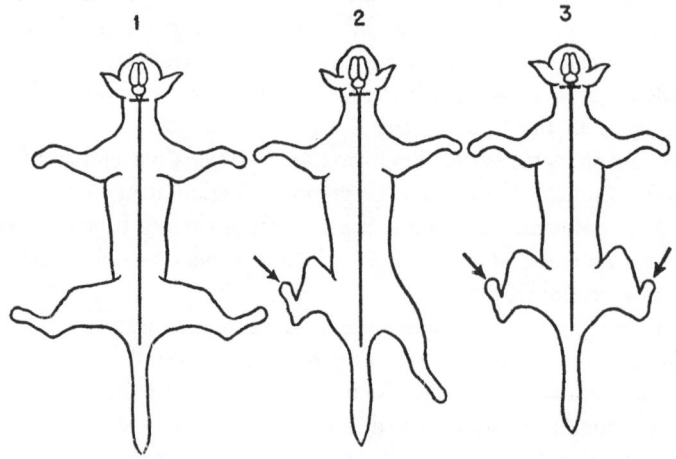

Fig. 66. Diagram (cat) of the predominant uncrossed flexor-reflex of the hind-limb inhibiting the crossed extensor-reflex otherwise obtainable by stimulation of the opposite limb

1. The initial pose of the spinal animal.
2. The pose assumed after stimulation of the left hind-foot; the flexors of the left hip, knee, and ankle, and the extensors of the right hip, knee, and ankle are in active contraction.
3. The pose assumed after simultaneous stimulation of both hind-feet. The extensor action of the hip, knee, and ankle that would appear from either side as a crossed reflex is bilaterally inhibited and the antagonistic flexor-reflexes bilaterally prevail.

of the final common paths at the expense of the less intense portion of the reflex. But if the intensity of the stimuli applied to the right and left feet be not closely enough balanced, the crossed extension of the reflex excited by the stronger stimulus is found to exclude even the homonymous flexion that the weaker stimulus should and would otherwise evoke from the leg to which it is applied.

It was pointed out above that in a number of cases the transference

Types of Skin Receptors

of control of the final common path *FC* (Fig. 44, p. 150) from one afferent arc to another is *reversible*. The direction of the transference can *ceteris paribus* be easily governed by making the stimulation of this receptor or that receptor the more intense. A factor largely determining whether a reflex succeed another or not is therefore intensity of stimulus.300

IV. SPECIES OF REFLEX

A fourth main determinant for the issue of the conflict between rival reflexes seems to be the functional *species* of the reflexes.300

Reflexes initiated from a species of receptor apparatus that may be termed *noci-ceptive*[252] appear to particularly dominate the majority of the final common paths issuing from the spinal cord. In the simpler sensations we experience from various kinds of stimuli applied to our skin there can be distinguished those of touch, of cold, of warmth, and of pain. The adequate stimuli for the first mentioned three of these are certainly different; mechanical stimuli, applied above a certain speed, which deform beyond a certain degree the resting contour of the skin surface, seem to constitute *adequate* stimuli for touch. Similarly the cooling or raising of the local temperature, whether by thermal conduction, radiation, etc., are *adequate* for the cold and warmth sensations. The organs for these three sensations have by stigmatic stimuli been traced to separate and discrete tiny spots in the skin. In regard to skin-pain it is held by competent observers, notably by v. Frey[148] and Kiesow,[270] that skin-pain likewise is referable to certain specific nerve-endings. In evidence of this it is urged that mechanical stimuli applied at certain places excite sensations which from their very threshold upward possess unpleasantness, and as the intensity of the stimulus is increased, culminate in 'physical pain'. The sensation excited by a mechanical stimulus applied to a touch-spot does not evoke pain, however intensely applied, so long as the stimulation is confined to the touch-spot. The threshold value of mechanical stimuli for touch-spots is in general lower than it is for pain-spots; and conversely the threshold value of electrical stimuli for touch-spots is in general higher than it is for the spots yielding pain. Similarly it is said that stimulation of a

Reflex Sequence

cold spot or of a warm spot does not, however intense, evoke, so long as confined to them, sensations of painful quality. But pain can be excited not only by strong mechanical stimuli and by electrical stimuli, but by cold and by warmth, though the threshold value of these latter stimuli is higher for pain than for cold and warm spots. If these observations prove correct there exist, therefore, numerous specific cutaneous nerve-fibres evoking pain.

A difficulty here is that sensory nerve-endings are usually provided with sense-organs which lower their threshold for stimuli of one particular kind while raising it for stimuli of all other kinds; but these pain-endings in the skin seem almost equally excited by stimuli of such different modes as mechanical, thermal conductive, thermal radiant, chemical, and electrical. That is, they appear *anelective* receptors. But it is to be remarked that these agents, regarded as excitants of skin-pain, have all a certain character in common, namely this, that they become *adequate* as excitants of pain when they are of such intensity as *threatens damage to the skin*. And we may note about these excitants that they are *all able to excite nerve* when applied to naked nerve *directly*. Now there are certain skin surfaces from which, according to most observers, pain is the *only* species of sensation that can be evoked. This is alleged, for instance, of the surface of the cornea—a modified piece of skin. The histology of the cornea reveals in its epithelium nerve-endings of but one morphological kind; that is, the ending by naked nerve-fibrils that pass up among the epithelial cells. Similar nerve-endings exist also in the epidermis generally. It may therefore be that the nerve-endings subserving skin-pain are free naked nerve-endings, and the absence of any highly evolved specialized end-organ in connexion with them may explain their fairly equal amenability to an unusually wide range of different kinds of stimuli. Instead of but one kind of stimulus being their adequate excitant, they may be regarded as adapted to a whole group of excitants, a group of excitants which has in relation to the organism one feature common to all its components, namely, a *nocuous* character.

With its liability to various kinds of mechanical and other damage in a world beset with dangers amid which the individual and species

Noci-ceptive Reflexes

have to win their way in the struggle for existence we may regard nocuous stimuli as part of a normal state of affairs. It does not seem improbable, therefore, that there should, under selective adaptation, attach to the skin a so-to-say *specific sense of its own injuries*. As psychical adjunct to the reactions of that apparatus we find a strong displeasurable affective quality in the sensations they evoke. This may perhaps be a means for branding upon memory, of however rudimentary kind, a feeling from past events that have been perilously critical for the existence of the individuals of the species. In other words, if we admit that damage to such an exposed sentient organ as the skin must in the evolutionary history of animal life have been sufficiently frequent in relation to its importance, then the existence of a specific set of nerves for skin-pain seems to offer no genetic difficulty, any more than does the clotting of blood or innate immunity to certain diseases. That these nerve-endings constitute a distinct species is argued by their all evoking not only the same species of sensation but the same species of reflex movement as regards 'purpose', intensity, resistance to 'shock', etc. And their evolution may well have been unaccompanied by evolution of any specialized end-organ, since the naked free nerve-endings would better suit the wide and peculiar range of stimuli, reaction to which is in this case required. A low threshold was *not* required because the stimuli were all intense, intensity constituting their harmfulness; but response to a wide range of stimuli of *different* kinds was required, because harm might come in various forms. That responsive *range* is supplied by naked nerve itself and would be cramped by the specialization of an end-organ. Hence these nerve-endings remained free.

It is those areas stimulation of which, as judged by analogy, can excite pain most intensely, and it is those stimuli which, as judged by analogy, are most fitted to excite pain, which, as a general rule, excite in the 'spinal' animal—where pain is of course non-existent— the *prepotent* reflexes. If these are reactions to specific pain-nerves, this may be expressed by saying that the nervous arcs of pain-nerves, broadly speaking, dominate the spinal centres in peculiar degree. Physical pain is thus the psychical adjunct of an imperative

Reflex Sequence

protective reflex. It is preferable, however, to avoid the term 'pain-nerves', since into the merely spinal and reflex aspect of the reaction of these nerves no sensation of any kind can be shown to enter. Remembering that the feature common to all this group of stimuli is that they threaten or actually commit damage to the tissue to which they are applied, a convenient term for application to them is *nocuous*. In that case, what from the point of view of *sense* are cutaneous pain-nerves, are from the point of view of *reflex reaction* conveniently termed *noci-ceptive* nerves.

In the competition between reflexes the noci-ceptive as a rule dominate with peculiar certainty and facility. This explains why such stimuli have been so much used to evoke reflexes in the spinal frog, and why, judging from them, such 'fatality' belongs to spinal reflexes.

One and the same skin surface will in the hind-limb of the spinal dog evoke one or other of two diametrically different reflexes according as the mechanical stimulus applied be of noxious quality or not, a harmful insult or a harmless touch.[252] A needle-prick to the planta causes invariably the drawing up of the limb—the flexion-reflex. A harmless smooth contact, on the other hand, causes extension—the extensor-thrust above described. This flexion is therefore a noci-ceptive reflex. But the scratch-reflex—which is so readily evoked by simple light irritation of the skin of the shoulder—is relatively mildly noci-ceptive. When the scratch-reflex and the flexion-reflex are in competition for the final neurone common to them, the flexion-reflex more easily dispossesses the scratch-reflex from the final neurone than does the scratch-reflex the flexion-reflex. If both reflexes are fresh, and the stimuli used are such as, when employed separately, evoke their reflexes respectively with some intensity, it is in my experience the flexion-reflex that is usually prepotent (Fig. 43). Yet if, while the flexion-reflex is being moderately evoked by an appropriate stimulus of weak intensity, a strong stimulus suitable for producing the scratch-reflex is applied, the steady flexion due to the flexion-reflex is replaced by the rhythmic scratching movement of the scratch-reflex (Fig. 51), and this occurs though the stimulus for the flexion-reflex is maintained unaltered. When the stimulus producing the scratch is discontinued the flexion-

Sexual Clasp Reflex

reflex reappears as before. The flexion-reflex seems more easily to dispossess the scratch-reflex from the final common paths than can the scratch-reflex dispossess the flexion-reflex. Yet the relation is reversible—by heightening the intensity of the stimulus for the scratch-reflex or lowering that of the stimulus for the flexion-reflex.

In decerebrate rigidity, where a tonic reflex is maintaining contraction in the extensor muscles of the knee, stimulation of the nociceptive arcs of the limb easily breaks down that reflex. The nociceptive reflex dominates the motor neurone previously held in activity by the postural reflex. And noci-ceptive reflexes are relatively little depressed by 'spinal shock'.

Noci-ceptive arcs are, however, not the only spinal arcs which in the intact animal, considered from the point of view of sensation, evoke reactions rich in affective quality. Beside those receptors attuned to react to direct *noxa*, the skin has others, concerned likewise with functions of vital importance to the species and colligate with sensations similarly of intense affective quality; for instance, those concerned with sexual functions. In the male frog sexual clasp is a spinal reflex.[6] The cord may be divided both in front and behind the brachial region without interrupting the reflex. Experiment shows that from the spinal male at the breeding-season, and also at other times, this reflex is elicited by any object that stimulates the skin of the sternal and adjacent region. In the intact animal, on the contrary, other objects than the female [40] are, when applied to that region, at once rejected, even though they be wrapped in the fresh skin of the female frog and in other ways made to resemble the female. The development of the reflex is not prevented by removal of the testes, but removal of the seminal reservoirs is said to depress it, and their distension, even by indifferent fluids, to exalt it. If the skin of the sternal region and arms is removed, the reflex does not occur. Severe mutilation of the limbs and internal organs does not inhibit the reflex, neither does stimulation of the sciatic nerve central to its section. The reflex is however depressed or extinguished by strong chemical and pathic stimuli to the sternal skin, at least in many cases. The tortoise exhibits a similar sexual reflex of great spinal potency.[112a, 112b]

Reflex Sequence

It would seem a general rule that *reflexes arising in species of receptors which considered as sense-organs provoke strongly affective sensation* ceteris paribus *prevail over reflexes of other species when in competition with them for the use of the 'final common path'*. Such reflexes override and set aside with peculiar facility reflexes belonging to touch organs, muscular sense-organs, etc. As the sensations evoked by these arcs, e.g. 'pains', exclude and dominate concurrent sensations, so do the reflexes of these arcs prevail in the competition for possession of the common paths. They seem capable of *preeminent intensity* of action.300

Of all reflexes it is the tonic reflexes, e.g. of ordinary posture, that are in my experience the most *easily* interrupted by other reflexes. Even a weak stimulation of the noci-ceptive arcs arising in the foot often suffices to lower or abolish the knee-jerk or the reflex extensor tonus of the elbow or knee. If various *species* of reflex are arranged, therefore, in their order of potency in regard to power to interrupt one another, the reflexes initiated in receptors which considered as sense-organs excite sensations of strong effective quality lie at the upper end of the scale, and the reflexes that are answerable for the postural tonus of skeletal muscles lie at the lower end of the scale. One great function of the tonic reflexes is to maintain habitual attitudes and postures. They form, therefore, a nervous background of active equilibrium. It is of obvious advantage that this equilibrium should be easily upset, so that the animal may respond agilely to the passing events that break upon it as intercurrent stimuli.

Therefore, intensity of stimulation, fatigue and freshness, spinal induction, functional species of reflex, all these are physiological factors influencing the result of the interaction of reflex-arcs at a common path. It is noticeable that they all resolve themselves ultimately *into intensity of reaction*. Thus, intensity of stimulus means as a rule intensity of reaction. Those species of reflexes which are habitually prepotent in interaction with others are those which are habitually intense; those specially impotent in competition are those habitually feeble in intensity, e.g. skeletal muscular tone. The tonic reflexes of attitude are of habitually low intensity, easily interfered with and temporarily suppressed by intercurrent reflexes, these latter

Variability of Reflex Reactions

having higher intensity. But these latter suffer fatigue relatively early, whereas the tonic reflexes of posture can persist hour after hour with little or no sign of fatigue. Fatigue, therefore, in the long run advantageously redresses the balance of an otherwise unequal conflict. We can recognize in it another agency working toward that plastic alternation of activities which is characteristic of animal life and increases in it with ascent of the animal scale.

The high variability of reflex reactions from experiment to experiment, and from observation to observation, is admittedly one of the difficulties that has retarded knowledge of them. Their variability, though often attributed to general conditions of nutrition, or to local blood-supply, etc., seems far more often due to changes produced in the central nervous organ by its own functional conductive activity apart from fatigue. This functional activity itself causes from moment to moment the temporary opening of some connexions and the closure of others. The chains of neurones, the conductive lines, have been, especially in recent years, by the methods of Golgi, Ehrlich, Apáthy, Cajal, and others, richly revealed to the microscope. Anatomical tracing of these may be likened, though more difficult to accomplish, to tracing the distribution of blood-vessels after Harvey's discovery had given them meaning, but before the vasomotor mechanism was discovered. The blood-vessels of an organ may be turgid at one time, constricted almost to obliteration at another. With the conductive network of the nervous system the temporal variations are even greater, for they extend to absolute withdrawal of nervous influence. Under reflex inhibition a skeletal muscle may relax to its post-mortem length,[304] i.e. there may then be no longer evidence of even a tonic influence on it by its motor neurone. The direction of the stream of liberation of energy along the pattern of the nervous web varies from minute to minute. The final common path is handed from some group of a *plus* class of afferent arcs to some group of a *minus* class, or of a rhythmic class, and then back to one of the previous groups again, and so on. The conductive web changes its functional pattern within certain limits to and fro. It changes its pattern at the entrances to common paths.[300] The changes in its pattern occur there in virtue of interaction between

Reflex Sequence

rival reflexes, 'interference'. As a tap to a kaleidoscope, so a new stimulus that strikes the receptive surface causes in the central organ a shift of functional pattern at various synapses. The central organ is a vast network whose lines of conduction follow a certain scheme of pattern, but within that pattern the details of connexion are, at the entrance to each common path, mutable. The grey matter may be compared with a telephone exchange, where, from moment to moment, though the end-points of the system are fixed, the connexions between starting points and terminal points are changed to suit passing requirements, as the functional points are shifted at a great railway junction. In order to realize the exchange at work, one must add to its purely spatial plan the temporal datum that within certain limits the connexions of the lines shift to and fro from minute to minute. An example is the 'reciprocal innervation' of antagonistic muscles—when one muscle of the antagonistic couple is thrown into action the other is thrown out of action. This is only a widely-spread case of the general rule that antagonistic reflexes interfere where they embouch upon the same final common paths. And that general rule is part of the general principle of the mutual interaction of reflexes that impinge upon the same common path. *Unlike reflexes have successive but not simultaneous use of the common path; like reflexes mutually reinforce each other on their common path.* Expressed teleologically, *the common path, although economically subservient for many and various purposes, is adapted to serve but one purpose at a time. Hence it is a co-ordinating mechanism and prevents confusion by restricting the use of the organ, its minister, to but one action at a time.*

In the case of simple antagonistic muscles, and in the instances of simple spinal reflexes, the shifts of conductive pattern due to interaction at the mouths of common paths are of but small extent. The co-ordination covers, for instance, one limb or a pair of limbs. But the same principle extended to the reaction of the great arcs arising in the projicient receptor organs of the head, e.g. the eye, which deal with wide tracts of musculature *as a whole*, operates with more multiplex shift of the conductive pattern. Releasing forces acting on the brain from moment to moment shut out from activity whole

Interference and Alliance of Reflexes

regions of the nervous system, as they conversely call vast other regions into play. *The resultant singleness of action from moment to moment is a keystone in the construction of the individual whose unity it is the specific office of the nervous system to perfect.* The interference of unlike reflexes and the alliance of like reflexes in their action upon their common paths seem to lie at the very root of the great psychical process of 'attention'.

Lecture VII

REFLEXES AS ADAPTED REACTIONS

ARGUMENT: Reflexes as adapted reactions. The purposes of various type-reflexes. Shock a difficulty in deciphering the purpose of reflexes. Characters of spinal shock. Its incidence confined to the aboral side of the transection. Its difference in severity in different reflexes and in different animals. Shock referable not to the irritation of the trauma but to the cutting off by the trauma of some supra-spinal influence. Pseudaffective reflexes afford opportunity for determining the pain-path in the spinal cord. This ascends both lateral columns, chiefly the one crossed from side of stimulation. The 'chloroform cry' in decerebrate animals. Mimesis of pleasure as compared with mimesis of pain. The bodily resonance of the emotions. The theory of James, Lange, and Sergi. Emotional expressions in dogs deprived of visceral and largely of bodily sensation.

IT is of course as impossible to disprove as to prove that psychical events accompany, or that they do not accompany, the nervous reactions of the 'spinal' animal. It is significant, however, that the best-known controversy (Pflüger, Lotze) as to the psychical powers of the spinal cord, occurred prior to the advent of the Darwinian theory of evolution. This latter suggests how purposive neural mechanisms may arise. It furnishes a key to the genesis and development of adapted reactions and, among these latter, reflexes.

That a reflex action should exhibit purpose is no longer considered evidence that a psychical process attaches to it; let alone that it represents any dictate of 'choice' or 'will'. In the light of the Darwinian theory every reflex *must* be purposive. We here trench upon a kind of teleology. It is widely and wisely held that natural knowledge pursues the question 'how' rather than the question 'why' The 'why' involves a judgement whose data lie so beyond present human experience and comprehension that self-abnegation in regard to the desire to attempt it is not only prudent, but to the unbiased judgement a necessity. Yet the question has its humbler forms as well as its more general and ambitious.

Older writings on reflex action concerned themselves boldly with

'Purpose' in Reflexes

the purpose of the reflexes they described. The language in which they are couched shows that for them the interest of the phenomena centred in their being regarded as manifestations of an informing spirit resident in the organism, lowly or mutilated though that might be. Progress of knowledge has tended more and more to unseat this anthropomorphic image of the observer himself which he projected into the object of his observations. The teleological speculations accompanying such observations have become proportionately discredited.

Self-wounded in this way physiology became for a time extremely reticent about purpose, remaining simply objectively descriptive.

The impetus given to biology by the doctrine of adaptation under natural selection, felt so strongly by morphological studies, seems hardly as yet to have begun its course as a motive force in physiology. But signs begin to be numerous that such an era is at hand.* The infinite fertility of the organism as a field for adapted reactions has become more apparent. The purpose of a reflex seems as legitimate and urgent an object for natural inquiry as the purpose of the colouring of an insect or a blossom. And the importance to physiology is, that the reflex reaction cannot be really intelligible to the physiologist until he knows its aim.

In general terms we may say that the effect of any reflex is to enable the organism in some particular respect to better dominate the environment. One often hears objection taken to the epithets—common in writings on biology—'lower' and 'higher' as applied to organisms, plant and animal. Such objection seems valid if the phrase assumes that the 'lower' organism any less perfectly fulfils its 'purpose' or 'design' than does the 'higher', or in those respects in which it has commerce with the environment is any less admirably adjusted than is the higher. But 'lower' and 'higher' may be used

---

* Such a 'motif' seems constantly present as an undercurrent in much recent writing in experimental pathology, notably that of Ehrlich in respect to his suggestive 'Antikörper' hypothesis. It is detectable as a principle in the fine researches by Bayliss & Starling. Most definitely and broadly it is expressed in the writings of A. Tschermak,298a especially in the remarkable essay, *Das Anpassungs-problem in der Physiologie der Gegenwart*, and in the contributions of v. Uexküll from the field of invertebrate physiology.

Reflexes as Adapted Reactions

without any connotation of that kind. In the course of evolution a number of organisms have become so adapted to the environment as to dominate it more variously and extensively than do other organisms. In that sense some organisms are higher and some are lower. In that sense man is the highest organism. And if evolution be a process of gradual and more or less uninterrupted course it is obvious that the highest form achieved will also be among the latest of the forms achieved. This grading of rank in the animal scale will be nowhere more apparent than in the nervous system in its office as integrator of the individual. The more numerous and extensive the responses made by a creature to the actions of the world around upon its receptors, the more completely will the bundle of reflexes, which from this standpoint the creature is, figure the complexity of the world around, mirroring it more completely than do the bundles of reflexes composing 'lower' creatures.

The study of reflexes as adapted reactions evidently, therefore, includes reactions of two ranks. With the nervous system intact the reactions of the various parts of that system, the 'simple reflexes', are ever combined into great unitary harmonies, actions which in their sequence one upon another constitute in their continuity what may be termed the 'behaviour' (Lloyd Morgan) of the individual as a whole. Into the intricate 'purposes' (adaptations) traceable in these total reactions which constitute the creature's behaviour as a social unit in the natural economy it is not our part to enter. Our part of the problem is a humbler one. In the analysis of the animal's life as a machine in action there can be split off from its total behaviour fractional pieces which may be treated conveniently, though artificially, apart, and among these are the reflexes we have been attempting to decipher. We cannot but feel that we do not obtain due profit from the study of any particular type-reflex unless we can discuss its immediate purpose as an adapted act.

When we try to assign what we may in this restricted sense call its 'purpose' to any particular reflex, the data for an answer are gathered in the main from one or other of the conditions attaching to the reaction. The *mode* of the adequate stimulus is one of these. The time-relations and spatial form of the response are others. The

Protective Reflexes

broad pressure applied under the foot-pad which seems the adequate stimulus[252] for the 'extensor-thrust' and the brief forcible straightening of the limb which constitutes the response suggest that that reflex has its purpose in the execution of an act in the series of movements of stepping in the animal's locomotion. And the recent analysis of Philippson[309] demonstrates that such an act occurs in the reflex trotting and galloping of the dog. Again, the connexion between the tickling irritative stimuli which seem 'adequate'[252] for the 'scratch-reflex', and the scratching movement itself which results, suggests that the purpose of that reflex is a grooming of the skin to protect that organ against parasites which infest it and would confuse its function as a receptive surface reacting to more significant environmental stimuli.

Grainger's[16] conclusion was that spinal cutaneous reflexes "are either of a preservative character or resemble the movements which the functions of the organ require". From the skin of the spinal creature reflex movements resembling those executed by the normal individual in preening or cleansing itself are of widespread occurrence. Together with the preening actions of the spinal fly,[84] grasshopper, *Astacus*,[178] etc., there fall into this category the movement by which the spinal frog wipes irritants from its back or head; the 'nettoyage' by the tortoise;[176] the posturing of the hind-limbs and tail of the spinal dog concurrently with reflex defecation,[252] tending to keep the body from being soiled; and the 'scratch-reflex' and the 'shake-reflex'[166a] of the spinal dog. The conjunctival reflex protecting the cornea, essentially a cutaneous and from the broad point of view a spinal reflex, is similarly preservative of the part whence it is initiated.

There are of course two modes of preservation, namely, escape and defence. Parts that can move themselves seem reflexly to employ the former. The spinal frog's foot is drawn out of harm's way when irritated; so also in the cat and dog. But parts that cannot of their own motion withdraw themselves effectively seem to invoke defensive movements from adjacent motile parts. The spinal frog's flank, when irritated, is defended by the hind-limb, which comes up and removes the irritant from the flank, the flank itself also

Reflexes as Adapted Reactions

shrinking away somewhat. Similarly in the scratch-reflex, the distant limb is brought up to the defence of the irritated shoulder or flank. There is indeed one, rarely exemplified, group of reflexes in which the organ is sacrificed for the preservation of the rest of the individual. In certain forms, e.g. *Asterias, Cometula, Ophiurus, Arachne, Carcinus*, a limb pulled upon violently or long suddenly ruptures itself and is shed. These actions have been shown by Fredericq to be reflexes, employing muscular contraction. Such reactions exhibit well how absolutely the nervous system is adapted to minister to the requirements of the organism as an integrated whole, and the position of that system as a keystone in the upbuilding of the solidarity of the individual.

But the assignment of a particular purpose to a particular reflex is often difficult and hazardous. The difficulty is inversely as the amplitude of the field covered by the reflex-effect. A slight movement confined to a single limb, or a transient rise of blood-pressure observed alone, is open to many interpretations and admits of no security of inference. It is a fractional reaction that may belong to any of many general reactions of varied aim.

When a reflex is elicited faintly in a spinal animal it occurs simply at the focus, so to say, of its area of distribution, and owing to the restricted character of its features its meaning may be difficult or impossible to read. It is in my experience only by repeated observations of a reflex under various circumstances of its development that as a rule its significance becomes clear. The accessory parts of it are often instructive concerning the whole. In the scratch-reflex of the dog, besides the rhythmic scratching movement of the hind-limb, say of the right, there is steady extension of the left hind-limb, and steady extension with some abduction of the two fore-limbs. The accessory parts of the reflex, namely those in the three limbs which are not scratching, are also contributory to the same effect as in the scratching movement in the right hind-limb itself. They steady the dog and secure the stability of its body during the performance of the scalptor act.

In the 'flexion-reflex' of the hind-limb excited by noxious stimuli, e.g. a prick or a faradic current, the limb itself is drawn up—

Spinal Shock

if weakly, chiefly by flexion at the knee; if strongly, by flexion at hip as strongly as at knee. At the same time the crossed hind-limb is thrown into action, primarily in extension, but this is soon followed by flexion, and alternating extension and flexion is the characteristic result. The rate of this alternation is about twice a second. That is to say, the foot which has stamped on the thorn is drawn up out of way of further wounding, and the fellow hind-limb runs away; and so do the fore-legs when—which is more difficult to arrange, owing to the height of the necessary spinal transection—they also are included, fairly free from shock, within the 'spinal' animal.

SPINAL SHOCK

One of the experimental difficulties in deciphering the purport of a spinal reflex is the phenomenon known as 'shock'. "If in a frog the spinal marrow be divided just behind the occiput, there are for a very short time no diastaltic actions in the extremities. The diastaltic actions speedily return. This phenomenon is 'shock'." (Marshall Hall.[23])

Whytt had, a century previous to Hall, drawn attention to the same phenomenon, although assigning to it no descriptive term. The whole of that depression or suppression of nervous functions which ensues forthwith upon a mechanical injury of some part of the nervous system and is of temporary nature may be conveniently included as 'shock'. Goltz considered it entirely a collection of inhibition phenomena. Among laboratory animals it is in the monkey that, on the whole, 'spinal shock' appears at maximum.

Spinal shock appears to take effect in the aboral direction only.[183,205] Section behind the brachial enlargement disturbs little if at all the reactions of the fore-limb, although the number of headward running channels of conduction ruptured by such a section is enormous. Striking instances of the absence of headward spread of the depression due to 'shock' are afforded by transections abutting on the lower edge of the fifth cervical segment; these depress the respiratory activity of the phrenic motor cells hardly at all, even momentarily. On the aboral side of the transection depression is

Reflexes as Adapted Reactions

profound. Analogously, the sudden cutting off of all that stream of centripetal impulses continually pouring for conscious and subconscious elaboration into the encephalon from the cutaneous, articular, and muscular sense-organs of the tail, limbs, trunk, and neck, and from the viscera, seems to disturb the reactions of the head and brain little or not at all.

After high cervical transection, 'shock' appears more severe in the fore-limbs than in the hind. For an hour or so it may be difficult to elicit any reflex movement from skin innervated behind the transection, whether by mechanical, thermal, or electrical stimuli.

The view of Goltz and his school that 'spinal shock' is a long lasting inhibition due to irritation by *trauma* is not, I think, really tenable. The argument implies, if it does not explicitly state, that the trauma, by its damage and by its subsequent processes of inflammatory reaction, formation of scar-tissue, etc., acts as a stimulus, exciting inhibition that depresses or suppresses reflex activity in adjacent and even remote arcs of the central nervous system. Against this explanation militate several facts. First, the shock takes effect almost exclusively in the aboral direction. Were the mere irritative action of the trauma the cause, it is not easy to see why the nervous centres near the trauma should not be depressed on either side of a spinal transection—for instance headward as well as backward. Secondly, experiments of the following kind give results difficult to reconcile with the view. When in the dog complete transection of the spinal cord through the eighth cervical segment is practised, a severe fall in the general arterial blood-pressure ensues, and vasomotor reflexes cannot be elicited. But in the course of some days this is largely recovered from, and after some weeks the blood-pressure will, with the animal in the horizontal position, often be found practically normal. When the animal is then anaesthetized and curarized, artificial respiration being maintained, it is usually easy to obtain good and often very large vasomotor reflexes, on stimulation of the central ends of divided afferent or mixed nerves, for instance of the internal saphenous nerve, the blood-pressure rising 50 mm. and more (Fig. 67). These reflexes upon the vascular musculature are purely spinal, since the cord has been divided just headward of the

Spinal Vasomotor Reflexes

thoracic region. Then, while these spinal vasomotor reflexes are regularly elicitable and serve as a guide to the reflex activity of the cord behind the transection, I have transected the cord again a couple of segments behind the original transection. This section excites an

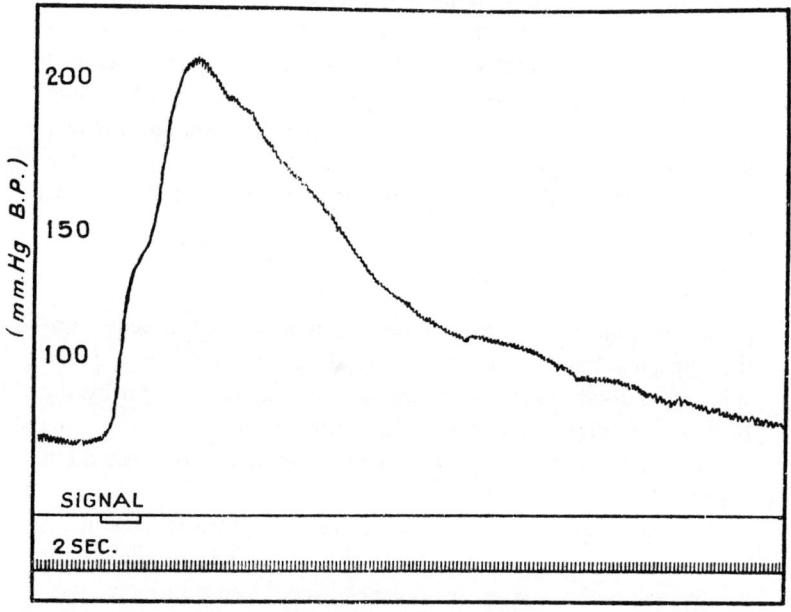

Fig. 67. Spinal vasomotor reflex

Dog: 300 days after spinal transection at 8th cervical level; chloroform and curare.
Records from above downwards:
    Arterial blood-pressure (carotid); scale in mm. Hg.
    Signal line indicates period of electrical stimulation of central end of a digital nerve of the hind-limb.
    Time in 2 sec.
The arterial pressure rises from 90 mm. Hg. to 208 mm. Hg.

immediate transient rise in the arterial pressure, lasting about a minute, and succeeded by a gradual fall. The arterial pressure, then, in my experience sinks to an equilibrium of pressure hardly lower than its mean prior to this second transection. There is none of that deep depression which ensued on the first trauma, though the second

Reflexes as Adapted Reactions

trauma has been practically *qua* trauma a complete repetition of the former one. If the fall of general blood-pressure be regarded as part, and a severe part, of the 'spinal' shock which ensues on spinal transection in the cervical region, the absence of that fall on repeating practically the same trauma must signify that the second trauma is not followed by the shock that followed the first trauma. Moreover, reflex heightenings of blood-pressure such as were regularly obtainable just prior to the second transection are obtainable immediately, i.e. 4 min., after the second spinal transection. The first trauma causes temporary deep depression of the spinal tonus of the vascular system and temporary abolition of vascular reflexes. The second trauma causes practically no depression, even transient, of the re-established tonus of the vascular system nor of the pressor spinal vascular reflexes that have become similarly re-established. It may perhaps be objected that the vascular tonus established subsequent to the first spinal transection is of peripheral mechanism and outside the spinal cord itself. That that is not its main factor is shown by the further deep depression of vascular tonus which occurs when the spinal cord in the thoracic region is itself not merely transected but destroyed.

The trauma *qua* trauma is as severe in the first instance as in the second. In these experiments, therefore, the 'shock' is not due to the trauma *qua* trauma. It seems to depend simply on solution of continuity of nervous channels, and this solution is practically equally great whether the actual trauma itself be relatively slight (a clean, sharply cut transection) or relatively severe (a contused and jagged transrupture), so long as in the two cases it involves an equal amount of the transverse area of the cord. The practical absence of spinal 'shock' on repetition of the trauma farther back is explicable by its then causing little further aggravation of the interruption of the nervous channels concerned with vascular tone and vascular reflexes, those channels having already been ruptured by the previous transection somewhat farther headward.

Similarly the flexion-reflex of the hind-limb, though it suffers considerably from shock after transection of the cord in the hinder cervical or thoracic region, when it has recovered is but little, and

Spinal Shock

but briefly, depressed by a second transection made behind the previous. In this case also trauma does not, therefore, account for the spinal shock. The shock following the trauma is proportioned not to the mere wound, but to the number and character of the descending nerve-paths through which the lesion breaks. Porter's[157a] well-known experiment on the respiratory intraspinal path from the bulb to the phrenic neurones points to the same conclusion.

There remains the further question as to whether spinal 'shock' is a phenomenon of inhibition. A reflex during its depression by spinal shock does not present the features it shows when reduced by inhibition so much as features resembling those characteristic of it when fatigued. The scratch-reflex under spinal shock (Figs. 68, 69) shows irregularity of rhythm, slow protracted relatively feeble beats, and speedy onset of temporary inexcitability, features which characterize it when nearly tired out (compare Figs. 62, 63, Lect. VI). So also with the flexion-reflex of the leg: in the period of depression by spinal shock the reflex is feeble even under strong excitation, is relatively short-lasting, and on cessation of the exciting stimulus shows little of the prolonged after-discharge that it is prone to show at other times: it also tires out then with abnormal rapidity. The scratch-reflex in spinal shock of pronounced degree fails to be elicitable by electrical stimulation at all, though still elicitable by rubbing. This indicates the greater efficacy of a stimulus more nearly like the adequate.

The condition of the spinal reflex-arcs in spinal shock appears to resemble a general spinal fatigue rather than an inhibition. It renders difficult and uncertain the process of conduction along the reflex-arc as judged by the discharge from the terminal neurone. This suggests a loosening of nexus between the links of the neurone-chain composing the arc; a defect of transmission at the synapse. Such a conception of the disorder accords well with the suggestion of v. Monakow[241] that a *diaschizis* takes place between the conducting cells, his 'schaltzellen' failing to perform their normal function as connecting elements.

I think, therefore, that spinal shock is neither due to irritation by trauma, nor in the main a phenomenon of inhibition. The rupture of

Reflexes as Adapted Reactions

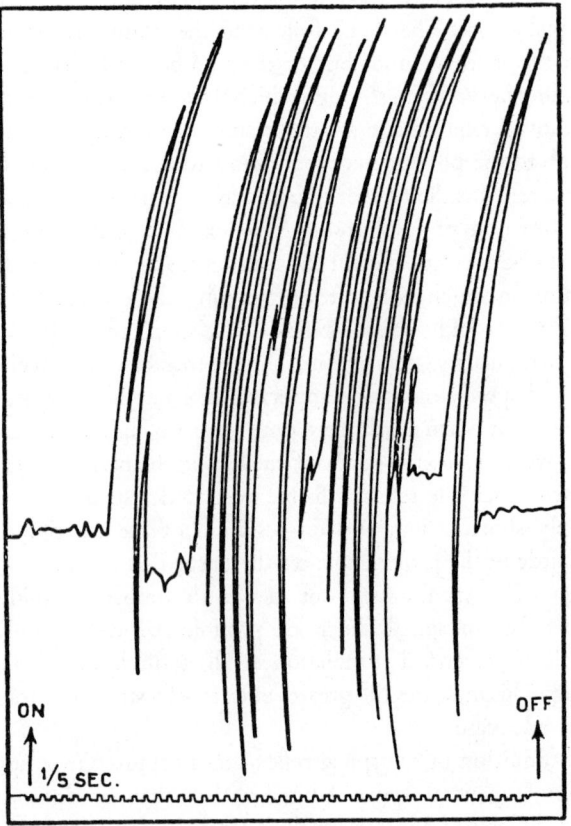

Fig. 68. Scratch-reflex under 'spinal shock'

Spinal transection 6 weeks previously. The reflex was elicited by vigorous mechanical stimulation, electrical stimulation being, as is usual under shock, unable to evoke it. The reflex is slow to appear, feeble and irregular, and lapses during the continuance of the stimulation. The small waves on the base line are due to the vigorous rubbing necessary to evoke the reflex at all, and are simply mechanically conveyed to the limb attached to the myograph. Arrows ON and OFF represent onset and cessation of stimulus for scratch-reflex.
Time in $\frac{1}{5}$ sec.

Spinal Shock

certain aborally conducting paths appears to induce it. Which these paths exactly are is matter for research. After cervical transection separating the cord from the bulbar vasomotor centre, the phenomenon might be attributable to the invariably severe fall of general arterial pressure. But this cannot be the chief explanation, for: (1) the head does not participate in the 'shock', although participating in the low blood-pressure; (2) with post-thoracic transection,

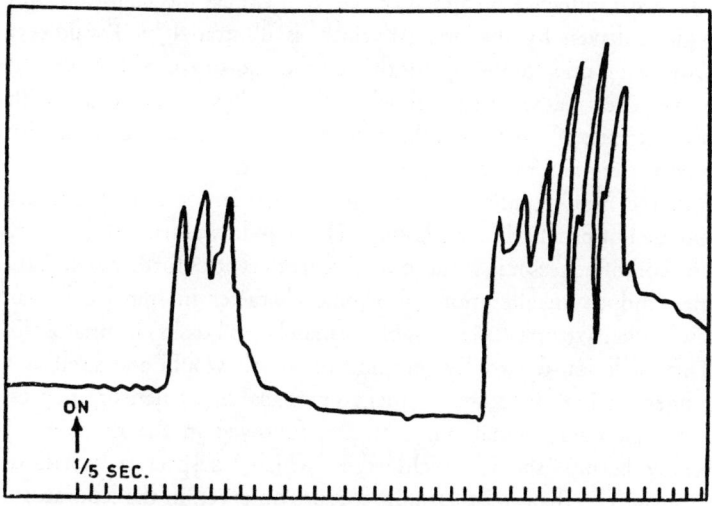

Fig. 69. Scratch-reflex under 'spinal shock'

The scratch-reflex, as in the previous figure, but obtained under still deeper depression of spinal shock.

Arrow ON indicates onset of period of mechanical excitation (to elicit scratch-reflex) which is continued throughout the time of the tracing.

Time in ⅕ sec.

the body region distal to the spinal lesion exhibits shock as severe as after cervical transection, though there is no fall of blood-pressure; (3) transection anterior to the bulbar vasomotor centre but posterior to the pons leaves the blood-pressure unreduced but the spinal shock severe.

The shock is more profound in the monkey than in other animals observed in the laboratory. This might suggest a cerebral origin for

Reflexes as Adapted Reactions

the paths implicated. But ablation of the hemispheres does not induce anything like the depth of spinal depression induced by transections behind the pons. The much severer character of the depression when the transection passes behind the pons indicates an aborally directed influence from some nucleus of the pontine or mid-brain system, driven probably by the great cranial receptors of otic labyrinth and eye, reinforced by impulses from the cord itself. The great influence on spinal centres of a cranial mechanism in this region, driven by the otic labyrinth, is illustrated by Ewald's[137] proposed name 'tonus labyrinth' for the end-organ of the octavus nerve. The great severity of shock in the monkey would accord with high exercise of function of this apparatus in an animal endowed with such variety and range of skeletal movement.

In the monkey and in man spinal shock is not only peculiarly intense but peculiarly long lasting. The withdrawal from the isolated cord of influences it is wont to receive from centres further headward may induce an alteration of trophic character in spinal cells—an 'isolation dystrophy'[183]—visible, it may be, as Nissl's chromatolysis. This 'isolation-dystrophy' ensuing on shock would add itself as a longer lasting in some elements perhaps a permanent, depression. Certainly spinal transection is followed in the monkey by longer lasting 'shock'—included in which I suspect is 'isolation-dystrophy'—than in other animal types observed in the laboratory. My results in monkeys bore out that which Bastian,[129] Bowlby,[131a] and Bruns,[140] contrary to previous observers, have described as the typical condition in man after spinal injury completely severing the cord. Thus, I found the knee-jerk sometimes inelicitable during a month or so after midthoracic transection in the monkey, whereas in the rabbit its abeyance lasts usually but ten minutes or a quarter of an hour.

It is noteworthy that spinal shock takes effect on just those tissues which *waste* when the synaptic nervous system is destroyed—namely the skeletal muscles. Where the primitive diffuse nervous system, the nerve-net, exists, as in the visceral and vascular musculature, neither 'spinal shock' nor atrophy occur consequently to spinal transection. In the skeletal muscles the 'spindles' do not waste.[153]

Spinal Shock

Jamin found that the disuse-wasting of the muscles in spinal dogs which had been daily exercised in reflex actions in my laboratory was much less than in other dogs he examined. The organs on which 'shock' falls least heavily are those which suffer least even after exsection of the spinal cord itself.

The deeper depression of reaction, into which the higher animal, as contrasted with the lower, sinks when made 'spinal', appears to me [194] significant of this, that in the higher types, more than in the lower, the great cerebral senses actuate the motor organs and impel the motions of the individual.

'Spinal shock' does not fall upon all reflexes with equal severity. Noci-ceptive reflexes suffer relatively slightly. In the dog, after spinal transection in the posterior part of the cervical region, the reflexes acting on the muscles of the hind-limb show less severe and shorter-lasting depression in regard to the flexion-reflex and in regard to the scratch-reflex than to the extensor-thrust. That may explain why a number of observers have not obtained any homonymous reflex of extension in the spinal mammal. The crossed extension-reflex, which is really a part of the great reflex of which homonymous flexion is the more prominent feature, recovers from spinal shock earlier than does the extensor-thrust.

There is variability in the order of recovery of the various spinal reflexes of the dog from spinal shock. Occasionally the scratch-reflex returns as early as the flexion-reflex. Although usually in the hind-limbs of the spinal dog no extensor rigidity develops, in some individuals it does so. The limbs are kept extended at knee and ankle even to a degree that it is difficult to break through by the inhibition accompanying elicitation of the flexion-reflex on stimulation of the foot. It is not difficult to see how this may come about. Some incidental circumstance determining the preponderance of some passive attitude of the limbs during the early days succeeding the lesion may, by its influence on the interaction of the recovering spinal arcs, impress an unwonted reflex habit upon the limbs. It is not uncommon to find, especially in the spinal monkey, I think, differences in the reflex condition of the right and left limbs, even although the spinal transection has given a perfectly symmetrical

Reflexes as Adapted Reactions

spinal lesion. Such inequality or dissimilarity of the spinal reflexes right and left does not necessarily afford any evidence that the spinal lesion is asymmetrical. Intercurrent circumstances suffice to impress slightly different reflex habits on the two limbs, and in one and the same individual the reflex habits of each limb may vary somewhat from period to period (cf. Lewandowsky on the production of hemiplegic contracture).

LOCAL SIGN IN REFLEXES

The *locus* of the stimulus plays an important part in determining the nature of the reflex evoked. This influence of the location of the stimulus on the resulting reflex movement has been one of the features most studied in reflex action. It furnishes a large part of the direct evidence of the 'purposive' character of spinal reflexes.*

The rule of spatial proximity given above partly expresses the influence of this factor. Much that was mentioned regarding long irradiation illustrates it further. Though the importance of the *locus* is high when broadly taken, it does not appear obvious as attaching to small differences of location in a more or less homogeneous receptive field or area. Yet in such a field the reflexes, though similar, are demonstrably not identical.[183] In the spinal monkey, excitation of the outer edge of the planta causes dorsi-flexion at ankle, and in doing so generally brings the peronei into play more than is the case when the flexion is excited from the inner edge of the planta; then tibialis anticus predominates, causing some inversion. In the frog, excitation of the skin of the dorsal aspect of the knee, and of the ventral aspect respectively, alike evoke flexion at hip, knee, and ankle, but in the former case the foot is somewhat everted, in the latter somewhat inverted. We must allow that the centripetal impulses, although they yield no sensation, yet possess, to borrow a term from the psychologist, 'local sign'. In the naked eye Medusa,

* The 'rule of spatial proximity' offers an explanation for many of those minor differences obtaining in broadly similar reflex movements, there being a tendency for the muscles belonging to the immediate spinal vicinity of the skin stimulated to respond in preponderant degree; similarly in the scratch-reflex.

Local Sign in Reflexes

called on account of its localizing reflexes *Tiaropsis indicans*,[72] the manubrium deflects itself towards the stimulated part of the nectocalyx; its tip is brought with precision to meet the concurrently contracted inbent portion of the nectocalyx. If one point of the nectocalyx be irritated, and while the manubrium is applied to that point, then another, the manubrium will leave the first point and move over to the second. In this way it may be made to indicate successively a number of points of irritation. "After a series of such irritations the manubrium subsequently continues for some time to visit first one and then another of the points which have been irritated."[72] A cut between the base of the manubrium and the point of irritation in the bell destroys the localization, though movement occurs toward some part of the quadrant of the bell containing the site of stimulus; but the accuracy of the localization is reduced. The reaction recalls the bending of the tentacles of *Drosera*[62] in the direction needful to reach the seat of stimulation on the leaf. The headless bee stings in response to stimulation of the under-surface pretty accurately at the site of irritation.[178] In the 'spinal' crayfish, if one leg is caught it is flexed and drawn up, and if the leg is not released, all the others are soon brought round it and push at the hand holding the limb.[79a] The yellow clover-fly will, after decapitation, stand cleaning its wings with its hind-legs, and clean its "three pairs of legs, rubbing them together in a determined manner, and raising its fore-legs vainly in air as if searching for its head to brush up".[84] But in *Astacus* the accuracy of localization is much impaired on the crossed side by cutting the cross commissures combining the ganglia most closely concerned with the reaction.[185] This recalls the effect of the tangential cut in the nectocalyx of *Tiaropsis*.[72]

In a reflex reaction exhibiting 'local sign' in the above sense, the afferent impulses involved are divisible into several groups according to their place of origin. There must be (1) a group originated at the seat of stimulus, (2) a group initiated in the motor and mobile organs reflexly set in action, and (3) in some cases a group arising at the distant spot to which the movement is directed. Regarding this last group, an experiment illustrates its extinction without extinction of the 'local sign'. Thus, in *Astacus*,[79a] after section of the nerve-cords behind the mouth, when, therefore, the hind creature without mouth has lost all nervous connexion with the front creature possessing the mouth, food given to the claws of the hind creature is still at once and accurately carried by them to the mouth, and this latter may refuse to take the morsel brought. In the grasshopper,[178a] after extirpation of the supra- and sub-oesophageal ganglia (entire brain), the front leg is protracted, and in the normal way catches the antenna, and the usual movements of cleaning the antenna go on, although the antenna has entirely lost its innervation owing to the destruction of the brain. Regarding the second mentioned group of afferent impulses, H. E. Hering[162] has made the interesting observation that the 'cleansing' reflex of the spinal frog which brings the foot to a seat of irritation on the dorsal or perineal skin is accurately executed after severance of the afferent spinal roots of the limb itself. In the same way the bulbo-spinal frog brings the fore-limb to the snout when the snout is stimulated after section of the afferent roots of the fore-limb. The scratch-reflex I find executed without obvious impairment of direction or rhythm when all the afferent roots of the scratching hind-limb have been cut through. In the execution of these spinal reflexes, therefore, the most important afferent factor as regards 'local sign' is the afferent channel from the place of *initiation* of the reflex.

PSEUDAFFECTIVE REFLEXES

If we turn to reflex-effects excited by nocuous stimulation of the skin but having for their field of development a wider conjunction of reflex-arcs and consequently a wider mechanism of reflex expression, the reflex response seems to indicate yet more clearly the 'purpose' of the reflex.

If from the cat under deep chloroform narcosis the cerebral hemispheres and part of the thalami be removed, on relaxing the narcosis a number of motor reactions can be observed against the background of *decerebrate rigidity*.[182] Among these reactions are some mimetic movements simulating expression of certain affective states. These 'pseudaffective' reflexes Woodworth and myself[275] have endeavoured to use for elucidation of the spinal path conducting

Pseudaffective Reflexes

those impulses that, were the brain intact, would, we may presume, evoke 'pain'. The search for such a path is, as regards channels from skin, a search for a path as specific as those of the special senses. The truncation of the brain of the mammal at the mesencephalon annihilates the neural mechanism to which the affective psychosis is adjunct. But it leaves fairly intact the reflex motor machinery whose concurrent action is habitually taken as outward expression of an inward feeling. When the expression occurs it may be assumed that, had the brain been present, the feeling would have occurred. Pain is the psychical adjunct of a protective reflex. A spinal translesion which prevents occurrence of the expression in response to a stimulus that previously excited the expression has therefore been regarded by us in the following experiments to be such as would, were the brain present, induce analgesia in regard to that stimulus. Even apart from that assumption, it is clear that such a lesion can be used for determining the conducting path of a noci-ceptive reaction. The spinal path concerned with the forward transmission of these impulses can therefore be designated not merely a headward path, but, having regard to the character of the reaction, the headward path for *nociceptive* (p. 227) reactions.

The reflex-effect observed has presented the following elements: diagonal cyclic movements of the limbs as in progression (sometimes producing progression), turning of head and neck toward the point stimulated; opening of the mouth, retraction of the lips and tongue, movement of the vibrissae; snapping of the jaw; lowering of the head; opening of the eye-lids, dilatation of the pupils; vocalization angry in tone (snarling), sometimes plaintive; and with these a transient increase of arterial blood-pressure. These reactions appear not only in combination, but sometimes singly or in small combinations. The most readily elicitable are movements of the vibrissae, opening of the mouth with retraction of the tongue, and lowering of the head; but though in some cases vigorous and prompt they never amount to an effective action of attack or escape. A characteristic feature of their ineffectiveness is their brief duration. The movement, even when most vigorous and prompt, dies away rapidly, to be succeeded in some cases by a few weaker repetitions, each in succession

Reflexes as Adapted Reactions

weaker and more transient than the last. Thus, the movements of the head may recur three or four times in response to a single stimulus, or the vocalization be repeated in a diminishing series for a minute or so.

Our method has been to compare by means of the above reaction the effect of two stimuli symmetrically but successively applied on opposite sides of the body, after a semisection or other lesion of the spinal cord headward of the entrance of the nerve-path stimulated.

After semisection at the 13th thoracic level the pseudaffective reaction was obtained by stimulation of either sciatic trunk, but more vigorously and promptly from the nerve of the side of the semisection: from this nerve also the reaction was evoked by weaker faradization. This indicates that the headward pathway taken by the impulses eliciting the vocal and other pseudaffective reactions is from the hind-limb both crossed and uncrossed, but is more largely crossed. From our experiments we are able to exclude the dorsal spinal column as the main path of conduction. Section of both dorsal columns made no appreciable difference in the reaction to the stimulus; neither did faradization of them evoke the reaction. The median portion of the ventral column has sometimes been trespassed on in making the semisection of the opposite side; this extension of the lesion has not prevented the reaction from occurring. In one case the whole grey matter of both halves of the cord was found at the autopsy to be heavily infiltrated and ploughed up with extravasated blood at the level of the semisection and for several millimetres both ahead and behind it. It must have been largely, if not completely, thrown out of function. Yet the pseudaffective reaction remained very brisk.

If, therefore, neither the dorsal nor the ventral column nor the grey matter affords the pathway for the noci-ceptive (algesia) impulses, the lateral column alone is left to them. This conclusion is confirmed by direct experiment. After transection of one lateral column alone the pseudaffective reaction is elicited from either lateral half of the body behind the lesion; after further section of the opposite lateral column, all pseudaffective reaction at once ceases to be elicitable from either half of the body behind the lesion. It is probable that in the posterior thoracic and lumbar segments this

Spinal Path for Pain

headward path is that already signalized by A. Fröhlich and myself[222] as inhibiting, under direct faradization, the rigidity of the triceps brachii in the decerebrate cat.

We concluded from our observations (1) that the *lateral* column furnishes the headward path in the spinal cord for noci-ceptive (algesic) arcs; (2) that each lateral column conveys such impulses from *both* lateral halves of the body, and somewhat preponderantly those from the crossed half; and (3) that this is true for these arcs whether they be traced from *skin, muscles,* or *viscera*.

It is noteworthy that the 'chloroform' or 'ether cry', that peculiar vocalization emitted by men and animals during certain stages of anaesthetization, was often uttered[275] by decerebrate cats during the continued administration of the anaesthetic after decerebration. This vocalization does not necessarily mean an imperfect anaesthetization or any persistence of consciousness, since in our animals the whole cerebrum and the "tween'-brain had been ablated when the administration of the vapour still evoked the vocalization typically.

The crying of the young infant has been noticed in hemicephalic children to be strong and of usual character even in total absence of the cerebrum and mid-brain (Sternberg & Latzko[267]). These malformed infants seem to react as do normal of the same age to stimuli that, judging from adult experience, are unpleasant. They cry or whimper, pucker the mouth, and retract the head. The drawing down of the angles of the mouth and the drawing down of the lower lip seem indicative of pain: pouting of the lips—a mimetic movement common also in the young gorilla, chimpanzee, and macaque—seems to indicate displeasure. Nothnagel and others incline to regard the optic thalamus as the seat of the nerve-centres of mimetic expression. Experiments on animals and the observations on hemicephalic children just referred to seem to contradict this. But we must remember that various *grades* of mimetic movements exist—and some seem phylogenetically much older than others. The congenital have to be distinguished from those that are acquired. The mimesis of the infant is not that of the adult. The latter may depend on the thalamic region; much of the former seems to be a reaction for which neither the fore-brain nor mid-brain are necessary. In the

Reflexes as Adapted Reactions

decerebrate cat we could never evoke such mimesis as might, had the cerebrum been present, have been indicative of pleasurable sensation. Never, for instance, could purring be elicited, although its opposite, snarling, was obtained so easily. The decerebrate dogs observed by Goltz[135] responded to almost all forms of skin stimulus by growling, as if in resentment. Thus, they did so when lifted from their cage to be fed each midday. No mimesis indicative of pleasure was ever obtained from them. Pain centres seem to lie lower than pleasure centres. As far as I can find from reference to books and the experience of colleagues, 'pain' is unknown as an *aura* in cortical epilepsy, or at least is of equivocal occurrence. No region of the cortex cerebri has been assigned to pain. Such negative evidence gives perhaps extraneous interest to the ancient view, represented in modern times by Schopenhauer, that pleasure is an absence of pain.

BODILY RESONANCE OF EMOTIONS

Some sensations are neutral or devoid of affective tone, while others are rich in affective tone. The development of these latter is closely connected with the origin of the coarser emotions. A physiological interest attaches to these states of emotion since certain reactions of the bodily organs are, as is well known, characteristic of them. That marked reactions of the nervous arcs regulating the thoracic and abdominal organs and the skin contribute characteristically to the phenomena of emotion has been common knowledge from time immemorial.

To this bodily resonance of the emotions has in recent years been assigned by some authorities a prominent role in the mechanism of the production of the emotional state itself in certain of the coarser emotions. Instead of the emotional state beginning, as Ladd[213] puts it, as "a sort of nerve storm in the brain, whence there descends an excitement which causes commotion in the viscera and vascular regions—thus secondarily inducing an organic reverberation"—the view has been advanced that the cerebral and psychological processes of emotion are secondary to an immediate reflex reaction of vascular and visceral organs of the body suddenly excited by certain stimuli of peculiar quality.

Bodily Resonance of Emotions

Of points where physiology and psychology touch, the place of one lies at 'emotion'. Built upon sense-feeling much as cognition is built upon sense-perception, emotion may be regarded almost *as* a 'feeling'—a feeling excited, not by a simple little-elaborated sensation, but by a group or train of ideas. To such compound ideas it holds relation much as does 'feeling' to certain species of simple sense-perceptions. It has a special physiological interest in that certain visceral reactions are peculiarly colligate with it. Heart, blood-vessels, respiratory muscles, and secretory glands take special and characteristic part in the various emotions. These viscera, though otherwise remote from the general play of psychical process, are affected vividly by the emotional. Hence many a picturesque metaphor of proverb and phrase and name—'the heart is better than the head', anger 'swells within the breast', 'Richard Cœur de Lion'. It was Descartes[1] who first promoted the emotions to the brain. Even last century Bichat wrote:[9] "The brain is the seat of cognition, and is never affected by the emotions, whose sole seat lies in the viscera." But the brain is now thought to be a factor necessary in all higher animals to every mechanism whose working has consciousness as an adjunct.

What is the meaning of the intimate linkage of visceral actions to emotional psychical states? To the ordinary day's consciousness in the healthy individual the life of the viscera contributes little at all, except under emotion. The perceptions of the normal consciousness are rather those of outlook upon the circumambient universe than inlook into the microcosm of the 'material me'. Yet heightened beating of the heart, blanching or flushing of the blood-vessels, the pallor of fear, the blush of shame, the Rabelaisian effect of fright upon the bowel, the secretion by the lachrymal gland in grief, all these are prominent characters in the pantomime of natural emotion. Visceral disturbance is evidently a part of the corporeal expression of emotion. The explanation is a particular case in the problem of movements of expression in general. The hypothesis of evolution afforded a new vantage point for study of that question. The bodily expressions of the 'coarser or animal emotions' are largely common to man and higher animals. This point of view is exemplified by

Reflexes as Adapted Reactions

Darwin's argument[50] concerning the contraction of the muscles round the eyes during screaming. "Children, when wanting food or when suffering in any way, cry out loudly, as do the young of most animals, partly as a call to their parents for aid, and partly from any great exertion serving as relief. Prolonged screaming inevitably leads to the engorging of the blood-vessels of the eye; and this will have led at first consciously and at last habitually to the contraction of the muscles round the eyes in order to protect them."[50] Herbert Spencer wrote:[85] "Fear, when strong, expresses itself in cries, in efforts to hide or escape, in palpitations and tremblings; and these are just the manifestations which would accompany an actual experience of the evil feared. The destructive passions are shown in a general tension of the muscular system, in gnashing of the teeth and protrusion of the claws, in dilated eyes and nostrils, in growls: and these are weaker forms of the actions that accompany the killing of prey." In short, the bodily expressions of emotion are instinctive actions reminiscent of ancestral ways of life.

They must have an explanation the same in kind as that of other instinctive movement. There is no real break between man and brute even in the matter of mental endowment. The instinctive bodily expressions of emotion arose, in the opinion of those quoted above, as attitudes and movements useful to the animal for defence, escape, seizure, embrace, etc. These as survivals have become symbolic for states of mind. Hence an intelligible nexus between the muscular attitude, the pose of feature, etc., and the emotional state of mind. But between action of the viscera and the psychical state the nexus is less obvious. This latter connexion adds a difficult corollary to the general problem.

The fact of the connexion is on all hands admitted, but as to the manner of it opinion is at issue. Does (1) the psychical part of the emotion arise and its correlate nervous action then excite the viscera? Or (2) does the same stimulus which excites the mind excite concurrently and *per se* the nervous centres ruling the viscera? Or (3) does the stimulus which is the exciting cause of the emotion act first on the nervous centres ruling the viscera, and *their* reaction then generate visceral sensations; and do these latter, laden with affective

Emotional Expression

quality as we know they will be, induce the emotion of the mind? On the first of the three hypotheses the visceral reaction will be secondary to the psychical, on the second the two will be collateral and concurrent, on the third the psychical process will be secondary to the visceral.

To examine the last supposition first. It is a view which in recent years has won notable adherents. Professor James[124] writes:* "Our natural way of thinking about these coarser emotions (e.g. 'grief, fear, rage, love') is that the mental perception of some fact excites the mental affection called the emotion, and that this latter state of mind gives rise to the bodily expression. My theory, on the contrary, is that *the bodily changes follow directly the perception of the exciting fact, and that our feeling of the same changes as they occur IS the emotion. ... Every one of the bodily changes, whatsoever it be, is FELT acutely or obscurely, the moment it occurs.* If the reader has never paid attention to this matter, he will be both interested and astonished to learn how many different local bodily feelings he can detect in himself as characteristic of his various emotional moods. ...If we fancy some strong emotion and then try to abstract from our consciousness of it all the feelings of its bodily symptoms we find we have nothing left behind, no 'mind-stuff' out of which the emotion can be constituted, and that a cold and neutral state of intellectual perception is all that remains. ...If I were to become corporeally anaesthetic, I should be excluded from the life of the affections, harsh and tender alike, and drag an existence of merely cognitive or intellectual form."

Professor Lange[106a] traces the whole psycho-physiology of emotion to certain excitations of the vasomotor centre. For him, as for Professor James, the emotion is the outcome and not the cause or the concomitant of the organic reaction; but for him the foundation and corner-stone of the organic reaction is as to physiological quality vascular, namely, vasomotor. Emotion is an outcome of vasomotor reaction to stimuli of a particular kind. This stimulus induces a vasomotor action in viscera, skin, and brain. The change thus induced in the circulatory condition of these organs induces changes in the actions of the organs themselves, and these latter evoke sensations

* The italics and emphasizing capitals are quoted as in the original.

Reflexes as Adapted Reactions

which constitute the essential part of emotion. It is by excitation of the vasomotor centre, therefore, that the exciting cause, whatever it chance to be, of emotion produces the organic phenomena which as felt constitute for Lange the whole essence of emotion. The teaching of Professor Sergi[152, 177] closely approaches to that of Lange.

The views of James, Lange, and Sergi have common to them this, that the psychical process of emotion is secondary to a discharge of nervous impulses into the vascular and visceral organs of the body suddenly excited by certain peculiar stimuli, and that it depends upon the reaction of those organs. Professor James's position in the matter is, however, not wholly like that of Professor Lange. In the first place, he does not consider vasomotor reaction to be primary to all the other organic and visceral disturbances that carry in their train the psychological appanage of emotion; and Professor Sergi, though more nearly in harmony with Lange, agrees with James so far. In the second place, Professor James seems to distinctly include other 'motor' sensations and centripetal impulses from musculature other than visceral and vascular, among those which causally contribute to emotion. Thirdly, he urges his theory as one completely competent only for the 'coarser' emotions, among which he instances 'fear, anger, love, and grief'. For Lange and Sergi the basis of apparition of all feeling and emotion is physiological, visceral, and organic, and has its seat for the former authority exclusively, and for the latter eminently, in the vasomotor system.

To obtain some test of this view is not difficult by experiment.[213a] Appropriate spinal and vagal transection removes completely and immediately the sensation of the viscera and of all the skin and muscles behind the shoulder (Fig. 70). The procedure at the same time cuts from connexion with the organs of consciousness the whole of the circulatory apparatus of the body. I have had under observation dogs in which this has been carried out. I will cite an animal selected because of markedly emotional temperament. Affectionate toward the laboratory attendants, one of whom had her in charge, toward some persons and toward several inmates of the animal house she frequently showed violent anger. Her ebullitions of rage were sudden. Their expression accorded with a description furnished by

Mechanism of Emotional State

Darwin.50 Besides the utterance of the growl, "the ears are pressed closely backwards, and the upper lip is retracted out of the way of the teeth, especially of the canines". The mouth was slightly opened and lifted, the eyelids widely parted, the pupils dilated. The hair along

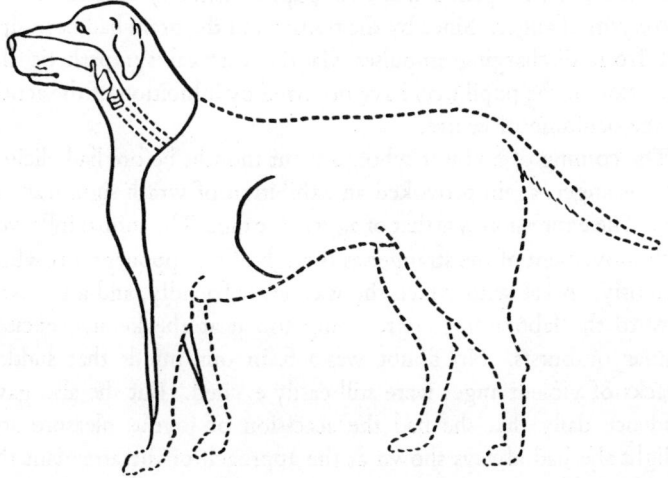

Fig. 70. Diagram to indicate the extent of the parts still retaining sensitivity after combined spinal and vagosympathetic nerve sections described in the text

The extent of skin surface left sentient is delimited by the continuous (not dotted) lines in the figure. The limit of 'deep', i.e. muscular, articular, etc., sensitivity also corresponds with this line. But the limit to which the respiratory and alimentary tracts still retained sensation is shown by dotted outlines of the larynx and upper part of oesophagus. From anatomical data it is presumed that the trachea and oesophagus had been deprived of all sensitivity somewhere about those levels. The curved line behind the chest indicates the diaphragm as the only muscle behind the shoulder still retaining afferent nerves.

the mid-dorsum, from close behind the head to a point more than half-way down the trunk, became rough and bristling.

The reduction of the field of sensation in this animal by the procedure above mentioned produced no obvious diminution of her emotional character. Her anger, her joy, her disgust, and when provocation arose, her fear, remained as evident as ever. Her joy

Reflexes as Adapted Reactions

at the approach or notice of the attendant, her rage at the intrusion of a cat with which she was unfriendly, remained as active and thorough. But among the signs expressive of rage the bristling of the coat along the back no longer occurred. On the other hand, the eyes were well opened and the pupils distinctly dilated in the paroxysm of anger. Since by the transection the brain had been shut out from discharging impulses via the cervical sympathetic the dilatation of the pupil may have occurred by inhibition of the action of the oculomotor centre.

The coming of a visitor whose advent months before had elicited violent anger, again provoked an exhibition of wrath significant as ever. The expression was that of aggressive rage. The animal followed each movement of the stranger as though of an opponent, growling viciously. A cat with which she was never friendly, and a monkey new to the laboratory, approaching too near the kennel, excited similar outbursts. No doubt was left in our minds that sudden attacks of violent anger were still easily excited. But she also gave evidence daily that she had the accession of joyous pleasure and delight she had always shown at the approach of the attendant the first thing of a morning, or at feeding time, or when caressed by him, or encouraged by his voice.

Few dogs, even when very hungry, can be prevailed upon to touch dog's flesh as food. Almost all turn from it with signs of repugnance and dislike. I had strictly refrained from testing this animal previously with regard to disgust at dog's flesh offered in her food. Flesh was given her daily in a bowl of milk, and this she took with relish. The meat was cut into pieces rather larger than the lumps of sugar usual for the breakfast table. It was generally horse-flesh, sometimes ox-flesh. We proceeded to the observation thus: the bowl was placed by the attendant in the corner of the stall with milk and meat in every way as usual; but the meat was flesh from a dog killed on the previous day. Our animal eagerly drew itself toward the food; it had seen the other dogs fed, and evidently was itself hungry. Its muzzle had almost dipped into the milk before it suddenly seemed to find something there amiss. It hesitated, moved its muzzle about above the milk, made a venture to take a piece of the meat, but

Disgust

before actually seizing it stopped short and withdrew again from it. Finally, after some further examination of the contents of the bowl (it usually commenced by taking out and eating the pieces of meat), without touching them, the creature turned away from the bowl and withdrew itself to the opposite side of the cage. Some minutes later, under encouragement from us to try the food again, it returned to the bowl. The same hesitant display of conflicting desire and disgust was once more gone through. The bowl was then removed by the attendant, emptied, washed, and horse-flesh similarly prepared and placed in a fresh quantity of milk was offered in it to the animal. The animal once more drew itself toward the bowl, and this time began to eat the meat, soon emptying the dish. To press dog's flesh upon our animal was of no real avail on any occasion; the coaxing only succeeded in getting her to, as it were, re-examine but not to touch the morsels. The impression made on all of us by the dog's behaviour was that something in the dog's flesh was repulsive to her, and excited disgust unconquerable by ordinary hunger. Some odour attaching to the flesh seemed the source of its recognition.

It would be instructive for judging the part played by the cerebral hemisphere in the reactions of coarser emotion did we know whether repugnance to dog's flesh as food would be exhibited by a dog after ablation of the cerebral hemispheres. Even the primitive emotions seem to involve perception—seem little other than sense-perceptions richly suffused with affective tone. Goltz's[135] dogs after ablation of the hemispheres evinced signs of hunger, namely restlessness when their feeding hour was deferred. When a little quinine (bitter) was added to the sop of meat and milk the morsels taken into the mouth were at once rejected. No inducement or scolding modified this unfailing and unhesitating rejection. Goltz adds that he threw to his own house dog a piece of the same doctored meat. The creature wagged its tail and took it eagerly, then pulled a wry face, and hesitated, astonished. But on a look of encouragement from its master the dog swallowed it. He overcame his instinctive rejection of it, and thus, as Goltz remarks, by his self-control gave proof of the intact cerebrum he possessed.

Fear appeared clearly elicitable (as also in dogs with spinal cervical

Reflexes as Adapted Reactions

transection only, Fig. 71). The attendant approaching from another room of which the door stood open, chid the dog in high scolding tones. The creature's head sank, her gaze turned away from her

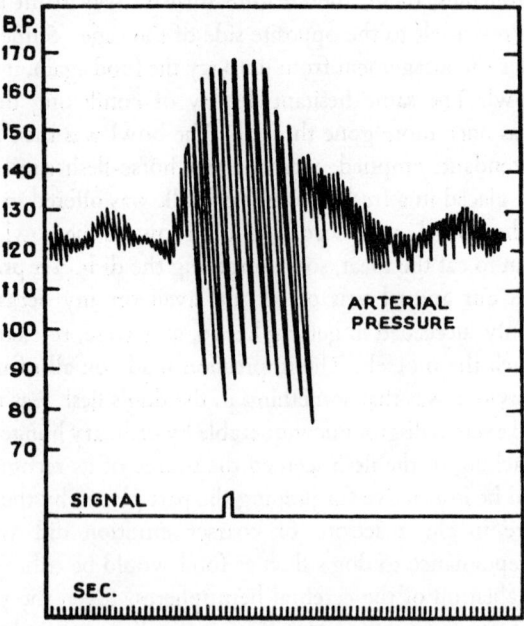

Fig. 71. Vascular reflexes under spinal shock

Record of the arterial pressure in a dog 41 days after spinal transection at the 7th cervical segment. The arterial pressure is high and good in spite of the transection, the period of vasomotor shock having passed by. For the short period marked by the signal the noise of the vibrator of an inductorium sounded and was heard by the animal. The point of the signal marked nearly 8 mm. farther to the right than did the kymograph pen. The inhibition of the heart is shown by the oscillations on the kymograph trace.

Scale on left indicates level of blood pressure in mm. Hg.

advancing master, and her face seemed to betray dejection and anxiety. The respiration became unquiet, but the pulse never changed its rate.

In the dog, after transection of the spinal cord, the regions of the body which have been thus made purely 'spinal' continue their life

Mechanism of Emotional State

in many respects normally. The hairy 'coat' changes in spring. The oestral periods recur even when the transection is performed in puppyhood, and altogether headward of the spinal origin of the sympathetic system, e.g. at the cervical segment. Goltz[58] observed successful impregnation, parturition and suckling completed without obvious abnormality. In my own observations[213a] the natural instinct of the female toward the male at oestrum was seen indubitably displayed after the spinal cord had been transected in the cervical region more than a year previously.

It may be objected to these experiments that although the animals expressed emotion they may yet have *felt* none. Had their expression been unaccompanied by, and had they not led on to, trains of acts logically consonant with their expressed emotion, that objection would have weight. Where the *facies* of anger is followed by actions of advance and attack with all appearance of set purpose, I find it difficult to think that the perception initiating the wrathful expression should bring in sequel angry conduct and yet have been impotent to produce 'angry feeling'.

A weaker point in such experimentation is that although the visceral and vascular and much of the muscular mechanism of emotional expression was cut off, a small but notable fraction of the latter, namely the facial, still remained open to react on the centres with which consciousness is colligate.

Nevertheless, in view of these observations the vasomotor theory of the production of emotion becomes, I think, untenable, also that visceral sensations or presentations are *necessary* to emotion. A mere remnant of all the non-projecting or affective senses was left, and yet emotion persisted. If I understand it aright, Professor James's and Lange's theory lays stress on organic and visceral presentations, but re-presentations of the same species might no doubt be put forward in their place. That would be a different matter. To exclude the latter hypothesis, the deprivation of vascular and organic sensation might have to date from a very early period of the individual life. Professor Lloyd Morgan writes[216a] in respect to the above experiments, "The avenues of connexion were closed *after* the motor and visceral effects had played their part in the *genesis* of the emotion on

Reflexes as Adapted Reactions

the hypothesis that the emotion is thus generated. Although new presentative data of this type were thus excluded, their re-presentative after-effects in the situation were not excluded." But it is noteworthy that one of the dogs under observation had been deprived of its sensation when only nine weeks old. Disgust for dog's flesh could hardly arise from the experience of 9 weeks of puppyhood in the kennel.

We are forced back toward the likelihood that the visceral expression of emotion is *secondary* to the cerebral action occurring with the psychical state. There is a strong bond between emotion and muscular action. Emotion 'moves' us, hence the word itself. If developed in intensity, it impels toward vigorous movement. Every vigorous movement of the body, though its more obvious instrument be the skeletal musculature of the limbs and trunk, involves also the less noticeable co-operation of the viscera, especially of the circulatory and respiratory. The extra demand made upon the muscles that move the frame involves a heightened action of the nutrient organs which supply to the muscles the material for their energy. This increased action of the viscera is colligate with this activity of muscles. We should expect visceral action to occur along with the muscular expression of emotion. The close tie between visceral action and states of emotion need not therefore surprise us.

That emotion is primarily a cerebral reaction obtains support from observations where the hemispheres of the brain have been removed. Goltz observed a dog kept many months in that condition. It on no occasion gave any evidence of joy or pleasure in commerce either with man or beast. Of sexual emotion it never gave a sign. Anger or displeasure, Goltz says, it repeatedly expressed, both by gesture and by voice. Save for these expressions of displeasure, it was indifferent and supremely neutral to its surroundings. We are, of course, in observations such as this, hopelessly cut off from introspective help. It can be urged that the expression of emotion might be provocable and nevertheless the psychical emotion remain absent. On such an hypothesis the same stimulus which excited the mind must excite concurrently and *per se* motor centres producing movement appropriate to an affective process in the mind. This is not

Bodily Reinforcement of Emotion

improbable. All sensations referred *to the body itself, rather than interpreted as qualities of objects in the external world*, tend to be tinged with 'feeling'. Sense-organs which initiate sensations tinged with feeling tend to excite motor centres directly and imperatively. Hence in animals reduced to merely spinal condition stimuli calculated to produce pain (although, of course, unable to do so in a spinal animal) evoke movements appropriate for escape from or removal of the stimulus applied. Now 'feeling' is implicit in the emotional state; the state is an 'affective state'. In the evolution of emotion the revival of 'feelings' pleasurable and painful must have played a large part. Hence the close relation of emotion with sense-organs that can initiate bodily pain or pleasure, and hence its connexion with impulsive or instinctive movement. There is no wide interval between the reflex movement of the spinal dog whose foot attempts to scratch away an irritant applied to its back—both leg and back absolutely detached from consciousness—and the reaction of the decerebrate dog that turns and growls and bites at the fingers holding his hind foot too roughly. In the former case the motor reaction occurs, although the mind is not even aware of the stimulus, far less percipient of it as an irritant. The action occurs, and plays the pantomime of feeling; but no feeling comes to pass. In the latter case the motor reaction occurs and is expressive of emotion; but it is probably the reaction of an organic machine which can be started working, though the mutilation precludes the psychosis.

And with the gesture and the attitude will occur the visceral concomitant. It would be consonant with what we know of reflex action, if the spur that started the muscular expression should simultaneously and of itself initiate also the visceral adjunct reaction. It is almost impossible to believe that with the mere stump of brain that remained to Goltz's dog there could be any elaboration of a percept. All trace of memory seemed lacking to the creature. Yet, though not evincing other emotion, anger it showed as far as expression can yield such revelation. Fear, joy, affection seem, therefore, in the experience of this skilled observer of animal behaviour, to demand higher nervous organization than does anger. Be that as it may, the retention of its expression by Goltz's dog

Reflexes as Adapted Reactions

indicates that by 'retrogradation' the complex movement of expression has in certain emotions passed into a simpler reflex-act: Under the canalizing force of habit the determining motives become, even in impulsive acts, weaker and more transient. The external stimulus originally aroused a strongly affective group of ideas, which operated as a motive, but now it causes a discharge of the act before it can be apprehended as an idea. The impulsive movement of a 'lower', 'coarser', so-called 'animal' emotion, has in this case become an automatic reflex no longer necessarily combined with the psychical state whence it arose, of which it is normally at once the adjunct and the symbol.

In view of these general considerations and of the above experiments, we may with James accept visceral and organic sensations and the memories and associations of them as contributory to primitive emotions, but we must regard them as reinforcing rather than initiating the psychosis. Organic and vascular reaction, though not the actual excitant of emotion, strengthen it. This is the kernel of the old contention about actuality of emotion in the art of the artist. Hamlet's description of the actor as really moved by his expression may be accepted as an answer.

Conversely, as Lloyd Morgan[216a] writes: "Whatever be the exact psychological nature of the emotions, it may be regarded as certain that they introduce into the conscious situation elements which contribute not a little to the energy of behaviour." A feeling of pain and a protective reflex movement—either of defence or escape—are concurrent in the reaction of an animal to a hurtful stimulus of the skin. Reflexes to which emotion is adjunct are not only prepotent (Lect. VI) but are imperative, that is, volition cannot easily suppress them. Now, the morphological disposition of the nervous channels is such that the physiologist can, by suitable severance of the spinal path to the brain, sunder the reflex movement from the sensation, leaving the former effect but perforce annulling the latter. The former is, however, in absence of the latter, not left unaltered; it is abnormally reduced, especially in duration (vide supra, p. 253). The pseudaffective reactions indicative of resentment and defence are, after ablation of the cerebral cortex, short-lived, the

Emotional Reaction

simulacra of mere flashes of mimetic passion. No cerebral reverberation descends to prolong and develop further the protective movement set going as a spinal reflex. This contrasts strongly with the fairly normal course that the headward part of the reflex, after loss of its vascular and visceral fields, runs. The difference argues that the reverberation from the trunk, limbs, and viscera counts for relatively little, even in the primitive emotions of the dog, as compared with the cerebral reverberation to which is adjunct the psychical component of emotional reaction.

Lecture VIII

SOME ASPECTS OF THE REACTIONS OF THE MOTOR CORTEX

ARGUMENT: Remarkable that electrical stimuli applied to the organ of mentality yield with regularity certain localized movements from certain restricted areas of its surface. Functional topography of 'motor' cortex in the chimpanzee, orang-utan, and gorilla. The cerebral fissures, not functional boundaries. The anthropoid ape has a direct pyramidal tract like that of man. Recovery of function not due to symmetrical part of opposite hemisphere taking on supplemental work. Inhibition as elicitable from the cortex. Reciprocal innervation of antagonistic eye-muscles. Reciprocal inhibition in other muscular groups. Seat of the inhibition subcortical in these cases. Reciprocal innervation in willed movements. Preponderant representation in the 'motor' cortex of the same movements as are preponderantly elicitable as local reflexes from the cord and bulb. Scanty representation of certain movements as cortical and local spinal reactions alike. Appearance under strychnine and tetanus toxin of these movements reversing the normal direction of the preponderance. This due to these agents transmuting reciprocal inhibition into excitation. *Decerebrate rigidity.* A system of tonic innervation in action. Strychnine and tetanus toxin augment this innervation. Hughlings Jackson's 'co-operative antagonism' of paired systems of innervation, one tonic, the other phasic. Decerebrate rigidity and hemiplegic rigidity. The relation of the cortex to receptor organs; the pre-eminent representation in it of the 'distance-receptors'.

WE shall now venture a glance at certain reactions of the cerebral hemisphere itself; our survey must be circumscript for several reasons. By use of such methods as we are employing, artificial excitation and so on, and under such observations as these allow, namely the initiation under narcosis of muscular movements or the recording of their immediate defects from normal movement, little light is given in regard to much that goes on in an organ whose chief function is mentality itself. Our expectation must be modest, for modest assuredly must be the achievement reached by such means in a problem of such a nature. The very poverty of the achievement is itself an indication that the methods pursued by the physiologist successfully in other spheres of his study are here confronted with

Functional Topography

problems to which they are far less suited. It is not that I esteem lightly the labours of the many distinguished workers in this field. As far as the methods referred to can avail, it is to the skill with which they have been used that we owe what knowledge we have of the topographical representation of movement in the various fields of cerebral cortex. We have only to remember how much more numerous the physiological facts concerning the cerebral cortex are to-day than prior to the experiments of Fritsch & Hitzig[47] and of Ferrier,[51] following on the observations of Broca,[29] Hughlings Jackson,[35] and Bastian.[46] Experiment had failed to get evidence of localization of function in the cortex of the hemispheres, though in microscopic structure that great sheet of grey matter presents such similarity to nervous formations regarded as nerve-centres elsewhere. Progress of knowledge in regard to the nervous system has been indissolubly linked with determination of localization of function in it. This has been so from the time of the Bell[10]-Magendie[11] discovery of the difference of function in the two spinal roots, and Flourens's[19] delimitation of the respiratory centre in the bulb. The discovery of localization of function in parts of the cortex has given the knowledge which now supplies to the student charts of the functional topography of the brain much as maps of continents are supplied in a geographical atlas. The student looking over the political map of a continent may little realize the complexity of the populations and states so simply represented. We looking at the brain chart of the textbook may never forget the unspeakable complexity of the reactions thus rudely symbolized and spatially indicated.

If we may be allowed an *a priori* consideration it is this—that although it is not surprising that such territorial subdivision of function should exist in the cerebral cortex, it is surprising that by our relatively imperfect artifices for stimulation we should be able to obtain clear evidence thereof. The neurone chains that together build up the nervous system are in the architecture of that system so arranged that the longest of them all tend to pass through the cerebral cortex. Every increase in the number of links composing a nerve-cell chain seems to increase greatly the uncertainty of its reactions under artificial excitation. With increase in number of links goes

Reactions of the Motor Cortex

increase in numbers of side branches and connexions. The difficulty of getting long chains of nerve-cells to react in a regular way under artificial stimulation seems greatly enhanced by the multiplication of the side connexions. The momentary condition of any cell-chain is in part a function of the condition at the moment of all the other cell-chains with which it is connected. The cortex cerebri might therefore well have been expected to yield under artificial stimulation only extraordinarily inconstant results. To Hitzig and Fritsch, and to Ferrier, we owe the pregnant demonstration that as regards the motor region this expectation is not well founded.

It is only of the reactions of the Rolandic area of the cortex that I shall venture to speak. Ferrier showed that the application of faradic currents to that cortex excites with great regularity movements which vary in distribution as the electrodes are moved from place to place, but remain within limits constant under repeated application of the stimulus to any one and the same spot. Ferrier's mode of indicating the topographical arrangement of the reactions he obtained is seen in his well-known diagrams of the cortex. His motor centres, as he termed them, were marked in his figures by circular areas. "The areas have no exact line of demarcation from each other, and where they adjoin stimulation is apt to produce conjointly the effect peculiar to each."[70] He showed these motor centres to extend forward over the frontal lobe, producing there movements of the eyeballs. Regarding their extension round and over the upper edge of the hemisphere and down upon the mesial surface he noted them in the marginal convolution. "This convolution in the parieto-frontal region gave rise to movements of the head and limbs apparently similar to those already obtained by stimulation of the corresponding regions on the external surface."[70]

This original research by Ferrier ranks among the classics of experimental neurology and physiology. It has been followed by a number of kindred contributions from workers whose names are familiar to us all: Albertoni, Schäfer, Munk, Luciani, Tamburini, Paneth, Beevor, Horsley, Mott, Ballance, Mann, and others. The detailed knowledge of the localization has been largely based on the cerebral cortex of the common ape, the macaque. It was an interesting

Anthropoid Motor Cortex

step further when Beevor and Horsley[127] published observations on the localization of the motor functions in the central cortex of an orang-utan. Their experiment long remained the single one for which an anthropoid species had been laid under contribution. It exercised a notable influence on the scheme of motor localization adopted as probably obtaining in the brain of man.

Of the three or four species of anthropoid apes that are known, most authorities agree that it is the gorilla which possesses the most highly developed cerebrum; next to it probably stands the chimpanzee, and a little below the chimpanzee comes *Simia satyrus*, the orang-utan. But there are great individual differences, and the simpler examples of chimpanzee brains seem inferior in development to well-developed examples of the brain of the orang.

A. S. Grünbaum[225,229] and myself have obtained observations on cerebral localization in the several species of anthropoid apes. In the chimpanzee the scheme of topography we find existent is illustrated by the accompanying Figs. 72 and 73.

The so-called motor area occupies unbrokenly the whole length of the precentral convolution, and in most places the greater part or the whole of its width. It extends into the depth of the central sulcus, occupying the anterior wall, and in some places the floor, and in some extends even into the deeper part of the posterior wall of the fissure. We have examined more than forty hemispheres, but have never found the motor area extend indubitably to the free face of the post-central convolution. This delimitation agrees remarkably with the original results obtained by Hitzig[53] on the brain of the monkey, *Innuus rhesus*.

At the upper mesial edge of the hemisphere the motor area extends round and down upon the mesial face of the hemisphere, but we have not found it reach the calloso-marginal fissure. The anterior limit of the motor region is in great part not coincident with any fissure. The front portion of the region usually dips into and across the upper part of the superior precentral fissure, and lower down it not infrequently dips into the inferior precentral fissure. Occasionally the front edge of the region dips into almost the whole length of the superior precentral sulcus. It is not the extent of the motor area which

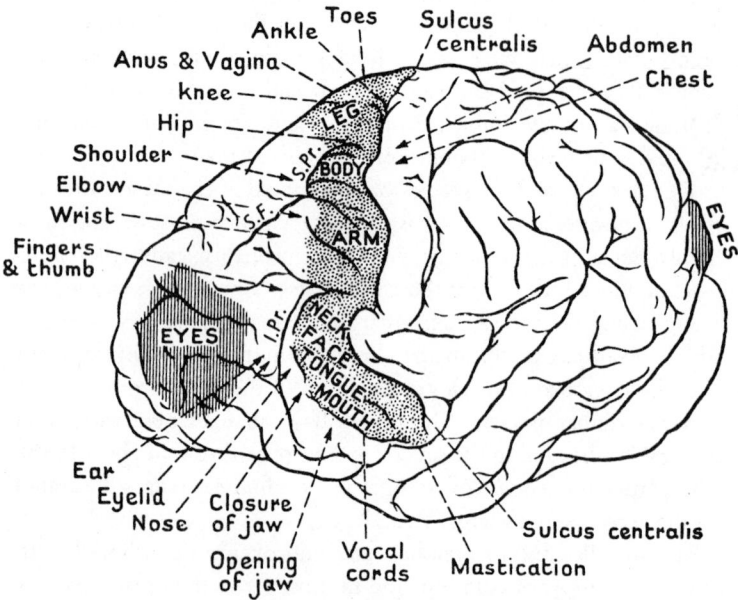

Fig. 72 (from Grünbaum & Sherrington). Brain of a chimpanzee (*Troglodytes niger*)

Left hemisphere viewed from side and above so as to obtain as far as possible the configuration of the *sulcus centralis* area. The figure involves, nevertheless, considerable foreshortening about the top and bottom of *sulcus centralis*. The extent of the 'motor' area on the free surface of the hemisphere is indicated by the black stippling, which extends back to the *sulcus centralis*. Much of the 'motor' area is hidden in sulci; for instance, the area extends into the *sulc. centralis* and the *sulc. precentralis*, also into occasional sulci which cross the precentral gyrus. The names printed large on the stippled area indicate the main regions of the 'motor' area; the names printed small outside the brain, indicate broadly by their pointing lines the relative topography of some of the chief subdivisions of the main regions of the 'motor' cortex. But there exists much overlapping of the areas and of their subdivisions which the diagram does not attempt to indicate.

The shaded regions, marked 'EYES', indicate in the frontal and occipital regions respectively the portions of cortex which, under faradization, yield conjugate movements of the eyeballs. But it is questionable whether these reactions sufficiently resemble those of the 'motor' area to be included with them. They are therefore marked in vertical shading instead of stippling (as is the 'motor' area).

S.F. = superior frontal sulcus. S.Pr. = superior precentral sulcus.
I.Pr. = inferior precentral sulcus.

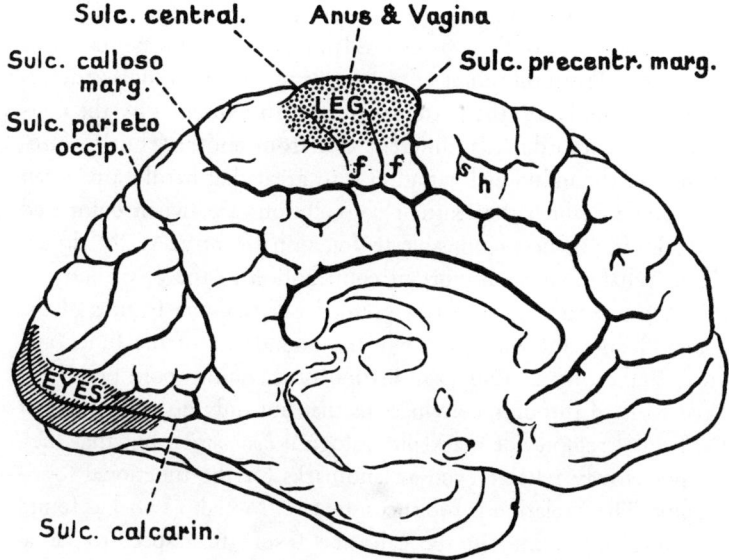

Fig. 73 (from Grünbaum & Sherrington). Brain of a chimpanzee (*Troglodytes niger*)

Left hemisphere; mesial surface. The extent of the 'motor' area on the free surface of the hemisphere is indicated by the black stippling. On the stippled area, 'LEG' indicates that movements of the lower limb are directly represented in all the regions of the 'motor' area visible from this aspect. So much mutual overlapping of the minuter subdivisions exists in this area that the diagram does not attempt to exhibit them. The pointing line from 'Anus, etc.', indicates broadly the position of the area whence perineal movements are primarily elicitable.

Sulc.central. = central fissure. *Sulc.calcarin.* = calcarine fissure. *Sulc.parieto occip.* = parieto-occipital fissure. *Sulc.calloso marg.* = calloso-marginal fissure. *Sulc.precentr. marg.* = precentral fissure.

The single italic letters mark spots whence, occasionally and irregularly, movements of the foot and leg (*f*), of the shoulder and chest (*s*), and of the thumb and fingers (*h*) have been evoked by strong faradization. Similarly the shaded area marked 'EYES' indicates a field of free surface of cortex which under faradization yields conjugate movements of the eyeballs. The conditions of obtainment of these reactions separates them from those characterizing the 'motor' area.

Reactions of the Motor Cortex

appears to be variable, the variant is the sulcus itself. The great variety of individual pattern exhibited by the convolutions and sulci in these richly convoluted brains gives opportunity for studying critically the claim of value of these fissures as landmarks in the topography of the cortex. From this point of view their use for strict localization is small. Not only are the extremes of pattern exhibited by the convolutions extraordinarily different one from another, but the frequency of the individual variation is so great that hardly a pair can be found in which the existent convolutions are, when compared with the minuteness applicable to functional centres, really closely alike. Schäfer, in his important contribution to the physiology of the motor cortex in 1887,[111a] pointed out that the fissures of the cortex do not mark in any sense the boundaries of the functional areas of the organ. Our examination of the anthropoid brains we have worked through, convinces us that not only do the fissures of the frontal region not mark physiological *boundaries*, but that they are not closely reliable even as landmarks for the functional topography. Their relation is too inconstant. v. Monakow[241] has found the same uncertainty in the calcarine fissure in respect to visual cortex. The degree to which these fissures are subject to individual variation and the frequency of their asymmetry in the two hemispheres stands in contrast with the constancy from individual to individual and greater bilateral symmetry which holds good for the arrangement of the functional centres. A practical outcome of this is that it is essential for accurately detailed localization, when the opening through the skull is of moderate size, not to trust to the anatomical details of the exposed cerebral surface, but to obtain orientation in the topography by application of the electrodes and observation of the movement, if any, which is excited. In our early experiments we thought to obtain much help by having at hand a brain of the same species already experimented upon and thought to save time in recording the results of the fresh experiment upon chart outlines prepared from the specimen already worked upon. But the variation of the convolutions from individual to individual has been too great to allow of these expedients. As an exception to the above general rule two landmarks of relative constancy are the genua of

Topography in the Chimpanzee

the sulcus centralis—the Rolandic fissure. In the chimpanzee and gorilla the genua are two (Fig. 72); the upper, opposite the junction between leg area and arm area, may be termed the cruro-brachial; the lower, between arm area and face area, may be termed the brachio-facial. In the orang there is in addition a third genu, which from its relation to the functional topography may be called the labio-lingual. In the orang the facial area of the cortex is considerably longer from above down than in the chimpanzee or gorilla.

It is a general belief that for excitation of the cortex in man there is needed an intensity of faradism much greater than that sufficing for the cortex of the monkey. Actually comparing the excitability of the cortex of the anthropoid with that of the bonnet monkey by employing exactly the same current in each case, we found the excitability as measured by the least intensity of current required to evoke motor reaction practically the same in the anthropoid and in the lower ape.[225] The motor cortex of the anthropoid, though undoubtedly far more complex in many ways than that of the lower ape, remains as readily amenable to electric stimulation. Cushing of Baltimore and Krause of Berlin find this holds good also for the human brain, and that it is not necessary to employ strong faradization. In the majority of the anthropoids upon which we have experimented cortical epilepsy has been quite easily provoked, just as it is in the small monkeys.

In the precentral gyrus, the sequence of representation of the musculature starting from below upward follows broadly that known for the lower apes. The sequence runs—tongue, jaw, mouth, nose, ear, eyelids, neck, hand, wrist, elbow, shoulder, chest, abdomen, hip, knee, ankle, toes, and perineal muscles. It is noticeable that movements of the eyeballs do not occur in this list. As did Beevor & Horsley[127] in their orang, so we in the chimpanzee, gorilla, and orang find a frontal area extending into the middle and inferior frontal convolutions excitation of which gives conjugate deviation of the eyeballs to the opposite side. We find this area separated by an intervening space from the area yielding the other movements. We find this intervening space broken, however, by small areas whence

Reactions of the Motor Cortex

movements of the eyeballs can be elicited, partially bridging between it and the upper facial region on the precentral convolution.

The sequence of representation of movement which we note follows a plan more in accordance with the order of the spinal series of segments than hitherto obtained. Between the place of representation of shoulder and that of hip is an area which, next to the shoulder, yields unilateral movement of the chest muscles, and, next to the hip, yields unilateral movement of the abdominal muscles, and furthest upward lies a focus for perineal muscles.

In our experience, in accord with the original observations by Hitzig[53] on the lower apes, the electrodes when placed upon the surface of the post-central convolution fail to evoke any obvious effect, though when placed with an even weaker current upon the precentral they evoke the regular reaction. In our experience, though small lesions in the precentral convolution caused marked paralyses and descending spinal degenerations, similar and larger lesions in the post-central did not produce even temporary paralysis nor any unequivocal degeneration.

With regard to the degenerations, it is noteworthy that from a hand-area lesion the spinal pyramidal degeneration shows in some chimpanzees a ventral direct pyramidal tract of size not obviously inferior to that of a man. But this ventral direct tract does not appear to be present in all individual chimpanzees—a fact agreeing with Flechsig's[70a] discovery of its variability in man. The hand-area lesion gives a heavy degeneration of the homolateral tract in the lateral column on the same side as the cerebral lesion.

As regards symptoms resulting from the cortical lesions, extirpation of a great part if not of the whole of the hand area from the right hemisphere caused an immediate severe crossed brachioplegia without the slightest sign of paresis in either face or leg. The paresis affected the fingers most; these were kept helplessly semi-extended, the wrist being dropped. The elbow seemed little if at all affected, but the shoulder seemed distinctly paretic, there being difficulty in raising or abducting the upper arm. The paresis diminished quite rapidly, and in six weeks' time the animal had in large measure recovered the usefulness of the limb.

Results of Lesions of Motor Cortex

A lesion in the leg-area similarly caused temporary paresis of the opposite leg, especially in the toes and at the ankle-joint. The lesion was smaller and the recovery more rapid than with the arm-area lesion. The knee-jerk, which showed no alteration under the arm-area lesion, here showed exaltation immediately, that is, a quarter of an hour after the leg-area lesion. Weeks later, when the paresis to inspection had passed off, the knee-jerk still exhibited greater briskness on the crossed side.

We have seen often confirmed what our predecessors[127] with the orang have well pointed out, namely, the greater integration of localized representation of movements in the anthropoid as compared with the lower ape. There is not one of the fingers that we have not seen move separately and alone under excitation of certain points of the cortex; again, isolated movement of the pinna of the ear, of the tip of the tongue, rare in the lower monkeys, are easily obtainable in the anthropoid.

As to the extent of the so-called motor area, from our observations we think it probable that in the anthropoid brain as much of that area lies hidden from the surface in the sulci as is actually exposed on the free surface on the convolutions. Nevertheless we endorse the opinion expressed by Beevor & Horsley that the so-called motor area in the anthropoid brain forms a smaller fraction of the total surface than it does in the lower types of monkey. If it has grown in extent—as undoubtedly it seems to have done—other regions belonging to those so-called 'silent' fields whence electric stimulation excites no obvious response have increased still more. It is especially with the exploration of that great inexcitable field that research has to deal. The discoveries of Flechsig, v. Monakow, Déjerine, Mott, Campbell, the Vogts, and others yearly advance further in the problem.

The results on the gorilla[225] confirm those we have obtained on the chimpanzee, though in the gorilla and orang in my experience eyeball movements have been elicited from a larger field of the frontal cortex than in the chimpanzee, an upper area yielding eye movement on a level with the hand area being more readily discoverable.

Reactions of the Motor Cortex

We have not found that the free surface of the post-central convolution belongs to the motor cortex. Brodmann[256a] and Campbell[272a] have since called attention to marked structural differences between the cortex respectively behind and in front of the central sulcus. The arrangement of the fibres and the character of the cells is different. Ramon-y-Cajal,[128a] using the Golgi method, and Flechsig[271a] following the myelinization, had also previously drawn distinction between the structure of the two convolutions divided by this great fissure; and observations by Mott, A. Tschermak, and others had indicated an especially close connexion of the post-central gyrus with ascending, presumably afferent, paths. Evidence of this last by excitation methods is of course difficult to obtain, but nothing in our experiments is contrary to it, and some occasional results that have come before me in experimenting by excitation lend themselves to such an explanation. To enter upon these here would lead too far from our main interest now.

It is natural to inquire whether reciprocal innervation is exemplified by reactions from the cortex. That inhibition of muscular contraction is obtainable by artificial excitation of the cortex was early noted by Bubnoff & Heidenhain[92] in the dog and by Exner[99] in the rabbit. I have myself worked chiefly with the monkey.[151, 304] In that animal the ocular axes are parallel, and the setting of the eyeball in the orbit is such that the tensions of its connexions, apart from unequal activity of its extrinsic muscles, are in equilibrium when the globes are approximately parallel. That is their primary position. This can be shown in various ways. Thus, if the III, IV, and VI nerves are all severed the eyeballs assume this primary position. If one eyeball be then rotated by the finger or fixation forceps to right or left, or up and down, a considerable resistance is felt, and on letting it go the globus springs back at once to the primary position. So also in chloroformization. In the early stage of chloroformization the eyes enter various positions of squint—in the monkey a very usual position is bilateral divergence upward and outward. When the narcosis has become profound, the eyes revert to approximate parallelism in the primary position. On being then displaced by the finger they at once swing into the primary median position

Reciprocal Innervation from Cortical Eyefields

again. So also immediately after death, before rigor mortis has set in.

If III and IV cranial nerves of one side, e.g. left, have been severed, so that rectus externus remains the only unparalysed ocular muscle, appropriate excitation of the cortex cerebri produces conjugate movement of both eyes towards the opposite side, i.e. from left toward right, the left eye travelling, however, only so far as the median line. Inhibition of the tonus and of the active contraction of rectus externus can thus be elicited from the cortex. The reaction is obtainable from all that portion of the cortex which on excitation gives conjugate lateral deviation of the eyes, i.e. from the area discovered by Ferrier[70] in the frontal region, and from that discovered by Schäfer & Brown[117a] in the occipital region.

This inhibition is obtainable from the frontal area after complete removal of the occipital lobe. It is conversely obtainable from the occipital area after complete removal of the frontal area. After a deep frontal section across the hemisphere and into the lateral ventricle (partly entering the internal capsule) so as to sever occipital from frontal cortex in the manner practised by Munk & Obregia,[128] the reaction is obtainable undiminished from both the frontal and from the occipital areas separately.

The cortex is not essential to the reaction. It is obtainable from the corona radiata underlying the frontal cortex after complete ablation of the frontal cortex itself. It is obtainable from the corona radiata running downwards and forwards from the occipital cortex after free removal of the latter. It is obtainable by direct excitation of the internal capsule itself. From the internal capsule it is elicitable at two distinct places, one in front, the other behind, the genu of the capsule. It is obtainable by excitation of the cross-section of corpus callosum about 3–5 mm. behind the genu; also from corpus callosum at the splenium. The section was laid bare as in Mott & Schäfer's[121a] second method. The reaction as obtained from corpus callosum has in my hands proved comparatively irregular. It is evident that the action of arrest may take place, in centres which are subcortical.

H. E. Hering & myself[173] made observations on limb movements

Reactions of the Motor Cortex

elicited from the cortex and found evidence of a similar co-ordination in regard to them. As in the experiments of Bubnoff & Heidenhain,[92] the degree of narcotization formed an important condition for the observations. The narcosis must not be too profound. It is best, starting with the animal in a condition of deep etherization, to allow that condition gradually to diminish. As this is done it almost constantly happens that at a certain stage of anaesthesia the limbs, instead of hanging slack and flaccid, assume and maintain a position of flexion at certain joints, notably at elbow and hip. This condition of tonic contraction having been assumed, the narcosis is as far as possible kept at that particular grade of intensity. The area of cortex cerebri previously ascertained to produce under faradization extension of the elbow-joint or hip-joint is then excited.

For clearness of description let us suppose the left hemisphere excited, and the affected limb the right. The result of excitation of the appropriate focus in the cortex, e.g. that presiding over extension of the elbow, is an immediate relaxation of the biceps with active contraction of the triceps. As regards the condition of the biceps, the relaxation is usually so striking that merely to place the finger on it is enough to convince the observer that the muscle relaxes. The following is however a good mode of studying the phenomenon: in a monkey with strongly developed musculature the forearm, maintained by the above-mentioned steady tonic flexion at an angle with the upper arm of somewhat less than 90° is lightly supported by the one hand of the observer, while with the finger and thumb of the other the belly of the contracted biceps is felt through the skin. On exciting the cortex the contracted mass becomes suddenly soft, melting under the observer's touch. At the same time the observer's hand supporting the animal's forearm tends to be pushed down with a force unmistakably greater than that which the mere weight of the limb would exert. If the triceps itself be felt at this time, it is easy to perceive that it enters contraction, becoming increasingly hard and tense, even when its points of attachment are allowed to approximate, and the passive tensile strain in it should lessen. If the limb be left unsupported the movement is one of simple extension at the elbow-joint. On discontinuing the excitation of the cortex the forearm usually immediately, or almost immediately, returns to its previous posture of flexion, which is again as before steadily maintained.

Conversely, when, as not infrequently occurs in conditions of narcosis resembling that referred to above, the arm has assumed a posture of extension and this is tonic and maintained, the opportunity may be taken to excite the appropriate focus in the cortex for flexion of forearm or upper arm. Triceps is then found to relax, and biceps at the same time to enter into active contraction. If the biceps be hindered from actually moving the arm, the prominence at the back of the upper arm due to the contracted triceps is seen simply to sink down and become flattened. When examined by palpation the muscle is felt to become more or less suddenly soft, and the biceps at the same time to become more tense than before. The movement of the limb, when allowed to proceed unhindered, is flexion with some supination. It is noteworthy that in this experiment not every part of the large triceps mass becomes relaxed; a part of the muscle which extends from the humerus to the scapula does not in this experiment relax with the rest of the muscle. This part, if the scapula be fixed, acts as a retractor of the upper arm, and is not necessarily an antagonist of the flexors of the elbow. This part of the triceps we observed sometimes enter active contraction at the same time as the flexors of the elbow. Under use of currents of moderate intensity we found that from one and the same spot in the cortex not only can relaxation and contraction of a given muscle be evoked at different times, but that the two effects are provocable at different, sometimes widely separate, points of the cortex, and are there found regularly.

We obtained analogous results in the muscles acting at the hip-joint. In the narcotized animal with the hip-joint maintained in flexion (the thighs being drawn up on the trunk) excitation of the region of the cortex which was previously ascertained to evoke extension of the hip when the limbs hang slack, now produces relaxation of the flexors of the hip combined with active contraction of the extensors of the thigh. We examined particularly the psoas-iliacus, and the tensor fasciæ femoris, also the short and long adductor

Reactions of the Motor Cortex

muscles. Each of these was found to relax under appropriate cortical excitation. If the knee were held by the observer it was found at the time of relaxation of the flexors of the hip to be forced downward by active extension of the hip.

Similarly with other groups of antagonistic muscles, both those of the small apical joints of the limb, e.g. flexors and extensors of the digits, and those of the large proximal joints, e.g. adductors and abductors of the shoulder. At these also instances of reciprocal innervation were obtained. By antagonistic muscles I mean only what are termed *true* antagonists; I do not include the cases where one muscle fixes a joint enabling another muscle thus to act better on *another* joint—H. E. Hering's pseudoantagonists.[168] Hering[169] has carefully analysed the co-ordination of such pseudoantagonists in the action of clenching the fist. He has shown that when that movement is evoked in the monkey by excitation of the cortex cerebri the extensors of the wrist are thrown into action simultaneously with the long flexor of the fingers. But there was no evidence that the *true* antagonists were ever thrown into simultaneous activity.

That a part of the triceps brachii (that retracting the upper arm) should actively contract exactly when another part (that extending the elbow) becomes relaxed is *exactly* comparable with a phenomenon which can be noted in the limb under spinal reflexes, both in triceps itself and in quadriceps femoris. Beevor and others have shown that different parts of what in gross anatomy is denominated one single muscle are used separately in various movements. And Hering and I similarly saw in the quadriceps femoris, on exciting the cortical region yielding extension of the hip, a relaxation of a part of the quadriceps (a part which flexes the hip) with contraction of another part (which extends the knee). I have also noted that in the monkey by stimulating the appropriate cortical area for flexion of the knee the knee-jerk is temporarily depressed or suppressed completely.

The results obtained from the internal capsule were as striking as those obtained from the cortex itself. From separate points of the cross-section of the capsula, relaxation of various muscles was evoked. Among the muscles whose inhibition was directly observed were supinator longus and biceps brachii, the triceps, the deltoid, the ex-

Reciprocal Innervation from Internal Capsule

tensor cruris, the hamstring group, the flexor muscles of the ankle-joint, and the sternomastoid.

The spots in the cross-section of the capsula which yielded the inhibitions were constant, that is, the position of each when observed remained constant throughout the experiment. The area of the capsular cross-section at which the inhibition of the activity of, e.g. the triceps, muscle can be evoked is separate from (that is to say not the same as) that area whence excitation evokes contraction of the triceps (or of that part of the triceps, inhibition of which is now referred to.) On the other hand, the area of the section of the internal capsule, whence inhibition of the muscle is elicited, corresponds with the area whence contraction of its antagonistic muscles can be evoked. Yet synchronous contraction of such pairs of muscles as gastrocnemius and peroneus longus is obtainable from the cortex. The observations make it clear that *reciprocal innervation* in antagonistic muscles is obtainable by excitation of the fibres of the internal capsule. Topolanski[184] observed them on exciting the corpora quadrigemina (rabbit). It is probable therefore that the inhibition elicitable from the cortex cerebri is not in these cases chiefly or at all due to an interaction of cortical neurones one with another.

Exner drew from his observations on the rabbit a similar inference that the inhibitory phenomena had their chief seat in the spinal mechanisms though elicited from the cortex. My own inference has been that the seat of inhibition in *these* reactions from the 'motor' cortex lies probably at the place of confluence of conducting channels in a common path, likely enough at their confluence upon the *final common path*, the motor neurone—that is at the ultimate synapse. But it may well be, indeed is in the highest degree likely, that in other fields of action one cortical element inhibits another cortical element.

In *willed* movements of the eyeballs of the monkey the same kind of co-ordination was revealed in some observations I obtained on this point. When the III and IV cranial nerves had been resected intracranially and the animals in 10 days or so had recovered completely from the surgical interference, the eye movements were examined.

In these animals if the gaze was attracted to an object, e.g. food,

Reactions of the Motor Cortex

held level with the eyes and to the right of the median plane, the left eye (left III and IV nerves cut) looked straight forward, the right looked to the right. If the object was then shifted more to the right or less to the right, the right eye followed it, moving as the object was moved, while the left eye remained motionless, looking straight forward all the time. But when the object was held to the left of the median plane both eyes were directed upon it, apparently quite accurately. When the object was shifted farther and farther to the left both eyes followed it with a steady conjugate movement not detectably different from the normal. When the object was carried from the left-hand verge of the field back toward the median plane both eyes followed it as accurately as before. If the object was moved suddenly from the extreme left-hand edge of the field up to the median plane both eyes immediately and apparently equally quickly reverted to parallelism with that plane. Or, if the object were suddenly brought back from the left edge of the visual field to some point intermediate between that and the median plane both eyes at once shifted apparently equally to a correspondingly diminished deviation from the primary position. These actions must mean that in the left eye relaxation of rectus externus kept accurate time and step with contraction of rectus externus of right eye. And the action of the left rectus externus gives presumably a faithful picture of a synchronous process going forward in the right rectus internus.

It is interesting to recall that in the seventeenth century Descartes in his *De Homine*,[2] discussing willed movements, suggested for the mechanism of the lateral movements of the eyeball, with which he deals in some detail, a co-ordination much resembling reciprocal innervation. He urged that the vital spirits were conducted into the external rectus by valved channels in that muscle, and at the same time were led out from the internal rectus by valved channels, so that as the one muscle became tense by distension the other became flaccid by emptying. He furnished with his own pencil a figure illustrating the mechanism as he conceived it (Fig. 74). There is an essential resemblance between his scheme and that of 'reciprocal innervation', except that he imagined the mechanism a peripheral

Descartes' Schema of Reciprocal Innervation

one, that is to say that the 'inhibition', as we now term it, had its seat in the muscle, not in the nerve-centres themselves.

Again, early last century (1823) Charles Bell, in a footnote to a paper in the *Philosophical Transactions*,[12] argued a similar kind of co-ordinate mechanism in the execution of willed movements. He wrote: "The nerves have been considered so generally as instruments

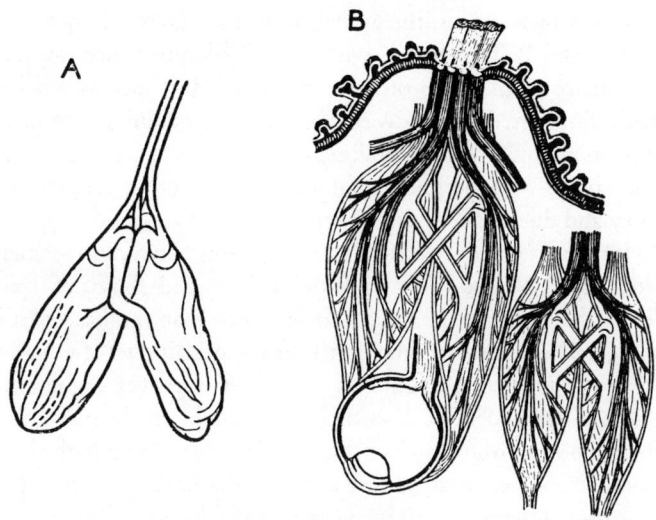

Fig. 74

A. Figure (slightly modified) from the *De Homine* of Descartes, edition of 1662, in which he illustrates his conception of the co-ordination of the antagonistic muscles of the eyeball by the above drawing from his own hand.

B. Figure illustrating the same text in *De Homine*, edition of 1677; in this the sketch by Descartes has been much elaborated.

for stimulating the muscles, without thought of their acting in the opposite capacity, that some additional illustration may be necessary here. Through the nerves is established the connexion between the muscles, not only that connexion by which muscles combine to one effort but also that relation between the classes of muscles by which the one relaxes and the other contracts. I appended a weight to a tendon of an extensor muscle which gently stretched it and drew out the muscle; and I found that the contraction of the opponent flexor

Reactions of the Motor Cortex

was attended with a descent of the weight, which indicated the relaxation of the extensor. ...If such a relationship be established, through the distribution of the nerves, between the muscles of the eyelids and the superior oblique muscles of the eyeball, the one will relax while the other contracts." But like Descartes he pictured a peripheral inhibition, for he says: "If we suppose that the influence of the 4th nerve is, on certain occasions, to cause a relaxation of the muscle to which it goes, the eyeball must then be rolled upwards." Descartes and Bell, therefore, with remarkable prescience imagined the existence of an action of nerve on muscle just such as was later actually discovered by the Webers[21] in the vagal inhibition of the heart—an inhibition which Volkmann[17] previous to the Webers met in the course of experiment, but unexpectant of it, rejected[18] as illusory and due to some experimental error.

As for salient objective differences observable between movements elicited from the so-called 'motor' cortex and those of spinal reflexes, these are for the most part less clear than might at first be supposed. The general statement that the co-ordination is of a 'higher' kind in the former has doubtless truth, but it proves vague when details are demanded. A co-ordination though simple may yet be perfect. The co-ordination by which the leg is drawn up in the spinal 'flexion-reflex' seems as perfect as when the limb is drawn up by stimulation of the cortex. It is true that in the dog's scratching movement elicited as a spinal reflex after transection of the cord the foot in my experience practically never attains accurately the site of the stimulation, although broadly directed toward it. Were the movement elicited from the cortex one would expect it to be more accurate in this respect. But I have never succeeded in eliciting this action from the cortex, and so am unable to institute the comparison.

If by higher co-ordination be meant that larger groups of reflex systems are simultaneously thrown into—or out of—action under cortical excitation than in merely spinal reflexes, that is more than probable. Yet we must admit that the field of musculature thrown into action by a focal stimulation of the cortex seems in some cases extremely limited. Thus A. S. Grünbaum and myself have seen that in the chimpanzee and gorilla any single manual digit can be moved

Cortical and Spinal Reactions Compared

isolatedly by stimulation of the cortex. We must not forget, however, that with even a small *movement* the field of inhibition may yet be wide, for I have on occasion noted inhibition of muscles of the shoulder when the thumb was moved under cortical excitation, the shoulder previously being unrelaxed.

There is the well-known clonic *after-discharge* following cortical stimulation. But a marked after-discharge is also usual in spinal reflexes, rhythmic in rhythmic reflexes, tetanoclonic in tetanic reflexes, e.g. in the 'flexion-reflex', and is sometimes enormously prolonged (Figs. 49 and 57). So that even this difference is less marked than is customarily thought. Certain other differences appear to me more significant. When a spinal reflex is prolonged under strong stimulation its discharge spreads, developing what Dr Hughlings Jackson[35] has termed a 'march'. The 'march' of the spinal reaction tends to *transgress the median line* more than does that of a cortical reaction, which tends rather to spread unilaterally. Also the progress of the spinal 'march' runs a more rapid course than does the cortical.

In the synthesis of movement in the animal it is obvious that these reactions elicitable from the motor cortex fall into three groups, like the three groups above distinguished in spinal reflexes (Lect. IV). In one group the movement evoked from the cortex of one hemisphere seems a fraction of a natural movement, the natural movement requiring in its completeness the co-operation of the symmetrical area of the cortex of the opposite hemisphere. Opening of the jaw as elicited from one hemisphere, e.g. the left, is seen after the jaw is split at the symphysis to be executed by the muscles of the crossed, i.e. right, half of the jaw, the muscles of the left half being very slightly activated or not at all. This cortical movement is evidently incomplete and fractional. The inference is unavoidable that in the natural undeviated opening of the mouth the actions of symmetrical areas of the right and left cortices are coupled as *allied* reactions. In a second group, instanced by conjugate lateral deviation of the eyeballs toward the opposite side, it is equally obvious that the reactions of symmetrical areas of the right and left cortices are related one to another as *antagonistic* reactions. Such reactions

Reactions of the Motor Cortex

have inhibitory relation one to another (pp. 153, 304). They must have this inhibitory relation even when combined, as Mott & Schäfer showed they can be, to yield convergence of the ocular axes under bilateral excitation of the right and left hemispheres. In a third group of cases the reactions of symmetrical cortical areas right and left seem neutral one to another. Thus, with the area which yields movement of the thumb that reaction seems neither to reinforce nor to interfere with the similar reaction evoked from the twin area of the opposite hemisphere. That the reactions are really wholly neutral one to another is of course difficult to say because the experimental observations are carried out under narcosis, and the narcosis probably sets in abeyance many co-ordinating mechanisms of the brain itself. It is clear, however, that the same broad groups of interrelationship (alliance, interference, neutrality) as were traced in bulbospinal reflexes reappear also between motor reactions of symmetrical areas of the cortex of the hemispheres.

It is striking that the complete, i.e. perfectly balanced, bilaterality of motor representation with which the Broca motor speech centre is credited, no doubt justly, is exceptional in the motor cortex. Beevor and Horsley pointed out that movements of perfectly balanced bilaterality are of much rarer distribution in the cortex of the hemisphere than was generally supposed. I incline to think that even the small category of such movements which they admit will have to be reduced further by the removal from it of 'mastication'. Certain it is that for a group of movements to be perfectly bilaterally represented in the area of one hemisphere and not equally in the corresponding area of the other hemisphere, the state of things generally supposed for the Broca centre, is an arrangement wholly unknown in the motor cortex. It shows how different must be the operations of the Broca area from those of the areas of the so-called motor cortex. Grünbaum and myself in excitation experiments could get no evidence of a Broca centre in the anthropoid apes.

One broad resemblance between the movements elicited from the motor cortex and spinal reflexes is striking, and yet is, I think, not insisted on by writers. We have seen that the movements elicitable in the various regions as local reflexes by stimulation of the afferent

Cortical and Spinal Reactions Compared

paths of those regions present regular and characteristic quality. Thus stimuli to a fore-limb induce lifting of that limb with flexion at elbow and retraction-flexion at shoulder; stimuli to a hind-limb induce drawing up of that limb with flexion at knee, hip, and dorsiflexion at ankle; stimuli to the mouth induce opening of the jaws, and so on. While these movements are emphatically evidenced as local spinal reactions the overwhelming predominance of their occurrence equally emphasizes the scarcity of occurrence of certain other movements as local spinal reactions. Extension of the hindlimb can, it is true, be evoked from that limb as a spinal reflex by a certain special form of stimulus, but that stimulus has to be applied to a special part of the foot and is successful only after 'spinal shock' has passed off; while the flexion-reflex can be evoked by various forms of stimuli applied practically to any point of the limb surface, and is elicitable almost from the very hour of spinal transection onward. So also I have occasionally succeeded in evoking closure instead of opening of the jaw by stimulation of a certain part of the lip in the decerebrate animal—but even then the reflex is not regularly elicitable. On the other hand reflex opening of the jaws is easily and regularly elicitable from various points of the oral surface. Similarly extension of the elbow as a local reflex elicitable by stimuli applied to the fore-limb itself is a reflex practically unknown to me.*

Now those movements that are practically wanting as local bulbospinal reflexes and strike the observer of the spinal or decerebrate animal by their default, are likewise practically absent, comparatively infrequent, or only limitedly and irregularly elicitable from the motor cortex itself.[304] On the other hand, the movements regularly and widely elicitable as local reflexes are liberally represented in the motor cortex.[304]

In the light of the observations mentioned above, which show that reciprocal innervation is a mode of co-ordination widely exhibited in the reactions elicitable through the motor cortex, this sparse occurrence of certain movements, e.g. extension of the knee

---

* Extension of elbow and of knee are of course easily obtainable as *crossed* reflexes and as parts of reflexes evoked from distant points. Such reflexes I do not include as *local* reflex reactions.

Reactions of the Motor Cortex

or closure of the jaw, does not mean that the extensor muscles of the knee or the muscles which close the jaws are unrepresented in the cortex. It does not mean that this cortex is in touch with the flexors alone and not with the extensors. It means that the usual effect of the cortex on these latter is *inhibition*. It means not that the extensors and the jaw-closers are unrepresented cortically, but that their normal representation in the cortex under the ordinary conditions of experiment has the form of inhibition, not excitation, and thus unless specially sought escapes observation.

Since, as above shown, strychnine and tetanus toxin transform certain inhibitions into excitations, we have a means of further testing this point. It is in my experience quite exceptional to obtain primary extension of the opposite knee as a motor reaction from the cerebral cortex of the cat—or even, indeed, as a secondary movement. In exploring the cortex with unipolar faradization I have often failed to elicit the movement at all throughout a series of observations. Flexion, on the other hand, is regularly obtainable. After exhibition of strychnine the extension of knee can be regularly excited from the cortex, and from the very points of it that yielded flexion previously. This conversion is not so facile as the conversion of the spinal reflex. The dose of strychnine has to be larger, or to operate longer. With doses additively given, there seems, early in the experiment, a period when reflex spinal inhibition of the extensors has been converted into excitation, but the cortex of the brain still yields knee-flexion, not knee-extension. The cortical reversal has required in my hands doses that evoke convulsive seizures from time to time. I have seen, immediately after a severe convulsion, the cortex either unable to evoke any movement of the knee or produce knee-flexion, though a short while before it gave knee-extension.

Tetanus toxin likewise converts the cortical flexion into extension. The effect is in its case the more marked, because, if the cortical examination be at an early stage of the progressive malady ensuing on inoculation by a moderate dose, or where the dose has been quite small, the tetanus is 'local' and confined to the inoculated limb, and then, if the tetanus be 'local' in one hind-limb, e.g. the

Action of Strychnine and Tetanus Toxin

left, the appropriate area of the right hemisphere yields knee-extension, whereas the corresponding of the left hemisphere yields knee-flexion.

But these effects are better studied in the monkey. There, in my experience, to obtain primary extension of the crossed knee from the cortex is, as in the cat, extremely unusual. A number of experiments can be made without obtaining it at all. Even as a secondary movement it is extremely poorly represented in the cortex. For twenty instances of flexion at knee it is, in my experience, often difficult to find one of extension at that joint. But after tetanus toxin or strychnine the whole 'leg-area' of the cortex, from all points of its surface, may yield nothing but leg-extension, in which extension of knee is prominent as an evident part of a primary combined movement. This is especially striking when the tetanus is still merely 'local', and confined to one hind-limb, e.g. left. The 'leg-area' of the right cortex then yields knee-extension everywhere; the 'leg-area' of the left cortex yields the normal flexion results. The 'leg-area' of the right cortex provokes moreover from many of its points extension of right knee and ankle, as well as of left, though less strongly. The 'leg-area' of left hemisphere does this little, if at all. Under moderate faradization the 'leg-area' in the monkey, in my experience, moves the homonymous hind-limb, in addition to the crossed, very slightly and rarely, much less easily than in the cat, though in both the movement is the same, namely, 'extension'. So localized may be the toxic influence in its early stage that reversal of the usual cortical effect at knee may obtain while in the same hemisphere that on hip and ankle may still remain flexion as usual.

Similarly with the 'arm-area'. In the cat, it is in my experience quite infrequent to obtain primary extension of the crossed elbow from the cortex. Flexion is readily and regularly obtained. Strychnine changes this: the very surface that yielded flexion then provokes extension, and strongly. But the dose of strychnine seems to be larger than for conversion of the spinal reflex, and the conversion shows the phases before mentioned in regard to the knee-inhibition, and its conversion in the case of the hamstring nerve. In the monkey, in my experience, the effect of strychnine and of tetanus toxin when

Reactions of the Motor Cortex

pushed to the general convulsive stage is often contrary to the effect in that stage in so many other animals. I have seen them, though producing extension at elbow at first, later produce flexion at elbow. In one case, in a monkey, in which the tetanus had become general in the sense that only one limb was unaffected, the affected arm was strongly extended and rigid at elbow with some retraction at shoulder. But in all my instances, where by introduction of the toxin into the trunk of the median or ulnar a 'local' tetanus of the arm has been produced, the limb has been extended rigidly at elbow and retracted at shoulder. In these cases faradic examination of the cortex showed that the small field of the 'arm-area' to which extension at elbow is restricted, was enlarged so as to include the whole 'arm-area'. Under the toxin the cortex that normally in the cat yields flexion of the crossed fore-limb and extension of the uncrossed, will yield extension of both when there is local tetanus in the crossed limb. Extension at elbow, sometimes alone, more often with retraction at shoulder, or with extension at wrist or fingers, sometimes as a leading movement, sometimes rapidly ensuent on retraction at shoulder or extension in the hand, according as higher or lower points in the area were stimulated, was prominently exhibited at all points of the entire surface of the 'arm-area'. That area, with this as its salient reaction, seemed particularly in evidence, for its extreme limits appeared traceable further than usual, and to encroach on or overlap more than is usual (under the feeble or moderate stimulation employed) the 'leg-area' above and the 'face-area' below, and to run exceptionally far forward above the precentral sulcus, though remaining undemonstrable in the free surface of the ascending parietal convolution. From no point in all this extensive 'arm-area', despite repeated trials, was any flexion at elbow or shoulder or hand obtained (Fig. 75). Various intensities of faradization were employed, and points known normally to yield it most regularly were tried: but extension, not flexion, always resulted.

This condition of the 'arm-area' can, in tetanus, exist in one hemisphere or even in both hemispheres, and yet the 'leg-area' of each hemisphere yield flexions at knee and hip and ankle, and its other normal forms of reaction. Tetanus produced by introduction of the

Action of Strychnine and Tetanus Toxin

toxin into the arm (e.g. median or ulnar trunk) affects subsequently to the inoculated limb, the fellow fore-limb first, and the jaw before the hind-limbs, although the knee-jerk on the homonymous side to the inoculation may be brisk.

Under decerebrate rigidity, e.g. in the cat, the closing muscles of the jaw are kept in tonic action, holding the mouth somewhat shut.[182] By stimulation of any point of a large 'skin-area' appropriate for the reflex, reflex opening of the mouth, including depression of the lower jaw, is easily and regularly elicited, or by faradization of an afferent twig of the trigeminus; or as was shown by Woodworth & myself,[275] even by stimulation of distant afferent nerves, e.g. plantar or saphenous. Here the action of the powerful closing muscles is reflexly inhibited while the weaker opening muscles are reflexly excited—it seems, in fact, a case of *Astacus* claw, except that the inhibition is central, not peripheral. This reflex 'opening' is in the decerebrate animal converted into reflex closure by tetanus toxin and by strychnine, the inhibition of the predominantly powerful closing muscles being converted into excitation of them.

Similarly, when the 'face-area' of the monkey's cortex is tested by faradization after exhibition of strychnine, the points of surface that previously yielded regularly the free opening of the jaw, yield strong closure of the jaw instead. Now closure of the jaw is a movement of very limited representation in the cortex of the monkey, even of the anthropoid. On the other hand, *opening* of the jaw is always readily and regularly elicitable from a large field of the 'face-area'. And adjoining and overlapping this large area whence steady opening of the jaw is obtained, is found an area whence, as Ferrier[70] first pointed out, 'rhythmic alternating opening and closing of the jaws", as in feeding, can be evoked. Under tetanus toxin (Fig. 75) and strychnine the whole of this combined area not only ceases to yield opening of the jaws, either maintained or rhythmic, but yields closing of them instead—often with visible retraction of the tongue For this conversion larger doses of strychnine have, in my hands, been required than for conversion of knee-flexion into extension. With tetanus toxin the conversion appears the more striking when examined early in the progress of the intoxication, because it may

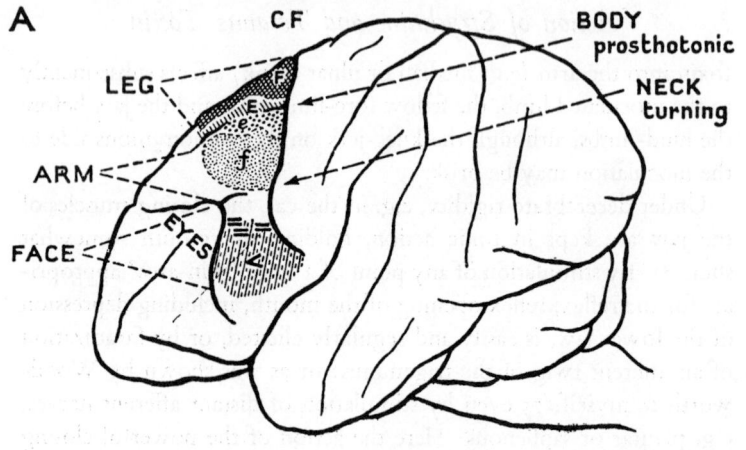
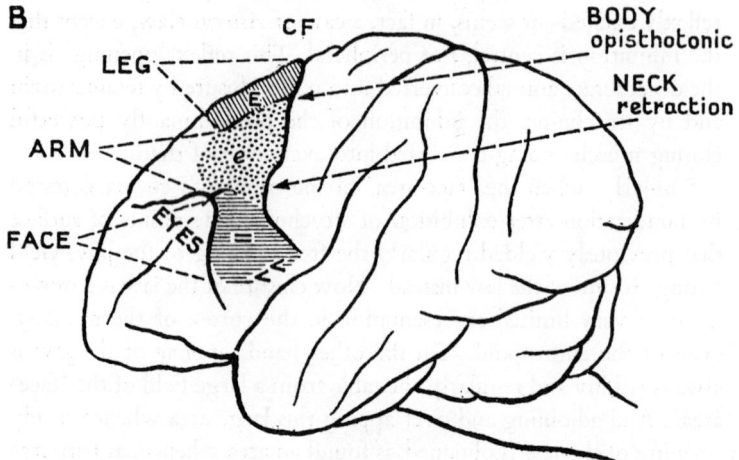

Fig. 75. Outline to illustrate the changes produced by tetanus-toxin in the functional topography of the motor-cortex of the monkey, *Cercopithecus callithrix*

CF = the central fissure. *F* indicates hip-knee flexion; *E* indicates hip-knee extension; *f* indicates elbow flexion, *e* indicates elbow extension; < indicates jaw opening; = indicates jaw closing; prosthotonic indicates in regard to 'body' ventral bending, opisthotonic indicates dorsal bending. The distribution of these symbols in the drawing indicates broadly the field whence could be elicited the movements that the symbols respectively stand for, in A *before* and in B *after* development of lockjaw. In B at the lowest part of the face-area a place still yielded opening of the mouth. In the experiment which furnished the specimen figured, the site of inoculation had been the leg, hence the toxic action reached the jaw comparatively late. Had the exploration of the cortex been deferred even longer the opening of the jaw might perhaps have been transformed to closure throughout the cortex.

Lockjaw

be found at a stage preceding altogether the occurrence of any general convulsions, and also because it can then sometimes be found to be unilateral, that is, to be present in the 'face-area' of one hemisphere* without or almost without any affection of the 'face-area' of the other hemisphere. The reactions of the normal field thus remain for comparison in the same individual with the reactions of the abnormal field.

Tetanus toxin shows marked predilection for the closure mechanism of the jaw. After inoculation in the hind-leg, even before the 'local' tetanus has obviously invaded the fellow limb of the opposite side, a slight tightness of jaw and an immobile pursing of the lips has several times given warning that general tetanus had really set in, before any trace of general convulsive seizures or any involvement of the arms was detected. Tetanus toxin had also certainly intensified the reactions of the cortical areas that give retraction of the neck and retraction of the abdominal wall (Fig. 75).

The progress of the change wrought by these agents in converting these reactions of the cortex from their usual form to the diametrically opposed seems to involve the same kind of steps as that noted above in their conversion of the inhibitory hamstring nerve effect on the knee-extensor. Stages can be found in which the inhibitory effect is less than normal, yet is not replaced by excitatory. With the cortical opening of jaw, in early tetanus a grade is discoverable when faradization of the cortex produces a slight opening of the jaw—a mere 'loosening' of the jaws, so to say—distinctly less than normal, and hardly effectively opening the mouth. Also with the 'leg-area' of the cortex, at an early stage of the tetanus it would seem that an undue but far from exclusive preponderance of plantar extension at ankle over dorsal flexion at that joint exists, while the symptomatic knee-extension is as yet not excitable though knee-flexion is almost in abeyance. Neither under tetanus toxin or strychnine have I at present observed conversion of the abducens inhibition into excitation.

The foregoing observations appear to give an insight into at least

* The hemisphere, the 'face-area' of which is earlier affected, is, in the case of inoculation in a limb, the hemisphere contralateral to the limb inoculated.

Reactions of the Motor Cortex

a part of the essential nature of the condition brought about by tetanus and by strychnine poisoning. These disorders work havoc with the co-ordinating mechanisms of the central nervous system because in regard to certain great groups of musculature they change the reciprocal inhibitions, normally assured by the central nervous mechanisms, into excitations. The sufferer is subjected to a disorder of co-ordination which, though not necessarily of itself accompanied by physical pain, inflicts on the mind, which still remains clear, a disability inexpressibly distressing. Each attempt to execute certain muscular acts of vital importance, such as the taking of food, is defeated because from the attempt results an act exactly the opposite to that intended. The endeavour to open the jaw to take food or drink induces closure of the jaw, because the normal inhibition of the stronger set of muscles—the closing muscles—is by the agent converted into excitation of them. Moreover, the various reflex-arcs that cause inhibition of these muscles not only cause excitation of them instead, but are, periodically or more or less constantly, in a state of super-excitement, and yet attempt on the part of the sufferer to restrain, to inhibit, their reflex reaction, instead of relaxing them, only heightens their excitation further, and thus exacerbates a rigidity or a convulsion already in progress.

It seems to me not improbable that the virus of rabies may similarly upset reciprocal innervation, though its field of operation, at least in man, lies not in the same group of mechanisms as are affected by strychnine and tetanus toxin but in an allied one, namely, that inter-regulating (by co-ordinations involving inhibition, as Meltzer & Kronecker showed) the acts of deglutition and respiration.

Little has met me in the course of observations on the reactions of the cortex under strychnine or tetanus toxin to indicate that the transformation of the motor effects of the reactions is due to action of these agents on the cortex itself. The change of result seems quite explicable by alteration produced in lower centres, e.g. spinal and bulbar, on which the cortex acts. This seems especially shown by the toxin when injected into the right arm and producing extensor rigidity at that elbow and rigid torticollis to the right, converting the flexion of arm-area of the *left* hemisphere into extension under

Decerebrate Rigidity

arm-area excitation, and in the *right* hemisphere torticollis movement to the right.

The vast role of inhibition in cerebral processes as evidenced by mental reactions, and the slightness of mental disorder in strychnine poisoning or tetanus indicates a difference between inhibition as it occurs in the bulbo-spinal arcs and in the arcs of purely sensual and perceptual level, a difference presumably of physicochemical nature.

We find therefore, these reactions changed in a like manner by strychnine and tetanus whether we excite them from the cortex or from reflex spinal arcs. And a further similarity between the representation of movement in the motor cortex and in the bulbo-spinal axis as a mechanism for local reflexes is the following. When the induced movement embraces both hind-limbs or both fore-limbs it is in an opposite sense in the two limbs. Thus the crossed accompaniment to the flexion-reflex of the limb is extension: and so also when cortical stimulation evokes (e.g. in cat) flexion, e.g. of the right fore-limb, not rarely it evokes movement, weaker it is true, in the left, and that movement, as Exner[99] noted in the rabbit, is extension.

The local reflex movements obtainable from the bulbo-spinal animal and the reactions elicitable from the motor cortex of the narcotized animal fall into line as similar series. Both consist of the same group. But in striking contrast to this group stands the motor innervation active in 'decerebrate rigidity'.

Decerebrate rigidity[182] is a condition which ensues on removal of the fore-brain by transection at any of the various levels in the mesencephalon or the thalamencephalon in its hinder part.

If in a monkey or cat transection below or in the lower half of the bulb has been performed, artificial respiration if necessary being kept up, the animal when suspended, hangs from the suspension points with deeply drooped neck, deeply drooped tail, and its pendent limbs flaccid and slightly flexed. The fore-limb is slightly flexed at shoulder, at elbow, and very slightly at wrist. The hind-limb is slightly flexed at hip, at knee, and at ankle. On giving the hand or foot a push forward and then releasing it, the limb swings back into and somewhat beyond the position of its equilibrium under gravity; and it oscillates a few times backward and forward before finally settling down to its original position.

To this condition of flaccid paralysis supervening upon transection in the lower half of the bulb the condition ensuing on removal of the cerebral hemispheres offers a great contrast. In the latter case the animal, on being suspended just as after the former operation, hangs with its fore-limbs thrust backward, with retraction at shoulder joint, straightened elbow, and some flexion at wrist. The hand of the monkey is turned with its palmar face somewhat inward. The hind-limbs are similarly straightened and thrust backward; the hip is extended, the knee very stiffly extended, and the ankle somewhat extended. The tail in spite of its own weight, and it is quite heavy in some species of monkey, is kept either straight and horizontal or often stiffly curved upward. There is a little opisthotonus of the lumbo-sacral vertebral region. The head is kept lifted against gravity and the chin is tilted upward under the retraction and backward rotation of the skull on the neck. The mouth is kept closed and there is some stiffness in the elevators of the jaw. When the limbs or tail or head or jaw are pushed from the pose they have assumed considerable resistance to the movement is felt, and unlike the condition after bulbar section, on being released they spring back at once to their former position and remain there for a time more rigid than before.

The rigidity is immediately due to prolonged spasm of certain groups of voluntary muscles. The chief of these are the retractor muscles of the head and the neck, the elevators of the jaw and tail, and the extensor muscles of the elbow and knee, and shoulder (i.e. deltoids) and hip. In the dog and cat, just as spinal shock is more severe in the fore- than in the hind-limbs, so decerebrate rigidity is more marked in the fore- than in the hind-limbs. This prolonged spasm may be maintained, with intermissions, for a period of four days. It is increased, and even when absent or very slight, may be soon developed by passive movement of the part. There is no obvious tremor in the spasm in the earlier hours of its continuance; later it does sometimes become tremulant.

Administration of chloroform and ether, if carried far, quite abolishes the rigidity. On interrupting the administration the rigidity again rapidly returns.

Section of the dorsal columns of the spinal cord does not abolish the rigidity. Section of one lateral column of the cord in the upper lumbar region abolishes the rigidity in the hind-limb of the same side as the section. Section of one ventro-lateral column of the cord in the cervical region destroys the rigidity in the fore- and hind-limbs of the same side.

The rigidity develops either very imperfectly or not at all in a limb the afferent roots of which have been severed some days prior to carrying out the operation which produces the rigidity.

If after ablation of both cerebral hemispheres, even when the rigidity is being maintained at its extreme height, the afferent roots previously laid bare and prepared, are carefully severed, the limb at once falls flaccid. The result is quite local, that is, confined to the one limb the afferent roots of which are severed.

Decerebrate rigidity exhibits reflex excitation in those very groups of muscles which the local reflexes and the motor cortex when stimulated excite but little. Not that the muscles exhibiting the rigidity are absolutely unamenable to transient spinal reflexes. The extensor-thrust and certain crossed reflexes are witness to the contrary. And they are not absolutely unamenable to cortical excitation. The extension of the elbow obtainable from the cortex refutes that. But these instances do not efface the broad fact that a wide system of musculature, including the extensors of the hip, knee, shoulder, and elbow, and the elevators of the tail, neck, and jaw, is inhibited by the overwhelming majority of local spinal reflexes and of reactions from the motor cortex, but on the contrary is excited in a set of reflex reactions which employ the local deep afferents (proprioceptive) and some cranial mechanism seated between cerebrum and bulb. The cerebellum at once rises to mind. But I found ablation of the cerebellum did not abolish the rigidity. It is significant that a vertical posture favours the appearance and development of the rigidity. The muscles it predominantly affects are those which in that attitude antagonize gravity. In standing, walking, running, the limbs would sink under the body's weight but for contraction of the extensors

Reactions of the Motor Cortex

of hip, knee, ankle, shoulder, elbow; the head would hang but for the retractors of the neck; the tail and jaw would drop but for their elevator muscles. These muscles counteract a force (gravity) that continually threatens to upset the natural posture. The force acts continuously and the muscles exhibit continued action, *tonus*. We seem to have here a field of muscles combined as a physiological entity. A characteristic reaction yielded by muscles of this field is the 'jerk', the 'tendon phenomenon', itself a sign of highly maintained reflex tonus.

Two separable systems of motor innervation appear thus controlling two sets of musculature: one system exhibits those transient phases of heightened reaction which constitute reflex movements; the other maintains that steady tonic response which supplies the muscular tension necessary to *attitude*. Starting from the tonic innervation as initial state the first step in movement tends to be flexion and involves under 'reciprocal innervation' an inhibition of the extensor excitation then in process. This will be involved whether the excitation be via local reflex or via the motor cortex. Hence the very muscles that to the observer are most obviously under excitation by the *tonic* system are those most obviously inhibited by the *phasic* reflex system. And the tonic system will, on inhibition of it passing off, contribute toward a return movement to the pre-existing pose, thus having its share in alternating movements and in compensatory reflexes. These two systems, the tonic and the phasic reflex systems, co-operate, exerting influences complemental to each other upon various units of the musculature. Drugs and other agents that act in a selective way upon nervous processes might be expected in some cases to throw into relief the operation of one or other member of this paired system. Strychnine and tetanus toxin administered to an animal in decerebrate rigidity increase that rigidity. The posture assumed by the limbs, neck, tail, head, etc., in strychnine poisoning and in tetanus resembles closely in many respects the attitude of decerebrate rigidity. There are differences—for instance, the ankle is often rigidly extended in tetanus whereas it is little affected in decerebrate rigidity; nevertheless there is much general resemblance.

And just as certain agents display their action more obviously in

Tonic and Phasic Systems

one member of these paired systems than in the other so processes of disease may be expected to deal with the two systems unequally and to reveal more obviously and affect more deeply one of them than the other. Hughlings Jackson[75, 78, 189] with characteristic penetration of thought argued nearly thirty years ago that rigidity ensuing in hemiplegia (hemiplegic contracture) is not owing to the cerebral lesion nor to the lateral sclerosis. He said: "Whilst the primary cerebral lesion can account for the paralytic element it cannot (nor can the sclerosis of the lateral column) account for the tonic condition of the muscles. My speculation is that the rigidity is owing to unantagonized influence of the cerebellum. Whilst the cerebrum innervates the muscles in the order of their action from the most voluntary movements (limbs) to the most automatic (trunk), the cerebellum innervates them in the opposite order. This is equivalent to saying that the cerebellum is the centre for continuous movements and the cerebrum for changing movements. Thus in 'walking' the cerebellum tends to stiffen all the muscles; the changing movements of walking are the result of cerebral discharges overcoming in a particular and orderly way the otherwise continuous influence. When the influence of the cerebrum is permanently taken off by disease of the cerebrum, as in hemiplegia, from the parts which it most specially governs (arm and leg) the cerebellar influence is no longer antagonized; there is unimpeded cerebellar influx and hence rigidity of the muscles which in health the cerebrum chiefly innervates. The spinal muscles are those which the cerebrum influences least and the cerebellum most. In health the whole of the muscles of the body are doubly innervated—innervated both by the cerebrum and cerebellum: there being a co-operation of antagonism between the two great centres."

This view of Hughlings Jackson seems supported and amplified by Luciani's and Stefani's work on the cerebellum. Wernicke,[119a] Mann,[153a] and Lewandowski[312] also point out that cerebral paresis selects one group of antagonistic groups of muscles in the limbs. We may very likely have to seek in the afferent nerves of muscles—especially of those antagonizing gravity—and in the nerve of the otic labyrinth—the 'tonus-labyrinth' of Ewald—the sources of the influence to which Hughlings Jackson refers as 'cerebellar', but that does not radically affect in its main feature the scheme he draws of a changeful 'clonic' (I would prefer to say 'phasic') innervation and a relatively unchanging tonic innervation as two systems in co-operative antagonism. Although we must also admit that the cortical innervation, pre-eminently phasic though it be, also is to some extent tonic; Lewandowski's[312] study of hemiplegic contracture seems to make this certain.

And here arises a question concerning the neural tonus of the skeletal musculature. Since Brondgeest's experiment neural tonus has been demonstrated to exist in various muscles and to be of reflex origin. It has however remained a question whether *all* skeletal muscles habitually exhibit a reflex tonus or only some of them. Various experiments (Heidenhain, Wundt) failed to discover reflex tonus in the muscles examined by them. If the reciprocal innervation of antagonistic muscles which obtains in so many reflexes obtains also in the tonic reflexes maintaining neural tonus in muscles, it is obvious that when one muscle of an antagonistic pair exhibits reflex tonus its antagonist will not exhibit reflex tonus, but on the contrary a slight degree of reflex inhibition. We have as yet no clear evidence on this. The feeble steady excitation which is the sign of reflex tonus is often difficult to demonstrate. Feeble steady inhibition would be even less easy to detect. But the selective distribution of the jerk-phenomena, under the ordinary conditions employed for their elicitation, to single members of antagonistic couples e.g. glutæus, vasto-crureus, masseter, and their absence, under those conditions, from the opposite members of the couples, is suggestive that, under the condition taken, reflex tonus may be confined to one member of each antagonistic pair, namely to that member which is then in reflex tonic operation, e.g. counteracting gravity for the preservation of an habitual pose of the animal.

I have laid some stress on the broad resemblance between the movements elicitable from the motor cortex and those of local spinal reflexes. There are broad differences as well.

Spinal reflex movements suggest fairly obviously protective, pro-creative, or visceral functions on the one hand, and on the other the

Combination of Cortical and Spinal Reactions

main movements of the progression habitual to the animal. They seem to refer to stimulation of noci-ceptive or sexual skin nerves or visceral afferent fibres, as though initiated by these. They carry little unequivocal reference to 'touch'. The existence of spinal reflexes elicited by pure 'touch'—apart from that noxious touch evoking scratching-reflexes or eye-blinking—appears to me not established in respect to the normal spinal cord. Similarly in the cat and dog after decerebration no purely auditory stimulus in my experience excites a reflex,* nor do visual, though the optic tracts and their midbrain connexions have been spared in the decerebration. On the other hand various movements elicitable from the motor cortex carry the significance of possible responses to tactual, auditory, or visual stimuli; for instance, the closure of the hand, the pricking of the ear, the opening of the eyes, and turning of the head in the direction of the gaze.

Combination of cortical reaction with spinal reflex seems patent in certain reactions of the dog. Thus, the normal dog can be seen to, as it were, release, direct, and cut short a scratching reflex (vide supra, p. 288). Darwin[50] draws attention to a phase of canine behaviour in regard to defecation. "Dogs after voiding their excrement often make with all four feet a few scratches backward, even on a bare stone pavement, as if for the purpose of covering up their excrement with earth, in nearly the same manner as do cats." In the spinal dog defecation is similarly followed by a number of vigorous backward kicks with the hind-limbs. The fore-limbs I have not been able to observe because the spinal transection has not lain far enough headward to liberate those limbs for free reflex action. But this movement in the hind-limb follows as a reflex in the spinal dog practically invariably in immediate sequence to reflex evacuation of the faeces. In the normal dog it is, as Darwin remarked, not invariable; and it is often not in *immediate* sequence to the evacuation. The reflex evidently shows modification by cerebral direction and control.

Finally, it seems to me that the number of reflex actions which are 'neutral' to each other, in the sense expressed in Lecture II, is less with

* I have only seen it do so when the decerebrate animal has been under large doses of atropin.

Reactions of the Motor Cortex

the cerebral cortex present than without it. This amounts to expressing concretely an inference that the cerebral cortex augments the motor solidarity of the creature. Since there is more solidarity as well as more diversity in those movements of an animal which are directed to its outer environment than to its inner—meaning by this latter the fraction of environment embraced within its own pulmono-digestive cavity—the representation of visceral movement in the cortex will be relatively slight, and chiefly concern parts where alimentary canal opens on outer surface.

The reactions of receptor-organs which respond to stimuli from a distance tend especially to have large cortical representation. These receptors tend more than others to control the skeletal musculature of the creature *as a whole*. The contribution made by the cerebral hemispheres to the solidarity of the motor creature is largely traceable to their bringing to bear on other reflexes the unifying influence of the reactions of the *distance-receptors*. This statement may in its baldness appear doctrinaire; of that character I hope to relieve it somewhat in the next Lecture.

As to the meaning of this whole class of movements elicitable from the so-called 'motor' cortex, whether they represent a step toward psychical integration or on the other hand express the motor result of psychical integration, or are participant in both, is a question of the highest interest, but one which does not seem as yet to admit of satisfactory answer. In regard to the relatively restricted problem in view in these lectures, namely, the simpler elements of the nervous integration of animal reaction, the motor reactions elicitable from the so-called 'motor' cortex furnish evidence confirmatory of points mentioned before in regard to lower reflex action. This is interesting, since they must be admitted to be movements of higher order than any of those others. Nevertheless, they are to my thinking merely fractional movements; movements which represent but parts of the nervous discharge which emanates from the brain under the normal working of its unmutilated whole. The results before you must appear a meagre contribution toward the greater problems of the working of the brain; their very poverty may help to emphasize the necessity for resorting to new methods of experimental inquiry in

Value of Experimental Psychology

order to advance in this field. New methods of promise seem to me those lately followed by Franz, Thorndyke, Yerkes, and others; for instance, the influence of experimental lesions of the cortex on skilled actions recently and individually, i.e. experimentally, acquired. Despite a protest ably voiced by v. Uexküll, comparative psychology seems not only a possible experimental science but an existent one. By combining methods of comparative psychology (e.g. the labyrinth test) with the methods of experimental physiology, investigation may be expected ere long to furnish new data of importance toward the knowledge of movement as an outcome of the working of the brain.

Lecture IX

THE PHYSIOLOGICAL POSITION AND DOMINANCE OF THE BRAIN

ARGUMENT: The primitive reflex-arc. The diffuse nervous system and the grey-centred nervous system; the central nervous system a part of the latter. Nervous integration of the segment. The three receptive fields. Richness of the extero-ceptive field. Special refinements of the receptor-organs of the 'leading' segments. The refined receptors of the leading segments are 'distance-receptors'. 'Distance-receptors'; the projicience of sensations. Extensive internuncial paths belonging to 'distance-receptors'. 'Distance-receptors' initiate precurrent reactions. Consummatory reactions; strong affective tone of the sensations adjunct to them. Receptive range and locomotion. The 'head' as physiologically conceived. Proprio-ceptive arcs excited secondarily to other arcs. Close functional connexion between the centripetal impulses from muscles and from the labyrinth. Tonic reflexes (of posture, etc.) and compensatory reflexes are characteristic reactions of this combined system. Nervous integration of the segmental series. Restriction of segmental distribution a factor in integration. The cerebellum is the main ganglion of the proprio-ceptive system. The cerebrum is the ganglion of the distance-receptors'.

WE may now attempt to gather from the various notions, however fragmentary, that have occupied us, some general conception of the neural architecture of an animal as a whole; though of course only in its motor aspect, for its truly sensorial aspects we have hardly had before us. The problem is too difficult for me to expect much success. Yet it will repay us if from the attempt we glean something at least of one cardinal feature of the scheme, namely, the dominance attained by one limited set of neural segments, the brain, over all the rest.

We must allow ourselves at certain points some repetition of considerations already urged, in order to draw from them now in new juxtaposition some further significance.

THE PRIMITIVE REFLEX-ARC

If we seek for a reflex-arc of simplest construction it is true we find in some unicellular organisms, e.g. *Vorticella*, a mechanism which resembles a nervous arc and is quite simple. This mechanism, com-

The Primitive Reflex-arc

posed from a single cell, shows differentiation into three parts respectively—*receptive, conductive,* and *effective.* In *Vorticella* the receptive element is the ciliated peristome; a stimulus reaching these cilia at the free end of the cell excites contraction of the myoid filament at the fixed end of the cell. Similarly with the individual cells of *Poteriodendron* (Verworn). In multicellular organisms of low organization like mechanisms occur. In *Actinia* there are ectoderm cells which have externally a receptive hairlet and internally a contractile fibre, and this latter contracts when the receptive hairlet is stimulated.

In view of such cases it might have seemed likely that in more highly developed organisms examples would have been forthcoming in which the differentiation of the parts of a single cell would have advanced further still and produced something yet more akin to a simple reflex-arc such as is considered typical of the true nervous system itself. That expectation is not realized. What we find as the simplest arc in the organisms which possess a true nervous system, is that the conductor mediating between receptor and effector is itself a separate cell intercalated between a receptive cell and an effector cell. At each end this separate conductive cell breaks up into branches. The branching at the receptive end places it in communication not with one but with several receptor cells. This must allow stimuli at a number of receptive points to combine by summation to a conjoint effect. By this means the threshold of reaction will be lowered and the organism in that respect become more sensitively reactive to the environment. At the deep, i.e. effector, end the branching of the conductive stem places it in touch not with one effective cell but with many. Thus, again, there must result lowering of the threshold —of what we may term the effective threshold. The contraction of a single muscle-fibre in a muscle is practically ineffective where the resistance and mass of the muscle and its load are great as compared with the power of a single muscle-fibre. But by its branching the motor neurone obtains hold of many muscle-fibres. This must tend to lower the effective threshold of reaction, and thus again the organism is rendered more delicately responsive to stimulation by its environment.

The Dominance of the Brain

But—and it is a striking fact—we do not know of any reflex-arc in which in fact the nervous conductor connecting receptor to effector is formed from end to end of one single neurone. The length of the conductor seems always to include *at least* two neurones in succession. A moment's reflexion reminds us that such arrangements as *Vorticella, Poteriodendron,* and the neuro-muscular cells of *Hydra* and *Actinia* do not exhibit the germ of a feature that we have already considered fundamental in the construction of the reflex nervous system. The cases cited do not exhibit even in germ the co-ordinative mechanism which is attained by the principle of the *common path*. Such cases confine each effector to the use of one receptor only, and confine each receptor to the use of one effector only. But we saw that a great principle in the plan of the nervous system is that an effector shall be at the behest of many receptors, and that one receptor shall be able to employ many effectors. We saw further in respect to this that there are two conditions which the nervous system satisfies. One is that the effector is at the behest of various receptors which can use it simultaneously and use it harmoniously all in more or less the same way. Thus an advantage accrues in that their reactions sum, even though the receptors may be of different modality; and by summation the threshold is lowered and the organism more sensitized to the environment. This arrangement cannot be obtained by the unicellular mechanisms instanced above. It can only be obtained by the formation of a common path, and the formation of a common path can only be rendered possible by having a conductor of pluricellular length. And there is another condition which the nervous system satisfies. The unicellular reflex-arc—if reflex-arc it can be called—not only admits no opportunity for *pluricellular summation* but also none for the second function of the jointed reflex-arc of pluricellular length, namely *interference*. In animals of complex organization the activity of one effector may interfere with the function of another, e.g. in the case of muscles which when contracting pull in opposite directions at the same lever. We have seen how this wasteful confusion is avoided by one receptor having power not only to throw a particular effector into action but also to throw the opposed effector out of action. We saw that this

Diffuse and Grey-Centred Nervous Systems

action it exercises not peripherally but within the nervous system, at the entrance to a common path. The unicellular reflex-arc allows no common path. It lacks, therefore, the mechanism which renders possible the two great co-ordinative processes of *plurireceptive summation* and of *interference*. Without these the nervous system is shorn of its chief powers to integrate a set of organs or an organism.

It is therefore a significant thing that in the nervous system there is not only no instance of the reflex triune—receptor, conductor, and effector—being formed of one cell only, but also no indubitable instance where the middle link, the conductor, is even itself formed of one cell (one neurone) only. In other words, we know of no instance in the nervous system of a reflex-arc so constructed as not to include a junction between one neurone and another neurone. And the rule is apparently always that at such junctions not only does one neurone meet another, but several neurones converge upon another and make of the latter a common path.

THE DIFFUSE NERVOUS SYSTEM, THE GREY-CENTRED NERVOUS SYSTEM, THE CENTRAL NERVOUS SYSTEM A PART OF THE LATTER

The term 'nerve-centre' is sometimes abused, yet seems in several ways apt. A keynote regarding that part of the nervous system which is termed 'the central' seems that it is wholly pieced together into one system. The nervous system in its simplest forms is diffuse—a number of scattered mechanisms performing merely local operations with much autonomy save that they have communication with their immediate neighbours across near boundaries. The co-ordination effected by the diffuse nervous system is not adapted to compass the quickly combined action of distant parts. It is slow, and it throws *en route* the effectors of intermediate regions into action. It is ill suited, therefore, to produce the integration of a large and complex individual as a whole, or even to integrate large differentiated portions of an individual. Yet the co-ordination it brings about in its own local field may be strikingly effective. A co-adjustment though simple and restricted may be not less perfect than one involving wide and complex neural mechanism. The co-ordination of a peristaltic

The Dominance of the Brain

movement of the bowel is, as shown by Bayliss & Starling, even when managed exclusively by the local diffuse nervous system, capable of the perfect taxis of two muscular coats arranged antagonistically in the viscus. It directs a relaxation of the one co-ordinately with a contraction of the other; it exhibits a primitive but none the less perfect form of 'reciprocal innervation'.

This diffuse system seems the only one in such an organism as Medusa. But in higher animals a system of longer direct connexions is developed. And this latter is 'synaptic', that is, possesses the adjustable junctions which belong characteristically to 'grey matter'. This *synaptic* system co-existing with the *diffuse* in various places dominates the latter. Thus it controls and oversees the actions of the local nervous system of the viscera, and heart, and blood-vessels, which even in the highest animal forms remain diffuse.

The synaptic nervous system has developed as its distinctive feature a central organ, a so-called *central nervous system*; it is through this that it brings into *rapport* one with another widely distant organs of the body, including the various portions of the diffuse nervous system itself.

That portion of the synaptic system which is termed 'central' is the portion where the nervous paths from the various peripheral organs meet and establish paths in common, i.e. *common paths*. It is therefore in accord with expectation that we find the organ in which this meeting occurs situated fairly midway among them all, i.e. centrally. In bilaterally symmetrical animals this organ would be expected to lie where it does, namely, equidistant from the two lateral surfaces of the animal, and to exhibit as it does, laterally symmetrical halves united by a number of nervous cross-ties bridging the median line. This central nervous organ contains almost all the junctions existent between the multitudinous arcs. In it the afferent paths from receptor-organs become connected with the efferent paths of effector-organs, not only those adjacent to their own receptors but, through *internuncial* (J. Hunter, 1778) paths, with efferent paths to effector-organs remote. This central 'exchange' organ is therefore well called the *central* nervous system. In the higher Invertebrata it is known as the longitudinal nerve-cord with ganglia, supraoesophageal, suboesopha-

Diffuse and Synaptic Nervous Systems

geal, etc.; in Vertebrata it is known as the spinal cord and brain. Under these different anatomical names the same physiological organ is designated. It would be more convenient for the biologist were one general term for it in use. We have seen that it is not merely a meeting place where afferent paths conjoin with efferent, but is, in virtue of its physiological properties, an organ of reflex reinforcements and interferences, and of refractory phases, and shifts of connective pattern; that it is, in short, an *organ of co-ordination* in which from a concourse of multitudinous excitations there result orderly acts, reactions adapted to the needs of the organism, and that these reactions occur in arrangements (*patterns*) marked by absence of confusion, and proceed in *sequences* likewise free from confusion.

By the development of these powers the synaptic system with its central organ is adapted to more speedy, wide, and delicate co-ordinations than the diffuse nervous system allows. Out of this potentiality for organizing complex integration there is evolved in the synaptic nervous system a functional grading of its reflex-arcs and centres. Thus, with allied reflexes, the mechanism of the common path knits together by plurireceptive summation not only the separate individual stimuli of similar kind, e.g. tangoreceptive or photoreceptive received from some agent as this latter becomes prepotent in the environment; but it knits together separate stimuli of even wholly different receptive species. C. J. Herrick has shown that in *Ameiurus nebulosus* (cat-fish) the reaction of the animal to stimulation of the barblets by meat is a reaction to a twofold stimulus, a chemical and a mechanical, and he finds that these two reactions mutually reinforce. Nagel reports a similar case with the tentacle of the Actinian, *Aiptasis saxicola*. v. Uexküll finds that the *Giftzangen* of *Echinus acutus* react only when a chemical and a mechanical stimulus are combined. The several qualitatively different properties of an object which is acting as stimulus are thus combined and reinforce each other in eliciting appropriate reaction. By this summation reflex complication in Herbart's sense is made possible. A touchstone for rank of a centre in this neural hierarchy is the degree to which paths from separate loci and of different receptive modality are confluent thither. Indicative of high rank is such functional position as relieves from 'local work' and involves general responsibility, e.g. for a series of segments or for the whole body. The 'three levels', of Hughlings Jackson is an expressive figure of this grading of rank in nerve-centres.

INTEGRATIVE ACTION OF THE NERVOUS SYSTEM IN THE SEGMENT AND IN THE SEGMENTAL SERIES

In animal organisms of any considerable complexity a division of the body into segments, metameres, is widely found. By the occurrence of separating constrictions or sepiments, or through the regular repetition of appendicular structures, subdivisions of the body are established which severally possess analogues of functions possessed more or less similarly by the other subdivisions but also severally possess functional unity. Such is this functional unity and completeness that in some instances a metamere comes to be independent of the total organism, and able to lead a separate existence. The nervous system it is which largely gives functional solidarity to the composite collection of unit lives and organs composing the individual metamere. Further, the linkage of the several metameres into one functional whole is largely of nervous nature. The integrative function of the nervous system is seen to perfection in the welding together of metameres into the unity of an animal individual. The kind of nervous system employed for this is the *synaptic* system. Although the nerve-net system is retained even in the highest vertebrates, it is then confined to unsegmentally arranged musculature, e.g. visceral and vascular. In the skeletal musculature, where segmental arrangement holds, the nervous system is *synaptic*. It is not surprising therefore that in metameric animals the nervous system, especially its synaptic part, should strikingly exhibit that metamerism.

Various schemes of metamerism have been evolved. Where it is radiate so that each segment bears exactly similar relations to the common axis and to the other segments, the opportunity for dominance of one segment over the rest is slight. The conditions of life for each segment are practically those which are the average for all. The mouth, for instance, lies equidistant from them all. Evolution

Segmental Arrangement in Nervous System

toward higher differentiation of the whole metameric individual and toward more intricate welding of its parts into one, is at a disadvantage in these radiate forms as compared with its opportunity in the great groups of Arthropoda and Vertebrata where the metameres are ranged serially along a single axis, the longitudinal axis of the organism. With fore and aft arrangement of its segments the animal body has its first opportunity for really high differentiation. Certain of the segments of necessity lie nearer to the mouth than do others; moreover certain segments come to habitually lead, that is to say go foremost, during the animal's active locomotion.

In the integrating function of the nervous system a segmental arrangement of its functions is frequently apparent. It makes itself felt in two ways. Firstly, the various separate and different elements of the segment are knit together by nervous ties. Secondly, where kindred functions are exercised in successive segments, so that throughout a series of segments one set of organs forms a more or less functionally homogeneous system, these organs are combined by interrelated nervous arcs. But particular systems of organs common to all or many metameres of an individual present special differentiation of their function in particular metameres. In this manner the organism is built up of component segments possessing resemblance one to another, but presenting also specializations peculiar to certain segments. Hence the segmental arrangement forms a convenient basis not merely for anatomical but for physiological description. And in dealing with the special problems of integration by the nervous system, especially those of the synaptic nervous system, analysis can employ two co-ordinate sets of descriptive factors—one the segment, the other the line of organs of analogous function scattered along the series of segments. In the two great animal groups just mentioned the latter ordinate is longitudinally extended, while the individual segment is extended transversely. The analysis thus proceeds formally somewhat in the same way as the analysis of a plane figure by rectangular co-ordinates.

The Dominance of the Brain

THE RECEPTIVE FIELDS

The *central* nervous system, though divisible into separate mechanisms, is yet one single harmoniously acting although complex whole. To analyse its action we turn to the receptor-organs, for to them is traceable the initiation of the reactions of the centres. These organs fall naturally into three main groups, distributed in three main fields, each field being differently circumstanced.

Multicellular animals regarded broadly throughout a vast range of animal types are cellular masses presenting to the environment a surface sheet of cells, and under that a cellular bulk more or less screened from the environment by the surface sheet. Many of the agencies by which the environment acts on the organism do not penetrate to the deep cells inside. Bedded in the surface sheet are numbers of *receptor* cells constituted in adaptation to the stimuli delivered by environmental agencies. The *underlying* tissues devoid of these receptors are not devoid of *all* receptor-organs; they have other kinds apparently specific to them. Some agencies act not only at the surface of the organism but penetratively through its mass. Of these there are for some apparently no receptors adapted, for instance, none for the Röntgen rays. For others of more usual occurrence receptors are adapted. The most important of these deep adequate agents seems to be mass acting in the mode of weight and mechanical inertia involving mechanical stresses and mechanical strain. Moreover, the organism, like the world surrounding it, is a field of ceaseless change, where internal energy is continually being liberated, whence chemical, thermal, mechanical, and electrical effects appear. It is a microcosm in which forces are at work as in the macrocosm around. In its depths lie receptor-organs adapted consonantly with the changes going on in the microcosm itself, particularly in its muscles and their accessory apparatus (tendons, joints, walls of blood-vessels, and the like).

There exist, therefore, two primary distributions of the receptor-organs, and each constitutes a field in certain respects fundamentally different from the other. The deep field we have called the *proprio-*

Classification of Receptors

ceptive field, because its stimuli are, properly speaking, events in the microcosm itself, and because that circumstance has important bearing upon the service of its receptors to the organism.

RICHNESS OF THE EXTERO-CEPTIVE FIELD IN RECEPTORS; COMPARATIVE POVERTY OF THE INTERO-CEPTIVE

The surface receptive field is again subdivisible. It presents two divisions. Of these one lies freely open to the numberless vicissitudes and agencies of the environment. That is to say, it is co-extensive with the so-called *external* surface of the animal. This subdivision may be termed the *extero-ceptive* field.

But the animal has another surface, its so-called *internal*, usually alimentary in function. This, though in contact with the environment, lies however less freely open to it. It is partly screened by the organism itself. For purposes of retaining food, digesting and absorbing it, an arrangement of common occurrence in animal forms is that a part of the free surface is deeply recessed. In this recess a fraction of the environment is more or less surrounded by the organism itself. Into that sequestered nook the organism by appropriate reactions gathers morsels of environmental material whence by chemical action and by absorption it draws nutriment. This surface of the animal may be termed the *intero-ceptive*. At its ingress several species of receptors are met with whose 'adequate' stimuli are chemical (e.g. taste organs). Lining this digestive chamber, this kitchen, the intero-ceptive surface is adapted to *chemical* agencies to a degree such as it exhibits nowhere else. Comparatively little is yet known of the receptor-organs of this surface, though we may suppose that they exhibit refined adaptations. But the body-surface in this recess, though possessed of certain receptors specific to it, is sparsely endowed as contrasted with that remainder of the surface (the *extero-ceptive* surface) lying open fully to the influences of the great outer environment. The afferent nerve-fibres in the sympathetic system as judged by their number in the white rami are comparatively few; Warrington's[298] recent observations show this conclusively. The poverty of afferent paths from the *intero-ceptive* field is broadly indicated by the fact that we know no wholly afferent

The Dominance of the Brain

nerve-trunk in the sympathetic (Langley's 'autonomic') system, though such are common enough in the nervous system subserving the extero-ceptive arcs; and that in the latter system we know no wholly efferent nerve-trunk, whereas in the sympathetic such exist, e.g. the cervical sympathetic trunk.

The extero-ceptive field far exceeds the intero-ceptive in its wealth of receptor-organs. This seems inevitable, for it is the extero-ceptive surface, facing outward on the general environment, that feels and has felt for countless ages the full stream of the varied agencies forever pouring upon it from the outside world. Mere enumeration of the different species of receptor-organs recognizable in it suffices to illustrate the importance of this great field. It contains specific receptors adapted to mechanical contact, cold and warmth, light, sound, and agencies inflicting injury (*noxa*). Almost all these species of receptors are distributed to the *extero-ceptive* field exclusively; they are not known to exist in the intero-ceptive or in the proprio-ceptive fields.

It is an instructive exercise to try to classify the stimuli adequate for the receptors of the extero-ceptive field. Each animal has experience only of those qualities of the environment which as stimuli excite its receptors; it analyses its environment in terms of them exclusively. Doubtless certain stimuli causing reactions in other animals are imperceptible to man; and in a large number of cases his reactions are different from theirs. Hence it is impossible for man to conceive the world in terms more than partially equivalent to those of other animals. Humanly, the classification of adequate stimuli can be made with various departments of natural knowledge as its basis. Physics and chemistry can be taken as basis usefully in a number of cases where the sources of stimulation are known to those more exact branches of experimental science. But in several ways a physico-chemical scheme of classification of stimuli lacks significance for physiology. Thus, in the case of the noci-ceptive organs of the skin, those receptors—probably naked nerve-endings—are *non-selective* in the meaning that they are excitable by physical and chemical stimuli of diverse kind, radiant, mechanical, acid, alkaline, electrical, and so on, so that a classification according to mode of exciting energy on the one hand fails to differentiate them from each of a number of more specialized other groups (tango-receptors, chemo-receptors, etc.) from which biologically they are quite different, and on the other hand that classification apportions them, though physiologically a single group, to a whole series of different classes. A physiological classification deals with them more satisfactorily. Physiological criteria can be applied which at once separate them from other receptors and yet show their affinity one to another. Thus, physiologically the stimulus which excites these end-organs must, whatever its physical or chemical nature, possess, in order to stimulate them, the quality of tending to do immediate harm to the skin. Further, the reflex they excite (i) is *prepotent*; (ii) tends to *protect* the threatened part by escape or defence; (iii) is *imperative*; and (iv) if we include psychical evidence and judge by analogy from introspection, is accompanied by *pain*.

Here what we may call the physiological scheme of classification proves the more useful at present. And similarly it proves useful with a group of stimuli that may be termed 'distance-stimuli', to which we must turn presently. The key to the physiological classification lies in the reaction which is produced. But the physico-chemical basis of classification also has its uses, and especially with those manifold receptors of the extero-ceptive field which possess highly developed accessory structures that render them selectively receptive —and among these are some of the most highly adapted and important receptors, e.g. photo-receptors, possessed by the organism. It is to the extero-ceptive field that these belong.

NERVOUS INTEGRATION OF THE SEGMENT

The edifice of the whole central nervous system is reared upon two neurones—the afferent root-cell and the efferent root-cell. These form the pillars of a fundamental reflex arch. And on the junction between these two are superposed and functionally set, mediately or immediately, all the other neural arcs, even those of the cortex of the cerebrum itself. The private receptor paths and the common effector paths are in the Chordata gathered up in a single nerve-trunk for each segment. Close to the central nervous organ, however, there occurs

The Dominance of the Brain

in the segmental nerves of many vertebrates a cleavage of the private receptor paths from the common effector paths. A dorsal spinal nerve of centripetal conduction and a ventral of centrifugal conduction results. Among the afferent root-cells (afferent spinal root of vertebrates) in each segment are quota from the *extero-ceptive* (cutaneous) and from the *proprio-ceptive* (deep) fields. In many segments there is a third quotum, *intero-ceptive*, from the visceral field. This visceral constituent of the spinal ganglion is not present in all segments and is probably, even in those segments in which it is present, numerically the weakest of the three components. Cranial, caudal, and other segments exist, therefore, in which the total afferent nerve of the segment is extero-ceptive and proprio-ceptive but not intero-ceptive. In the remaining segments it is intero-ceptive as well as extero-ceptive and proprio-ceptive, and in these its function is therefore fundamentally threefold.

The efferent segmental nerve conversely radiates outward from the central end of the afferent nerve and the central nervous organ to the various effector organs at the surface and in the depth of the segment. Function does not, however, strictly respect the ancestral boundaries of segments. Among the efferent fibres in the ventral root are a number that extend quite beyond the boundaries of the segment in which the spinal root is placed. These pass to the viscera and muscles of the skin. They embouch not directly into their effector organs, e.g. intestinal muscle-wall, pilomotor muscle, etc., but into ganglia of the sympathetic system. In these ganglia, although not grey matter in the same sense as spinal cord and brain, axone-endings, perikarya, and dendrites are nevertheless found. By its distribution to the cells in such a ganglion and by being distributed in many cases to more than one such ganglion, a single constituent efferent path in the ventral spinal root obtains access to a very large number of effector organs. These ganglia seem, therefore, mechanisms for the *distribution* of nerve-impulses. We have seen (p. 309) how by such widening of distribution the threshold of effective reaction is lowered. But though adapted for distribution of nerve-impulses there is no evidence that these ganglia can serve for the *regulation* of them in the same sense as does the grey matter of the

Nervous Integration of Segment

spinal cord with its synapses of *variable* resistance and connexion. Prominent among the integrating connexions intrinsic to each segment itself are conducting paths from the extero-ceptive field to the 'final common paths' for the skeletal musculature. Thus, in the mammal we laid it down (Lect. V, p. 160) as a general rule that "for each afferent root there exists in immediate proximity to its own place of entrance into the cord, i.e. in its own segment, a reflex motor path from skin to muscle of as low resistance as any open to it anywhere".

The extero-ceptive arcs appear in most segments less closely connected with the visceral musculature than with the skeletal musculature. The intero-ceptive arcs appear in most segments less closely connected with the skeletal musculature than with the visceral. In physiological parlance a resistance to conduction seems intercalated between the two. But both extero-ceptive and intero-ceptive fields easily influence through their nervous arcs the musculature of the blood-vascular organs. So also do the receptors of the proprioceptive field itself; and these latter are in particularly close touch with the skeletal musculature, exerting tonic influence on it. In certain segments these general relations are modified in special ways. Thus, in those segments where the intero-ceptive and extero-ceptive fields conjoin, e.g. at the mouth and the cloaca, closer nervous connexions exist between the intero-ceptive arcs and the skeletal musculature, and conversely between the extero-ceptive arcs and the visceral musculature. Thus stimuli acting on the pharyngeal receptors evoke or inhibit activity of skeletal muscles subserving respiration and deglutition; stimuli to the cloacal mucosa evoke movements of the caudal skeletal muscles; and so forth.

It is not merely specific difference between the receptors of the extero-ceptive field and those of the intero-ceptive which brings the former into closer relationship with the skeletal musculature. Receptors of the one and the same species, if they lie in the extero-ceptive field, work skeletal musculature; if they lie in the intero-ceptive, work visceral musculature. Thus the chemo-receptors on the outer surface of the head (gustatory of the barblets of fish) excite reflexes which move the body round, bringing the mouth to the morsel;

The Dominance of the Brain

while the similar chemo-receptors within the mouth excite reflex swallowing without outward movement of the animal (C. J. Herrick).

Receptors of the *same* specific system, where they lie close together, mutually reinforce reaction. On the contrary, where members of two *different* systems lie close together, e.g. tango-receptor and noci-ceptor, in one and the same piece of skin, they, as mentioned above, often have conflicting mutual relation. One relationship between receptor arcs of the same species may be particularly noted. Receptors symmetrically placed on opposite sides of the segment, especially if distant from the median plane, excite reactions which mutually 'conflict'. Thus, when a noci-ceptor is stimulated on the right side of the tail of the spinal dog or cat or lizard, the reaction moves the organ to the left. The symmetrical receptor on the left side does the converse. The two reactions thus conflict. And the like holds true for many right and left symmetrical receptors which initiate exactly converse reactions.

But a group of special cases is formed by reactions initiated from receptors distributed at or near to the median line. Stimulation of such a small group of receptors at the median line in many cases evokes a bilateral movement which is symmetrical, e.g. a touch on the decerebrate frog's lip in the median line causes both fore-limbs to sweep forward synchronously over the spot. The median overlap of the distribution of the afferent fibres of the dorsal spinal roots may be connected with this.

SPECIAL REFINEMENTS OF THE RECEPTORS OF THE 'LEADING' SEGMENTS

As the receptors that are excitable by the various adequate agencies, e.g. mechanical impact, noxa, radiant energy, chemical solutions, etc., are traced along the series of segments, it is found that in one region of the longitudinal segmental series remarkable developments exist.

In motile animals constituted of segments ranged along a single axis, e.g. Vertebrata, when locomotion of the animal goes on, it

Refinements of Receptors of Leading Segments

proceeds for the most part along a line continuous with the long axis of the animal itself, and more frequently in one direction of that line than in the other. The animal's locomotor appendages and their musculature are favourably adapted for locomotion in that habitual direction. In the animal's progression certain of its segments therefore *lead*. The receptors of these leading segments predominate in the motor taxis of the animal. They are specially developed. Thus, in the earthworm, while all parts of the external surface are responsive to light, the directive influence of light is greatest at the anterior end of the animal. The leading segments are exposed to external influences more than are the rest. Not only do they receive *more* stimuli, meet *more* 'objects' demanding pursuit or avoidance, but it is they which usually *first* encounter the agents beneficial or hurtful of the environment as related to the individual. Pre-eminent advantage accrues if the receptors of these leading segments react sensitively and differentially to the agencies of the environment. And it is in these leading segments that remarkable developments of the receptors, especially those of the extero-ceptive field, arise. Some of them are specialized in such degree as almost obscures their fundamental affinity to others distributed in other segments. Thus, among the system of receptors for which radiation is the adequate agent, there are developed in one of the leading segments a certain group, the *retinal*, particularly and solely, and extraordinarily highly, amenable to radiations of a certain limited range of wave-length. These are the *photo-receptors*, for which light and only light, e.g. not heat, is the adequate stimulus. In like manner a certain group belonging to the system receptive of mechanical impacts attains such susceptibility for these as to react to the vibrations of water and air that constitute physical sounds. The retina is thus a group of glorified 'warm-spots', the cochlea a group of glorified 'touch-spots'. Again, a group belonging to the system adapted to chemical stimuli reach in one of the leading segments such a pitch of delicacy that particles in quantity unweighable by the chemist, emanating from substances called odorous, excite reaction from them.

The Dominance of the Brain

THE REFINED RECEPTORS OF THE LEADING SEGMENTS ARE 'DISTANCE-RECEPTORS.' THE AFTER-COMING SEGMENTS FORM A MOTOR TRAIN ACTUATED CHIEFLY BY THE 'DISTANCE-RECEPTORS'

It is in the leading segments that we find the *distance-receptors*. For so may be called the receptors which react to *objects* at a distance. These are the same receptors which, acting as sense-organs, initiate sensations having the psychical quality termed *projicience*. The receptor-organs adapted to odours, light, and sound, though stimulated by the external matter in direct contact with them—as the vibrating ether, the vibrating water or air, or odorous particles,—yet generate reactions which show 'adaptation', e.g. in direction of movements, etc., to the environmental *objects* at a distance, the *sources* of those changes impinging on and acting as stimuli at the organism's surface. We know that in ourselves sensations initiated through these receptors are forthwith 'projected' into the world outside the 'material me'. The projicience refers them, without elaboration by any reasoned mental process, to directions and distances in the environment fairly accurately corresponding with the 'real' directions and distances of their actual sources. None of the sensations initiated in the proprio-ceptive or intero-ceptive fields possess this property of projicience. And with the distance-receptors considered simply as originators of reflex actions, their reflexes are found to be appropriate to the stimuli as regards the direction and distance of the sources of these latter. Thus, the patch of light constituting a retinal image excites a reflex movement which turns the eyeball toward the source of the image and adjusts ocular accommodation to the distance of that source from the animal itself. Even a negative stimulus suffices. The shadow of the hand put out to seize the tortoise excites, as it blots the retinal illumination, withdrawal of the animal's head to within the shelter of the shell.

How this result of 'distance' has been acquired is hard to say. The net effect is reached in various ways, and with very various gain in the degree of 'distance' acquired. By long vibrissae certain tango-receptors obtain excitation from objects still at a distance from the

Role of Distance Receptors

general surface of the organism. By reduction of their threshold value of stimulus, certain other receptors akin to tactual, inasmuch as their adequate stimuli are mechanical, become responsive to vibratory movements of water and air so as to react to physical sounds whose sources lie remote from the animal. Certain chemo-receptors acquire so low a threshold that they react not merely to food and other substances in contact with them in mass, but react to almost inconceivably diluted traces of such, traces which drift off from the objects and permeate the environment through long distances, as so-called odours, before impinging upon the delicate receptors in question. The leading segments thus come to possess not only taste, but taste at a distance, namely smell. In such cases it seems chiefly by lowering of their threshold that these receptors of the leading segments have been brought to react to objects still remote from the organism.

The 'distance-receptors' seem to have peculiar importance for the construction and evolution of the nervous system. In the higher grades of the animal scale one part of the nervous system has, as Gaskell insists, evolved with singular constancy a dominant importance to the individual. That is the part which is called the brain. *The brain is always the part of the nervous system which is constructed upon and evolved upon the 'distance-receptor' organs.* Their effector reactions and sensations are evidently of paramount importance in the functioning of the nervous system and of the individual. This seems explicable, at least partly, in the following manner.

An animal organism is not a machine which merely transforms a quantum of energy given it in potential form at the outset of its career. It has to replenish its potential energy by continued acquisition of suitable energy-containing material from the environment, and this material it has to incorporate in itself. Moreover, since death cuts short the career of the individual organism, the species has to be maintained, and for that in most higher organisms there is required accession of material (gametic) from another organism (of like species) to rejuvenesce a portion of the adult, which portion then cast off leads a new individual existence. To satisfy, therefore, the primary vital requirements of an animal species, actual material

The Dominance of the Brain

contact with certain objects is necessary; thus, for feeding, and in many cases for sexual reproduction.

In these processes of feeding and conjugation the non-distance-receptors play an important and essential part. But ability on the part of an organism to react to an object when still distant from it allows an interval for preparatory reactive steps which can go far to influence the success of attempt either to obtain actual contact or to avoid actual contact with the object. Thus, we may take in illustration the two sets of selective chemo-receptors, the gustatory and the olfactory. Both are responsive to certain chemical stimuli which reach them through solution in the moist mucous membranes of the mouth and nose. No odorous substance appears to be tasteless, and if the threshold value for olfaction and for taste be measured respectively, the threshold for the former as determined in weight of dissolved material is lower than for the latter. The former is the distance-receptor. Animal behaviour shows clearly that in regard to these two groups of receptors the one subserves differentiation of reaction, i.e. swallowing or rejection, of material already found and acquired, e.g. within the mouth. The other, the distance-receptor, smell, initiates and subserves far-reaching complex reactions of the animal anticipatory to swallowing, namely, all that train of reaction which may be comprehensively termed the quest for food. The latter foreruns and leads up to the former. This precurrent relation of the reaction of the distance-receptor to the non-distance-receptor is typical.

The 'distance-receptors' initiate anticipatory, i.e. precurrent, reactions. I ventured above to use the word 'attempt'. Just as a salient character of most of the reactions of the non-projicient receptors taken as sense-organs is *affective tone*, i.e. physical pain or physical pleasure, so *conative feeling* is salient as a psychical character of the reactions which the projicient or distance-receptors, taken as sense-organs, guide. As initiators of reflex movements the action of these latter is characterized by tendency to work or control the musculature of the animal as a *whole*—as a single machine—to impel locomotion or to cut it short by the assumption of some *total* posture, some attitude which involves steady posture not of one limb or one

Whole-Body Control by Distance Receptors

appendage alone, but of all, so as to maintain an attitude of the body as a whole. Take, for instance, the flight of a moth toward a candle, the dash of a pike toward a minnow, and the tense steadiness of a frog about to seize an insect. These reactions are all of them excited by distance-receptors, though in the one case the musculature is impelled to locomotion toward the stimulus (positive phototropism), in the other restrained (inhibited) from locomotion. Whether the reaction be movement toward or movement away from (positive or negative) or whether it be motion or its restraint (excito-motor or inhibito-motor) does not matter here. The point here is that in both reactions the skeletal musculature is treated practically as a *whole* and in a manner suitably anticipatory of a later event. That is far less the case with the non-projicient receptors. The decerebrate frog changes the whole direction of its path of locomotion when a visual obstacle is set in its way, but a skin impact excites a movement in a small field of musculature only, e.g. the eyelid blinks on corneal contact, the foot flexes at a digital *noxa*; where the part itself cannot well move itself, musculature accessory to it but distant from it is moved. Thus the hind-limb is swept over the flank on irritation there, or the fore-limb over the snout on irritation there. But in these cases the movement induced is merely local and does not affect the body as a whole. Sufficient intensity (we may include summation under intensity) of a stimulus can of course impel the whole creature to movement even through a non-projicient receptor. A decerebrate frog touched lightly between the scapulae will lower its head at first touch, and again more so at a second; at a third will, besides lowering the head, draw the front half of its trunk slightly backward; at a fourth the same movement with stronger retraction; at a fifth give an ineffectual sweep with its hind- or fore-foot; at a sixth a stronger sweep; at a seventh a feeble jump; at an eighth a free jump, and so forth. Considerable intensity or summation is required to evoke a reflex action of the skeletal musculature as a whole from these cutaneous receptors. The projicient receptors and their reflexes once gone, even intense stimuli do not *readily* move or arrest the creature as a whole. It is relatively difficult to get the 'spinal' frog to spring or swim. Co-ordinate movement of the creature as a whole is *then*

The Dominance of the Brain

obtained by general stimulation (i.e. plurireceptive summation), or if by localized stimulation the stimulus must be intense. Thus the spinal frog will swim when placed in water at 36° C. The warm water forms a noci-ceptive stimulus to the receptors of the immersed body-surface generally.

EXTENSIVE INTERNUNCIAL PATHS OF 'DISTANCE-RECEPTORS'

Conformably with the power of the 'distance-receptors' to induce movements or postures of the individual as a whole we find the neural arcs from these receptors particularly wide and far-reaching. The nerve-fibre that starts from the receptor does not in many of these cases itself extend to, or send processes to, the mouths of the *final common paths*. Instead of doing so it ends often far short of them, and forms connexion with other nerve-fibres (internuncial paths), which in their turn reach distant 'final common paths'. This arrangement involves an intercalation of grey matter between the 'private receptor' path and the 'final common path' not only at the mouth of the latter, but also where the internuncial path itself commences. The *significance of this seems that the internuncial path is itself a 'common path,' and therefore a mechanism of accommodation.* Its community of function is not so extensive as that of a 'final common path', not co-extensive for instance with all the receptors of the body, as would appear the case with a motor-nerve to a skeletal muscle. Yet it furnishes a path for use by certain sets of receptors in common. In *Mustelus* the nerve paths from the retinal and from the olfactory receptors converge toward the roof-nucleus of the mid-brain, whence passes the long mesencephalo-spinal path to the spinal motor nuclei. The inference is that conjoint stimulation of eye and nose exert a combined influence and impinge together on the spinal motor machinery. Similarly the Reissner fibre[290] may serve as an internuncial path between paths coming in from olfactory and visual receptors on the one hand and the spinal motor common paths from the spinal cord to the muscles on the other. Another instance of an internuncial path is the so-called 'pyramidal tract' characteristic of the mammalian nervous system. It furnishes a path of internuncial

Precurrent and Consummatory Reactions

character common to certain arcs that have arisen indirectly from various receptors of various species and are knitted together in the cerebral hemisphere. Another instance is the path from the thalamus to the post-central convolution (Mott, Tschermak, and others).

PRECURRENT REACTIONS. CONSUMMATORY REACTIONS

It might seem at first that all motor reflexes may be grouped into those that tend to prolong the stimulus and those that tend to cut it short. Consideration shows that such a grouping expresses the truth but partially. We argued above that the 'distance-receptors' induce anticipatory or precurrent reactions, that is, precurrent to *final* or consummatory reactions. The reflexes of certain non-projicient receptors stand in very close relation to 'consummatory' events. Thus the tango-receptors of the lips and mouth initiate reflex movements that immediately precede the act which for the individual creature viewed as a *conative and a sentient agent* is the final consummatory one in respect to nutriment as a stimulus, namely, swallowing. Similarly with the gustato-receptors and their reactions. The sequence of action initiated by these non-projicient receptors is a short one: their reflex leads immediately to another which is consummatory. Those receptors of the chelae of *Astacus, Homarus*, etc., which initiate the carrying of objects to the mouth, or again the tango-receptors of the hand of the monkey when it plucks fruit and carries it to the lips, give reactions a step further from the consummatory than those just instanced. *These reactions are all steps toward final adjustments, and are not themselves end-points.* The series of actions of which the distance-receptors initiate the earlier steps form series much longer than those initiated by the non-projicient. Their stages, moreover, continue to be guided by the projicient organs for a longer period between initiation and consummation. Thus in a positive phototropic reaction the eye continues to be the starting place of the excitation, and in many cases guides change in the direction not only of the eyeball but of the whole animal in locomotion as the reflex proceeds. The mere length of their series of steps and the vicissitudes of relation between bodies in motion reacting on one another at a distance conspire to give to these precurrent reflexes a multiformity and complexity un-

The Dominance of the Brain

paralleled by the reflexes from the non-projicient receptors. The reaction started by 'distance-receptors' where positive not only leads up to the consummatory reactions of the non-projicient, but on the way thither associates with it stimulation of other projicient receptors, as when, for instance, a phototropic reaction on the part of a Selachian brings the olfactory organs into range of an odorous prey, or, conversely, when the beagle sees the hare after running it by scent. In such a case the visual and olfactory receptor arcs would be related as 'allied' arcs (Lect. IV), and reinforce each other in regard to the mesencephalo-spinal path, or in higher mammals the 'pyramidal' or other pallio-spinal path. It is easy to see what copious opportunity for adjustment and of side connexion such a reaction demands, consisting as it does of a number of events in serial chain, each link a modification of its predecessor.

STRONG AFFECTIVE TONE AN ACCOMPANIMENT OF CONSUMMATORY REACTIONS

We may venture to turn briefly to the psychical aspect of such sequences. To consummatory reactions affective tone seems adjunct much more than to the anticipatory, especially the remotely anticipatory of the projicient sense-organs. Thus the affective tone of 'tastes' is strong. The reaction initiated by a *noci-ceptor* (pp. 227-32) is to be regarded as consummatory. The application of an irritant to the flank of a frog evokes a movement of the leg adapted to remove at once that stimulus from the skin of the flank. Or again, an irritant applied to the skin of the foot evokes a movement of the foot away from that stimulus. In both cases the reaction is a consummatory one, because it is calculated of itself to be final. To judge by our own introspection the affective tone adjunct to these reactions is strong. They instance strong affective tone pertaining to consummatory reactions. The affective tone of the reactions of the projicient receptors is less marked: physical pleasure or pain can hardly be said to accompany them. Not of course that they are wholly unrelated to affective tone. The relative haste with which an animal when hungry approaches food offered to the visual field suggests that conation attaches to the visual reaction by association through

Affective Tone in Consummatory Reactions

memory with affective tone. By associative memory a tinge of the affective tone of the consummatory reaction may suffuse the anticipatory. The latter becomes indirectly a pleasure-pain reaction. The neutral tango-receptive reactions of the feet of the tortoise hastening stumblingly towards its food may in this way be imbued with a tinge of affective tone derived from the affective tint of the leading reflex, namely the visual, which itself has thus memorial association with a consummatory reflex of strong affective tone. Examples of this type of reaction furnished by new-born animals are given by Lloyd Morgan.[165] When "after a few days the new-born chick leaves ladybirds unmolested while he seizes wasp-larvae with increased energy" he affords evidence that reactions of his projicient receptors have acquired a new value, and that value is made up *mediately* of affective tone. How they have acquired it or what exact nature their new attribute has is not our question. It is enough here that in regard to certain stimuli the new value—the meaning—which the projicient sensation has obtained has reinforced greatly the conative intensity of the reaction to the stimulus. It has given the stimulus increased force as a spring of precurrent actions aimed at a final consummatory one. It has given this not by altering the external stimulus, nor the receptor-organ, but by, among other alterations, altering internal connexions of the receptor arc. Thus it is that, be it by associative memory or other processes, the reactions of the 'distance-receptors' come in higher animals to reveal a conative driving force which is perhaps the end for which these psychoses exist.

Nor are the series of reactions, short though they be, which the non-projicient receptors initiate wholly *devoid* of conative appearance. They show adaptation as executive of steps toward an end. Food, sexual consummation, suitable posture, preservation from injury, are ends to which their direction leads, as with the longer series of actions due to projicient receptors reacting to objects at a wider horizon. It is rather that the latter afford a freer field for the winning of more subtle adjustments with wider application of associative memory. In the latter there is more scope for the play of mind—mind it may be of such elementary grade as to be difficult for us to picture in its operations.

The Dominance of the Brain

We may suppose that in the time run through by a course of action focussed upon a final consummatory event, opportunity is given for instinct, with its germ of memory however rudimentary and its germ of anticipation however slight, to evolve under selection that mental extension of the present backward into the past and forward into the future which in the highest animals forms the prerogative of more developed mind. Nothing, it would seem, could better ensure the course of action taken in that interval being the right one than memory and anticipatory forecast: and nothing, it would seem, could tend to select more potently the individuals taking the right course than the success which crowns that course, since the consummatory acts led up to are such—e.g. the seizure of prey, escape from enemies, attainment of sexual conjugation, etc.—as involve the very existence of the individual and the species. The problem before the lowlier organism is in some slight measure shadowed to us by the difficulties of adjustment of reaction shown by the human child. The child, although his reactions are perfect within a certain sphere of his surroundings, shows himself at the confines of that sphere a little blunderer in a world of overwhelming meaning. Hence indeed half the pathos and humour derivable from childhood.

It is the long serial reactions of the 'distance-receptors' that allow most scope for the selection of those brute organisms that are fittest for survival in respect to elements of mind. *The 'distance-receptors' hence contribute most to the uprearing of the cerebrum.* Swallowing was above termed a consummatory reaction. Once through the maw, the morsel is, we know by introspection, under normal circumstances lost for consciousness. But it nevertheless continues to excite receptors and their nervous arcs. The significant point is that the object has passed into such a relation with the surface of the organism that 'conation' is no longer of advantage. The naive notion that when we have eaten and drunken we have *fed* is justified *practically*. No *effort* can help us to incorporate the food further. Conation has then done its all and has no further utility in respect to that food taken. It is significant that all direct psychical accompaniment of the reactions ceases abruptly at this very point. The immediately precedent reactions that were psychically suffused with strong affective

Receptive Range of Receptors

colour pass abruptly over into reactions not merely affectively neutral but void—normally—of psychical existence altogether. The concomitance between certain nervous reactions and psychosis seems an alliance that strengthens the restless striving of the individual animal which is the passport of its species to continuance of existence.

RECEPTIVE RANGE

The ascendency of 'distance-receptors' in the organization of neural function may be partly traceable to the relative *frequency* of their use. Although it would be incorrect to assess the value of an organ by the mere frequency with which it is of service, yet *ceteris paribus* that seems a fair criterion. The frequency with which a receptor meets its stimuli is, other things being equal, proportionate to the size of the slice of the external world which lies within its *receptive range*. Although in a fish, for instance, the skin with its tango-receptors is much larger in area than are the retinae with their photo-receptors, the restricted 'receptive-range'—the adequate stimulus requiring actual proximity—of the former gives a far smaller slice of the stimulus-containing world to the skin than pertains to the eyes. In the case of the eye not only is the slice of environment pertaining to it at even a short distance more wide and high than that of the skin, but it is at each moment multiplied by the third dimension. There arise in it, therefore (*ceteris paribus*), in unit of time many more stimulations, with the result that the receptor-organ of 'distant' species receives many more fresh stimuli per unit of time than does the receptor-organ of restricted receptive range. The greater richness of the neural construction of the photo-receptive system than of the tango-receptive accords with this. Thus in the photo-receptive system the so-called 'optic nerve' (which since it is the second neural link and therefore to some extent a 'common path', presents numerical reduction from the first or private path in the retina itself) contains more conductive channels (nerve-fibres) in man (1,000,000, Krause) than are contained in the whole series of afferent spinal roots of one side of the body put together (634,000, Ingbert[264, 265]), and of these latter the cutaneous afferent fibres form only a part, and of that part the tango-receptive fibres themselves form only a fraction. The large number of the channels in the retinal path is no doubt primarily indicative of spatial differentiations of the receptive surface, but that spatial differentiation is itself indicative of the numbers of the stimuli frequenting that receptive field.

LOCOMOTION AND 'RECEPTIVE RANGE'

Locomotive progression and distance receptivity are two phenomena so fundamentally correlated that the physiology of neither can be comprehended without recognition of the correlation of the two. Evidence is forthcoming from ontogeny and phylogeny. The elaborateness of the photo-receptive organs of the flying Insecta corresponds with the great power of these forms to traverse space. When the Brachiopod passes from a motile wandering life to a fixed sedentary one its 'eyes' degenerate and go. The free-swimming *Ascidia* with fin-like motor organs and semi-rigid axial notochord, affording elasticity and leverage, bears at its anterior end a well-formed photo-receptor organ (eye) and a well-formed otocyst (head proprioceptor). Connected with the nerves of these, the anterior end of its truly vertebrate central nervous system has a relatively large 'brain'. Thence extends backward along the body a spinal cord. Suddenly its free-swimming habit is exchanged for a sedentary; by adhesive projections from its head, it attaches itself permanently to some fixed object. At once there ensues a readaptive metamorphosis. Degeneration sets in concurrently in its locomotive musculature, its eye, its otocyst, its brain, and its cord. These vanish as by magic save that a fraction of the brain remains as a small ganglion near the mouth. The sessile creature retains, so far as can be judged from their microscopic structure, only some gustatory (?) receptors round the mouth, and some tango-receptors (? noci-ceptors) in the tegument, connected doubtless with an irregular diffuse subtegumental layer of unstriped muscle-tissue. Experimental observations seem wanting on the point, but we may presume that in this metamorphosis the *receptive range* of *Ascidia* dwindles from dimensions measurable by all the distance through which its free motile individual floats and swims, to a mere film of the external world, say 1 mm. deep, at its

Receptive Range and Locomotion

own surface, especially round its mouth, and unextended by succession of time, save passively by the mere flowing of the water. Such instances illustrate the fundamental connexion between the function of the skeletal musculature and that of the 'distance-receptors'. Did we know better the sensual aspects of these cases the more significant doubtless would be the comparison.

THE 'HEAD' AS PHYSIOLOGICALLY CONCEIVED

As regards the objects acting on the organism at any moment through its receptors, the extension of environmental space—the animal's *receptive range*—is not equal in all directions as measured from the organism itself. The extension is greater in the direction about the 'leading' pole. Thus, the reactions initiated at the eye precede reactions (cf. Loeb's *Ketten-reflexe*) that will in due time come to pass through other receptor-organs. The visual receptors are usually near the leading pole, and so placed that they see into the field whither progression goes. And similarly with the olfactory receptors. The motor train behind, the elongated motor machinery of the rest of the body, is therefore from this point of view a motor appendage at the behest of the distance-receptor organs in front. The segments lying at the leading pole of the animal, armed as they are with the great 'distance' sense-organs, constitute what is termed the 'head'.

THE PROPRIO-CEPTIVE SYSTEM AND THE HEAD

We may now attempt to enquire whether this dominance of the leading segments which is traceable in the receptors of the exteroceptive field applies in the field of reception which we termed the proprio-ceptive. We arrived earlier at the notion that the field of reception which extends through the depth of each segment is differentiated from the surface field by two main characters. One of these was that while many agents which act on the body surface are excluded from the deep field as stimuli, an agency which does act there is mass, with all its mechanical consequences, such as weight, mechanical inertia, etc., giving rise to pressures, strains, etc., and that the receptors of this deep field are adapted for these as stimuli. The other character of the stimulations in this field we held to be that the stimuli are given in much greater measure than in the surface field of reception, by actions of the organism itself, especially by mass movements of its parts. Since these movements are themselves for the most part reactions to stimuli received by the animal's free surface from the environment, the proprio-ceptive reactions themselves are results in large degree habitually secondary to surface stimuli. The immediate stimulus for the reflex started at the deep receptor is thus supplied by some part of the organism itself as agent.

In many forms of animals, e.g. in vertebrates, there lies in one of the leading segments a receptor-organ (the labyrinth) derived from the extero-ceptive field, but later recessed off from it; and this is combined in action with receptors of the proprio-ceptive field of the remaining segments. This receptive organ, like those of the proprioceptive field, is adapted to mechanical stimuli. It consists of two parts, both endowed with low receptive threshold and with refined selective differentiation. One part, the otolith organ, is adapted to react to changes in the incidence and degree of pressure exerted on its nerve-endings by a little weight of higher specific gravity than the fluid otherwise filling the organ. The other part, the semicircular canals, reacts to minute mass movements of fluid contained within it. These two parts constitute the labyrinth. The incidence and degree of pressure of the otoliths upon their receptive bed change with changes in the *position* of the segments in which the labyrinth lies, relatively to the horizon line. *Movements* of the segment likewise stimulate the labyrinthine receptors through the inertia of the labyrinthine fluid and the otoliths. By the labyrinth are excited reflexes which adjust the segment (and with it the head is usually immovably conjoined) to the horizon line. And other parts are similarly reflexly adjusted by it. Thus, the refined photo-receptive patches in the head—the retinae—which conduct reflexes delicately differential in regard to space, appropriate for stimuli higher or lower or to right or to left in the photo-receptive patch, depend in their conduct of these upon a more or less constant standardization of their own normals of

The Proprio-ceptive System

direction in regard to the horizon line. These photo-receptive patches are set movably in the head; by the action of muscles they can retain their bearing to the horizon, although the head itself shifts its relation to the horizon. The control of these muscles lies largely with the labyrinth. The labyrinth produces a compensatory eyeball reflex. Thus in the head segments the labyrinth effects reflex movements analogous to that which the proprio-receptive nerves from the extensor muscles of the knee excites in the leg segments, reflexes restoring an habitual posture that has been departed from.

And from the above it seems clear that there is another feature of resemblance between the labyrinthine receptor and the proprio-ceptors of the limb. Stimulation of the labyrinth must in preponderant measure be given not by external agents directly but by the reaction of the organism itself. Posture and movement of the head are the immediate causes which stimulate the labyrinth, whether or not they be part of a total movement or posture of the whole individual. Such movement is most frequently an active one on the part of the animal itself. Thus, when *Ascidia* becomes sedentary and its locomotor musculature atrophies its otocyst disappears. But an animal's active movement is in its turn usually traceable as a reaction to an environmental stimulus affecting the receptors at the surface of the animal. Thus the labyrinthine receptors like the proprio-ceptors in other segments, are stimulated by the animal itself as agent, though secondarily to stimulation of the animal itself via some extero-ceptor.

And there is another point of likeness between labyrinth reflexes and those of the proprio-ceptors of the limb and other segments. The proprio-ceptors of the limbs appear productive of certain continuous, that is *tonic*, reflexes. Thus, in the decerebrate dog the tonic extensor rigidity of the leg appears reflexly maintained by afferent neurones reaching the cord from the deep structures of the leg itself. Similarly, if the knee-jerk be accepted as evidence in the spinal animal of a spinal tonus in the extensor muscle, this tonus seems maintained by afferent fibres from the extensor muscle itself, since the knee-jerk is extinguished by severance of those fibres. Again, the rapidity of onset of rigor mortis in a muscle is speedier when its tonus prior to death has been high. Section of the afferent roots of the

The Dominance of the Brain

limb prior to death delays onset of rigor mortis[304] in that limb as judged by stiffness at the knee; but that delay is not observable when skin-nerves only have been severed. The labyrinthine receptors appear likewise to be the source of certain maintained, that is tonic, reflexes. Destruction of the labyrinth also delays the onset of rigor mortis in the muscles to which its field of tonus can be traced. Ewald has shown that each labyrinth maintains tonus especially in the neck and trunk muscles and in the extensor-abductor limb-muscles of the homonymous side.

In regard to these tonic reflexes it is difficult to see how a steady mechanical stimulus can continue to elicit a reflex constantly for long periods. If we take sensation as a guide, a touch excited by constant mechanical pressure of slight intensity fades quickly below the threshold of sensation. It is said that a spinal frog may even be crushed by mechanical pressure without exciting from it a reflex movement provided that the pressure be applied by very slowly progressive increments. The office of a receptor would seem to be, placed across the line of a stream of energy, to react under the transference of energy across it, as for instance from the environment to the organism, or vice versa. We have many instances in which the living material adapts itself to, and maintains its own equilibrium under, different grades of environmental stress, treating each fairly continuous or slowly altering grade as a normal zero. The slow changes of barometric pressure on the body surface originate no skin-sensation, though they are much above the threshold value for touch. There constantly streams from the body through the skin a current of thermal energy much above the threshold value of stimuli for warmth sensations; yet this current evokes under ordinary circumstances no sensation. It is the stationary condition, the fact that the transference of energy continues at constant speed, which makes it unperceived. The receptor apparatus is not stimulated unless there is a change of rate in the transference, and that change of rate must occur in most cases with considerable quickness, otherwise there is a mere unperceived shift in the stationary equilibrium which forms the resting zero of the sensual apparatus. Over and over in the elicitation of reflexes as well as in the artificial excitation of nerve or muscle we meet this same

Reflex Tonus and Attitude

feature. Both for sensation and for reflex action a function in the threshold value of stimulus is time, as well as intensity and quantity. If a weak agent is to stimulate, its application must be abrupt. But in the tonic reflexes whose source lies at the proprio-ceptors and the labyrinth, a weak stimulus, although apparently unchanging, seems to continue to be an effective stimulus.

The proprio-ceptors and the labyrinthine receptors seem to have in common this, that they both originate and maintain tonic reflexes in the skeletal muscles. And they, at least in some instances, reinforce one another in this action. Thus the tonus of the extensor muscle of the knee in the cat and dog appears to have a combined source in the proprio-ceptors of that muscle itself and in the receptors of the homonymous labyrinth. The tonus of skeletal muscles is an obscure problem. Its mode of production, its distribution in the musculature, its purposive significance, are all debatable. The steadiness and slight intensity of the contraction constituting the tonus render its detection difficult. Part of the discrepancy between the experimental findings may be traced to the supposition that a reflex tonus if present is present in all muscles at all times. A single muscle examined for reflex tonus has been taken to represent all muscles under all conditions, although the answer has been sometimes positive and sometimes negative.

It appears to me likely that reflex tonus is the expression of a neural discharge concerned with the maintenance of *attitude*. In many reflex reactions the effect is movement and the muscles are dealt with as organs of motion. In these cases the stimuli and the reactions both of them are short-lived events. But much of the reflex reaction expressed by the skeletal musculature is postural. The bony and other levers of the body are maintained in certain attitudes both in regard to the horizon, to the vertical, and to one another. The frog as it rests squatting in its tank has an attitude far different from that which gravitation would give it were its musculature not in action. Evidently the greater part of the skeletal musculature is all the time steadily active, antagonizing gravity in maintaining the head raised, the trunk semi-erect, and the hind-legs tautly flexed. Innervation and co-ordination are as fully demanded for the

The Dominance of the Brain

maintenance of a posture as for the execution of a movement. This steady co-ordinate innervation antagonizes gravitation and other forces, e.g. as in currents of water. In these tonic as in other reflexes, antagonistic muscles co-operate co-ordinately. There is nothing to show that reciprocal innervation does not obtain in the one class of reflex as in the other. If so, it becomes easily intelligible that the slight reflex contraction termed *skeletal tonus* should under given conditions be found in some muscles and not in others. The slight reflex contraction will be accompanied by reflex inhibition of the antagonistic muscles. For reflex tonus to be the expression of a neural discharge which maintains attitude accords well with the ascription of its source to the proprio-ceptors, including the labyrinth. Those are exactly the receptors which, functioning as sense-organs, initiate sensations of posture and of attitude (Bonnier). And it accords also with the share in the production and regulation of skeletal tonus which the cerebellum has (Luciani's *atonia*) and the cerebrum.

Naturally, the distinction between reflexes of attitude and reflexes of movement is not in all cases sharp and abrupt. Between a short lasting attitude and a slowly progressing movement the difference is hardly more than one of degree. Moreover, each posture is introduced by a movement of assumption, and after each departure from the posture, if it is resumed, it is reverted to by a movement of compensation. Hence the taxis of attitude must involve not only static reactions of tonic maintenance of contraction, but innervations which execute reinforcing movements and compensatory movements. In all this kind of function the proprio-ceptors of the body generally and the labyrinthine receptors in the head, appear to co-operate together and form functionally one receptive system.

This system as a whole may be embraced within the one term 'proprio-ceptive'. Our inquiry regarding it is now, whether that part of it which is situate in the leading segments, namely its labyrinthine part, exerts preponderance in the system as do the extero-ceptors situate in the leading segments in the extero-ceptive system. It must be remembered of the extero-ceptive system that even in the segments which are not the leading segments its receptors considered

Role of Labyrinth in Total Posture

as sense organs produce sensations that have *some* projicience; and that in animals provided with outstanding skin appendages, e.g. hair, the tango-reflexes are to a slight extent reactions to objects at a distance. This germ of distance reaction and projicience of sensation in the extero-ceptors of the ordinary body-segments is developed in the extero-ceptors of the leading segments into the vast distance-reactions of the eye and the absolute projicience of vision. But the proprio-ceptors of the limb and body segments exhibit no germ of distance-reaction nor of projicience of sensation. And the specialized proprio-ceptor organ of the leading segment (the labyrinth) is similarly not a distance-receptor: although some of its sensations seem projected into the environment as well as referred to the organism itself, to the 'material me'. Any predominance this proprio-ceptor in the leading segments may exhibit in the proprio-ceptive system is not therefore in virtue of the quality of reaction at a distance. If pre-eminently important to the organism as a whole, its pre-eminence of importance rests on other grounds than does the importance of the great distance-receptors—the olfactory, the visual, and the auditory.

A posture of the animal as a whole—a total posture—is as much a complex built up of postures of portions of the animal—segmental postures (Bonnier)—as is the total movement of the animal—its locomotion—compounded of segmental movements. With the hinder part of its spinal cord alone intact the frog maintains a posture in its hind-limbs. These limbs are kept flexed at hip, knee, and ankle. When displaced from that posture they return to it. But if the animal be rolled over on its back it makes no attempt to right itself. The decerebrate frog with its labyrinths intact and their arcs still in connexion with the skeletal musculature maintains the well-known attitude before mentioned. If inverted it at once reverts to that. The labyrinth keeps the world right-side up for the organism by keeping the organism right-side up to its external world. The cranial receptors control the animal's *total* posture as do receptors of the hinder musculature the *segmental* posture of the hind-limbs when but the hind end of the spinal cord remains.

Thus the labyrinthine proprio-ceptors are largely the equilibrators

The Dominance of the Brain

of the head, and since the retinal patches are movably attached (in mobile eyeballs) to the head, and since each retina has its normals of direction conforming with those of the head, these equilibrators of the head are closely connected by nervous arcs with the musculature maintaining the postures of the eyeballs. The posture of the head in many animals is dependent on the musculature not of the head segments themselves but of a long series of segments behind the head. In many forms the motor organs that steadily maintain or passingly modify the position of the head in regard to the external world—conveniently indexed by the line of direction of gravitation—are contributed to by the skeletal musculature of many post-cranial segments. Hence the labyrinthine receptor is in touch with all the segments of the body, and these in a measure may be regarded as appended to the otic segment. Destruction of the labyrinth in the fish, the frog, the pigeon, and the dog produces not only malposture of the eyeball and the head, but of the limbs and body as a whole. The 'knock-out blow', where the lower jaw conveys concussion to the otocyst, reduces in a moment a vigorous athlete to an unstrung bulk of flesh whose weight alone determines its attitude, if indeed a reactionless mass can be described as possessing attitude at all.

The labyrinthine receptors and their arcs give the animal its definite attitude to the external world. The muscular receptors give to the segment—e.g. hind-limb—a definite attitude less in reference to the external world than in reference to other segments, e.g. the rest of the animal. Our own sensations from the *labyrinth* refer to some extent, as said above, to this environment, that is, have some projected quality; our *muscular* sensations refer to the body itself, e.g. contribute to perceptions of the relative flexions or extensions of our limbs. The arcs of the proprio-receptor of the leading segments control vast fields of the skeletal musculature, and deal with it as a whole, while the arcs of the proprio-ceptors of the other segments work with only limited regions of the musculature. Hence, in conformity with this the proprio-ceptor of the leading segments possesses long internuncial paths, for instance, bulbo-spinal from Deiter's nucleus proceeding to all levels of the spinal cord.

We traced the reactions of proprio-ceptors of the limb to bear

Nervous Integration of Segmental Series

habitually a secondary relation to the reactions of the extero-ceptors of the limb. Similar secondary relation is evident also between the reactions of the proprio-ceptor of the leading segments (the labyrinth) and the reactions of the extero-ceptors of those segments. These latter extero-ceptors were seen to be distance-receptors, and the reactions of distance-receptors were seen to be signalized by their anticipatory character. From secondary association with these distance-receptors the reactions of the labyrinth come in their turn to have anticipatory character. They retain, however, their own special features of equilibration and tonus. The locomotion of an animal impelled by its eye toward its prey involves co-operation of the labyrinth with the retina. And the tonic labyrinthine reflex which maintains an attitude may be just as truly an anticipatory reaction as any movement is. The steady flexed posture of the frog directed toward a fly seen on the aquarium wall is a co-ordinate innervation securing preparedness for the seizure of the food. Its character is as truly anticipatory as is that of any movement. We might speak of the animal as 'at rest', but it is the tense quietude of the hunter watching quarry rather than rest, such as supervenes in sleep and other conditions where active innervation is actually relaxed or reflex action is truly in abeyance.

NERVOUS INTEGRATION OF A SEGMENTAL SERIES

By longitudinal integration *short* series of adjoining segments become in respect to some one character combined together, so as to form in respect to that character practically a single organ. It is convenient to speak of such reflex reactions, confined from start to finish to a single integrated set of segments, as 'short reflexes' giving '*local reactions*'. Thus the vertebrate appendages called limbs are plurisegmental, but the individual segments constituting the limb form in respect of the limb a functional group of such solidarity that their reactions in the limb are at any one time unitary.

The reflexes that extend beyond the limit of such a group are on the other hand conveniently termed '*long reflexes*'. And it is in the integration of long series, or of the *whole* series, of segments one with

The Dominance of the Brain

another, that. apart from psychical phenomena, the nervous system seems to reach its acme of achievement. Here it is that we see eminently what Herbert Spencer has insisted on, namely, that integration keeps pace with differentiation.

In the segmental series the nervous concatenation of the segments repeats broadly the kind of association evidenced within each segment taken singly. Broadly taken, each segment has on the one hand a piece of the extero-ceptive field, a piece of the proprio-ceptive field, and a piece of the intero-ceptive field, though this last is wanting in not a few segments. On the other, it has fractions of the skeletal, of the vascular, and of the visceral effector organs. Each segment has musculature and glands on its outer and visceral surfaces. Some segments have also secretors discharging into body spaces. Each of these sets of features of the segments has in the series of segments a nervous system of some functional homogeneity. With these plurisegmental systems as with their unisegmental pieces in the single segment the same harmonies of interconnexion are observable. Thus, the nervous arcs embouching into the skeletal musculature start chiefly in the extero-ceptive field in so far as concerns execution of passing movements, in the proprio-ceptive field in so far as concerns tonic postures; and so on, as sketched above. If the receptors of the extero-ceptive field are regarded from the point of view of the nature of the agency adequate for each of their species, representatives of each species are found in almost every segment. In this way the functional properties of the extero-ceptive field form not one but several multisegmental organs or systems of organs. In each segment exist receptors responsive to mechanical, chemical, and radiant agencies respectively. There is thus formed a tango-ceptive system to which practically every segment contributes, a thermo-ceptive system, a noci-ceptive system; so also a musculo-ceptive system, and probably the receptors of the intero-ceptive surface similarly constitute a homogeneous system, prominent among their adequate agencies being those of chemical quality. These systems of receptive arcs present, though more or less compound, a solidarity of action in each system that gives each some rank as a physiological entity.

Position of Receptor as Factor in Differentiation

RESTRICTION OF SEGMENTAL DISTRIBUTION A FACTOR IN INTEGRATION

The impulse to nervous integration given by regional restriction of a peculiar species of organ to a single segment has especial force where that organ is of especial importance. This is the case with effector organs subserving important actions of consummatory (vide supra pp. 326, 329) type, e.g. a sexual appendage, or the mouth. Such organs as these are of restricted regional distribution and subserve important reactions of consummatory type. With the mouth is associated differentiation of organs around it. Many postures and movements of the organism are advantageous or disadvantageous to the animal's existence mainly inasmuch as they improve or disimprove the position or attitude of the mouth in regard to objects in the external world. Much of the long series of movements and other reactions initiated and guided by 'distance-receptors' themselves is by-play on the way to a consummatory reaction which requires an appropriate placing and attitude of the mouth. That there is only one mouth and that of limited segmental extent involves co-ordination of the activities of many other segments with the oral. Integration of plurisegmental activity is effected here, as in the other cases, mainly by the synaptic nervous system. The fact that the mouth is usually placed near the leading segments of the anterior pole is therefore a further factor in differentiating the segments at that end from the after-coming train. Thus it comes about that in many cases the animal consists of two portions broadly different in character but complemental the one to the other, the *head* and the *trunk*.

It is noteworthy that the increase of susceptibility instanced by the distance-receptors is in each case restricted to a special patch, quite limited in area. Given a synaptic nervous system, no single item of functional arrangement more enforces integration of an individual from its segments than the restriction of a special kind of receptor to a single area or segment in the whole series. The motor apparatus of many segments has then to subserve a single segment, since that segment is provided with a receptor of a species not otherwise possessed by the individual at all. For integrative co-ordination of

The Dominance of the Brain

that kind, the synaptic nervous system affords the only instrument in the animal economy. Only by the formation of common paths can due advantage be reaped from a specially refined recipient path (private path) of locally restricted situation.

Further, the condensed setting of a group of specialized receptors favours their simultaneous stimulation in groups together. Stimuli even of small area then cover a number of receptive points in the receptive sheet. Thus, ocular images of various two-dimensional shape tend to be better differentiated by the photo-receptors the more closely the individual photo-receptors lie together. More data are thus gained as a basis for differential reaction.

Further, the juxtaposition of groups of specially refined receptors in one set of segments, the leading or head segments, conduces toward their simultaneous stimulation by several agencies emanating from one and the same environmental object. Thus, the property of brightness and the property of odour belonging to an object of prey may then better excite in unison a reaction in the distant reagent, or excite more potently than would either property alone. And movements of the reagent itself are then more apt to intensify simultaneously the reactions of its two kinds of receptors. The collocation of the disparate receptors in one region will favour that which psychologists in describing sensations term 'complication', a process which in reflex action has a counterpart in the conjunction of reflexes excited by receptors of separate species but of allied reaction. This alliance of reaction we have seen finds expression as mutual reinforcement in action upon a final common path. Thus a reaction is synthesized which deals with the environmental object not merely as a stimulus possessing one property but as a 'thing' built up of properties. A reflex is attained which has its psychological analogue in a sense percept.

THE CEREBELLUM IS THE HEAD GANGLION OF THE PROPRIO-CEPTIVE SYSTEM

If the basis taken for classification of receptors be a physiological one with, as its criterion, the type of reaction which the receptors induce, separate receptive systems may be traced running throughout the

Cerebellum is Head-Ganglion of Proprio-ceptive System

whole series of segments composing the total organism. We have seen that such separate receptive systems may be treated as functional unities, extending through the segmental series. In any such system there is evident a tendency for its central nervous mechanisms, that is to say, the components of the central nervous organ which specially accrue to the system in question, to be gathered chiefly where the most important contribution to its receptive paths enters the central nervous system. The receptive system in question has as it were its focus at that place. Thus receptive neurones which can influence respiratory movement enter the central nervous organ at various segments, but the chief respiratory centre lies in the bulb where the receptive neurones from the lung itself make entrance and central connexion, the vagal receptors being preponderantly regulative in that function. And we have seen that a proprio-ceptive organ (the labyrinth) in the head segments seems preponderantly regulative in those functions which the proprio-ceptive system subserves. The central neural mechanism belonging to the proprio-ceptive system is preponderantly built up over the central connexions of this proprio-ceptive organ (the labyrinth) belonging to the head. Thither converge internuncial paths stretching to this mechanism from the central endings of various proprio-ceptive neurones situate in all the segments of the body. There afferent contributions from the receptors of joints, muscles, ligaments, tendons, viscera, etc., combine with those from the muscular organs of the head and with those of the labyrinthine receptors themselves. A central nervous organ of high complexity results. Its size from animal species to animal species strikingly accords with the range and complexity of the habitual movements of the species; in other words, with the range and complexity of the habitual taxis of the skeletal musculature. This central organ is the cerebellum.

The symptoms produced by its destruction or injury in whole or in part in many ways resemble, therefore, the disturbances produced by injury of the labyrinth itself. It also influences tonus very much as do the simple proprio-ceptive arcs themselves. It is closely connected structurally and functionally with the so-called motor region of the cerebral hemisphere, just as the simpler proprio-ceptive arcs and reflexes are closely associated with the mechanisms of exteroceptive reactions. Knowledge is not ripe as yet for an adequate definition of the function of the cerebellum. Many authorities have defined it as the centre for the maintenance of the mechanical equilibrium of the body. Others regard it as the organ for co-ordination of volitional movement. Spencer suggested that it was the organ of co-ordination of bodily action in regard to space, the cerebrum he suggested being the organ of co-ordination of bodily action in respect of time. Lewandowski considers it the central organ for the 'muscular sense'. Luciani, the universally acknowledged authority on the physiology of the cerebellum, describes it as the organ which by unconscious processes exerts a continual reinforcing action on the activity of all other nerve-centres.

It is instructive to note how all these separate pronouncements harmonize with the supposition that the organ is the chief co-ordinative centre or rather group of centres of the reflex system of proprioception. The cerebellum may indeed be described as the head ganglion of the proprio-ceptive system, and the head ganglion here, as in other systems, is the main ganglion.

THE CEREBRUM IS THE GANGLION OF THE 'DISTANCE-RECEPTORS'

By the 'distance-receptors' are initiated and guided long series of reactions of the animal as a whole. Other receptive reactions integrate individual segments; the reactions of the distance-receptors integrate the whole series of segments. It is in the sphere of reactions of these 'distance-receptors' that the most subtle and complex adjustments of the animal therefore arise. In their neural machinery not only short arcs but long arcs, involving extensive internuncial tracts, figure largely. Chains of reaction conducive to a final reaction relatively remote are more evident with them than with other arcs. If appeal to psychical evidence be ventured on, it is to the field of operation of the arcs of these distance-receptors that higher feats of associative memory accrue, and, though the phrase is hardly permissible here except with curtailed scope, conation becomes more intelligent. Finally, in harmony with the last inference, it is over

Cerebrum is Ganglion of 'Distance-Receptors'

these 'distance-receptors' and in connexion with their reflexes and arcs that the cerebrum itself is found. The cerebrum constitutes, so to say, the ganglion of the 'distance-receptors'. Langendorff[74, 74a] has pointed out that a blinded frog resembles in its reactions a frog with the cerebrum removed: the elasmobranch without its olfactory lobes behaves as if it had lost its fore-brain. Edinger traces the genesis of the cerebral cortex to a distance-receptor, namely the olfactory organ.

The integration of the animal associated with these 'distance-receptors' of the leading segments can be briefly with partial justice expressed by saying that the rest of the animal, so far as its motor machinery goes, is but the servant of them. We might imagine the form of the individual and the disposition of the sense-organs as primitively very simple; for instance, a spheroid with a digestive cavity and sense-organs distributed especially over the external surface. Such an imaginary form we should expect under evolution to become modified. If a motile organism, its contractile mechanisms would obtain mechanical advantage (leverage) by its elongation in certain directions. The lengthwise extension of the vertebrate body and of its lateral motor appendages, e.g. limbs, are in so far such as might be argued *a priori*. Under evolution in motile animals adaptations securing appropriate leverage for the contractile apparatus appear, and length along certain axes is always a consideration in them. In animals with segments ranged along a single axis, the animal for the greater part of its length comes to be one great motor organ, complex and able to execute movements in various ways, but still a unity. The pole at which the great 'distance-receptors' (visual, olfactory, auditory) lie is that which, in the habitual locomotion of the animal under the action of the motor train attached, 'leads'. The animal therefore moves habitually into that part of environmental space which has been already explored by the distance-receptors of its own leading segments.

The head is in many ways the individual's greater part. It is the more so the higher the individual stands in the animal scale. It has the mouth, it takes in the food, including water and air, it has the main receptive organs providing data for the rapid and accurate

The Dominance of the Brain

adjustment of the animal to time and space. To it the trunk, an elongated motor organ with a share of the digestive surface and the skin, is appended as an apparatus for locomotion and nutrition. The trunk must of necessity lie at the command of the great receptor-organs of the head. The co-ordination of the activities of the trunk with the requirements of the head is a cardinal function of the synaptic nervous system. Conducting arcs must pass from the cephalic receptors to the contractile masses of the body as a whole. The spinal cord contains these strands of conductors in vertebrates and is from this point of view a mere appendage of the brain. A salient feature of these conducting arcs is that the nerve-fibres from the cephalic receptors do not run, as might perhaps *a priori* have been thought natural, direct from their cephalic segment backwards to reach the common effector paths upon which they embouch. Instead of having that arrangement, these fibres, starting in the cephalic receptors, end in the gray matter of the central nervous axis not far from their own segment. Thence the conducting arc is continued backward by another strand of fibres, and these reach (perhaps directly) the mouths of the final common paths in the grey matter of segments of the spinal cord. This is the arrangement exemplified by the pulmono-phrenic and other respiratory arcs, the depresso-splanchnic arcs, the olfacto-phrenic respiratory arcs, the arcs between the otic labyrinth and the muscles maintaining posture in the trunk. and practically that of the retino-motor arcs connecting the retina with the muscles of the neck. It gives at least one synapsis more than the first alternative would do. And each *synapse is an apparatus for co-ordination*; it introduces a '*common path*'. And it is in the exercise of the distance-receptors with their extensive range overlapping that of other receptors that the reflexes which relate to 'objects' in the sense that they are reflexes synthesized from receptors of separate species, become chiefly established. The ramifications of the central neurones attached to these receptors are so extensive and the reactions they excite are so far spreading in the organism that their association with the reactions and central mechanisms of other receptors is especially frequent and wide.

The distance-receptors are the great inaugurators of reaction. The

Cerebrum is Ganglion of 'Distance-Receptors'

reduced initiation of action which ensues on ablation of the cerebrum seems explicable by that reason. The curtailment which ensues is indicative of damage which their removal inflicts on reactions generated by the distance-receptor organs. By a high spinal transection the splendid motor machinery of the vertebrate is practically as a whole and at one stroke severed from all the universe except its own microcosm and an environmental film some millimetres thick immediately next its body. The deeper depression of reaction into which the higher animal as contrasted with the lower sinks when made spinal signifies that in the higher types more than in the lower the great distance-receptors actuate the motor organ and impel the actions of the individual. The deeper depression shows that as the individual ascends the scale of being, the more reactive does it become as an individual to the circumambient universe outside itself. It is significant that spinal shock hardly at all affects the nervous reactions of the intero-ceptors (visceral system); and that it does not affect the interoceptive arcs appreciably more in the monkey than in the frog. Its brunt falls, as we have seen before, on the reactions of the skeletal musculature. Not that in the highest animal forms the 'distance-receptor' merely *per se* has necessarily reached more perfection or more competence than in the lower. In the lower types, as in fish, are found 'distance-receptors' of high perfection, but their ablation does not in lower types cripple in the *same way* as in higher types. It is that in the higher types there is based upon the 'distance-receptors' a relatively enormous neural superstructure possessing million-sided connexions with multitudinous other nervous arcs and representing untold potentialities for redistribution of so-to-say stored stimuli by *associative recall*. The development and elaboration of this internal nervous mechanism attached to the organs of distance-reception has, so far as we can judge, far outstripped progressive elaboration of the peripheral receptive organs themselves. Adaptation and improvement would seem to have been more precious assets in the former than in the latter. And, as related to the former rather than to the latter, must be regarded the parallelism of the ocular axes and the overlapping of the uniocular fields of photo-reception which in mammals has gradually reached its acme in the monkey and in man.

The Dominance of the Brain

This overlapping yields, in virtue one would think of some process akin to Herbart's 'complication', an important additional datum for visual space. This, together with promotion of the fore-limb from a simple locomotor prop to a delicate explorer of space in manifold directions, together also with the organization of mimetic movement to express thoughts by sounds, have, with the developments of central nervous function which they connote and promote, been probably the chief factors in man's outstripping other competitors in progress toward that aim which seems the universal goal of animal behaviour, namely to dominate more completely the environment. Remembering these conditions, it need not surprise us that the distance-receptors more and more exert preponderant directive influence over the whole nervous system. To say this is to say no more than that the motile and consolidated individual is driven, guided, and controlled by, above all organs, its cerebrum. The integrating power of the nervous system has in fact in the higher animal, more than in the lower, constructed from a mere collection of organs and segments a functional unity, an individual of more perfected solidarity. We see that the distance-receptors integrate the individual not merely because of the wide ramification of their arcs to the effector organs through the lower centres; they integrate especially because of their great connexions in the high cerebral centres. Briefly expressed, their special potency is because they integrate the animal through its brain. The cerebrum itself may be indeed regarded as the ganglion of the distance-receptors.

Lecture X

SENSUAL FUSION

ARGUMENT: Nervous integration in relation to bodily movement and to sensation compared. Sensual fusion in a relatively simple instance of binocular vision. The rotating binocular lantern. Flicker sensations generated at 'corresponding retinal points'; absence of evidence of their summation or interference either with synchronous or asynchronous flicker of similar frequency. Their interference when the flicker is of dissimilar frequency. Talbot's law not applicable to 'corresponding points'. Fechner's paradox. Prevalence of contours under Weber's law and under binocular summation compared. The physiological initial stages of the reaction generated in either of a pair of corresponding retinal points proceeds without touching the apparatus of the twin point. Only after the sensations initiated from the right and left 'points' have been elaborated so far as to be well amenable to introspection does interference between the reactions of the two (right and left) eye-systems occur. The convergence of nerve-paths from the right and left retinae respectively toward one cerebral region is significant of union for co-ordination of motor reaction rather than for synthesis of sensation. Resemblances between motor and sensual reactions. The cerebrum pre-eminently the organ of and for the adaptation of reactions.

THE animal whose nervous construction we have been attempting to follow thus far, we have supposed merely a puppet moved by the external world in which it is immersed; and we have supposed it a puppet without passions, memory, feelings, sensations, let alone ideas concrete or abstract. From time to time we have purposely invoked appeal to sensations and feelings such as our own experience of ourselves provides in order to see better whither lead the blind reactions of the thing that we have been imagining a fatal mechanism. Whether such sensations or feelings accompany or do not accompany the reactions we have been studying we have left open. We have tacitly consented that our point of study of those reactions leaves that question, to which the present time gives no clear answer, as one with which we are not concerned. But we may agree that if such sensations and feelings or anything at all closely like them do accompany the reactions we have studied, the neural machinery to whose working *they* are adjunct lies not confined in the nervous arcs we have so far traced but in fields of nervous apparatus that,

Sensual Fusion

though connected with those arcs, lie beyond them, in the cerebral hemispheres.

In the attempt to trace the integrative work of the nervous system on its motor side, one of our leading principles has been that of the *correlation of reflexes about a final common path*. Owing to the convergence of many various reflex-arcs toward and their confluence in a common efferent path, co-ordination in their use of that path obtains and is demonstrable.

It has been shown that some reflexes are so correlated in regard to a final common path that their actions on it coalesce and reinforce each other. These are *allied* reflexes and have allied arcs. Good examples of allied reflexes and arcs are those which arise in receptors of one species distributed in one regional locality and subserving one and the same type-reflex; such are the arcs from the shoulder region of the dog subserving the scratch-reflex. We have also seen that reflexes which use the same 'final common path' but use it to different or opposed effect are so correlated in regard to it that one reflex can temporarily inhibit the other from use of the path. These reflexes we termed in regard to each other *antagonistic*.

From these motor reactions it is natural to attempt to cross the gulf from movement to sensation. In the bulbo-spinal dog we may produce a flexion of the fore-limb by stigmatic stimulation of the outer digit. We may also provoke a reflex, in its motor expression to all outward appearance like the preceding, by simultaneous stimulation of the skin of the innermost together with that of the outermost digit. Or we may evoke a similar reflex in the limb by stimulating simultaneously with the fore-foot the opposite hind-foot. Here there is no conflict between the reactions to the component stimuli. We may add further the simultaneous stimulation of the same side pinna. The reflex is then of more compound origin, but its component reflexes are so correlated about their *final common paths* to the fore-limb that their actions there coalesce and reinforce. Further, we may add to these stimuli others applied to receptors of species actually different from any of the cutaneous and thus still further add to the sources of the total reflex; and we may choose sources which are harmonious and the impulses from them flow together and combine.

Nervous Synthesis underlying Simple Sense Perception

On the other hand, instead of adding factors that tend to combine in the production of a particular reflex we may excite simultaneously with other sources a source whose reaction is incompatible with theirs. Then struggle and rivalry ensue and the result may be inhibition of that particular reflex movement and appearance of some other.

It appears to follow from such considerations that when we find electrical excitation of certain spots of the cerebral hemisphere regularly evoke certain movements, e.g. of a limb, the probability is that we have there a nodal point where various harmoniously acting neural arcs are tied together and can be there reached and driven as a unit—though a highly synthesized one—and produce the effect which is the common resultant of them all.

The receptive points and organs which under stimulation initiate reflex movements also initiate, in the intact animal with unmutilated brain, sensations. As each reflex has a reflex action attributive to it, so it has potentially at least a sensual reaction. These sensual reactions, like the motor reflexes, are of various grades of complexity. The simple perceptual image of an object is usually a resultant as regards external stimulation of stimuli applied jointly to several sense-organs. It has direct sensual factors traceable from various sources. The cigar taken from its box may be simultaneously sensed through eye and hand and nose and ear. The object experimentally regarded as a single object excites a neural reaction that has its starting points in many spatially and qualitatively distinct receptive points, each point the commencement of separate nervous arcs. In the psychical result of the reactions thus set going there is amplification and modification by conditions memorial, affective, judicial, conative, etc., obtaining in the mind and not due immediately to the stimulus. The neural process resulting from the nervous impulses initiated by the retinal, olfactory, cutaneous, and muscular receptors is therefore internally modified in the nervous system by processes and states already existent there or evoked there by itself as a reverberation of its action. Can we at all compare with the simultaneous co-ordination of the nervous factors in a motor reflex the synthesis of the nervous elements whose combination underlies a simple sense-perception?

Sensual Fusion

We may somewhat reduce the complexity of the sense-percept by limiting its paths of initiation to those of a single sense, namely the visual, excluding the object, e.g. the *seen* cigar, from directly stimulating other sense channels, tactual, olfactory, auditory, muscular, etc. The cigar may be offered only to the eye. Then we have left as regards the external stimulation merely the fusion of the right-eye and the left-eye images. This fusion is so complete that we cannot by introspection discriminate in the visual image the right-eye image from the left-eye image. Moreover, this fusion is so elemental that introspection cannot detect in it any effort of memory, judgement, or reason. It appears innate—a datum ready provided even at dawn of individual human consciousness. We can further strip the problem of some of its complexity by substituting for the three-dimensional object, e.g. the cigar, with its perspective shading and its patches of colour and its characteristic associations, etc., a simple and relatively meaningless discoid patch of moderate, even, and uncoloured brightness, small enough to lie wholly on the central area of each retina. We can then test to what degree the visual singleness of the observed surface, sensed through right eye and left eye together, is due to direct confluence of the sensory paths excited by the right-eye and left-eye images respectively. We can attempt this in the following way.[299]

A double sheet of thick milk-glass is observed by transmitted light given by a lamp. This lamp is set in the axis of a rotating cylinder (Fig. 76). In the side of the cylinder are three horizontal rows of rectangular windows, tier above tier. The lamp, though fixed in the axis of rotation of this revolving cylindrical screen, is entirely free from all attachment to it. The milk-glass plate is fixed between the lamp and the inner face of the tiers of windows, close to the latter.

Outside the moving cylindrical screen is a fixed semi-cylindrical screen concentric with the revolving one, and just wide enough to allow the inner revolving one to turn within it freely (Fig. 76). In the fixed cylindrical screen four circular holes are arranged so that two are centred on the same horizontal line, and of the other two one is centred just so far above the left-hand hole of the just mentioned pair as the other is below the right-hand member of the pair. The

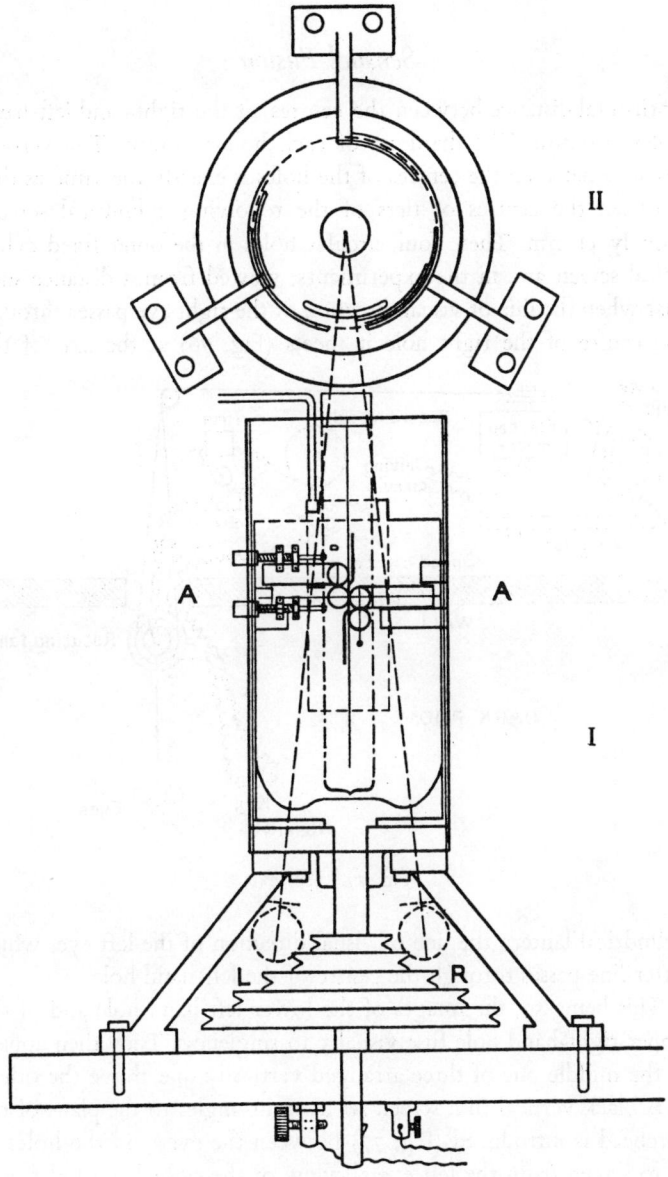

Fig. 76. Rotating Lantern
I. Elevation seen from front. II. Horizontal plan, through level of A–A of I. Supports seen in perspective. The eyeballs, pupil screens, and convergent visual axes are indicated belonging to II, but carried through I. The plan of the lantern is given one-fourth actual size. Description in text.

Sensual Fusion

horizontal distance between the centres of the right- and left-hand holes is 9 mm. The diameter of each hole is 8 mm. The vertical distance between the centres of the holes is exactly the same as that between the centres of tiers of the revolving cylindrical screen, namely 11 mm. These four circular holes in the outer fixed cylindrical screen are, in the experiments, viewed from a distance such that when the line of visual direction of the right eye passes through the centre of the right hole it meets (Fig. 76) at the axis of the

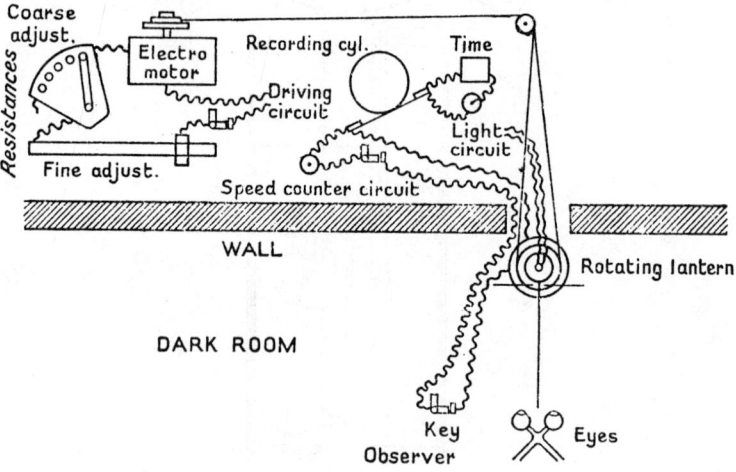

Fig. 77. See text

cylindrical lantern the line of visual direction of the left eye, which latter line passes through the centre of the left-hand hole.

This being so, the images of the lower left-hand hole and of the upper right-hand hole fuse visually to singleness. They then appear as the middle one of three arranged vertically one above the other.

A black vertical thin screen set at right-angles to the plane of the forehead is introduced (Fig. 77) between the eyes and the holes so as to screen from the left eye all view of the right-hand holes, and from the right eye all view of the left-hand holes.

The revolving screen is driven by an electromotor. The speed of revolution of this motor is controlled by a coarse adjustment and by

The Rotating Binocular Lamp

a fine adjustment. The speed of rotation of the cylindrical screen is recorded by marking the completion of each revolution of its spindle by an electromagnetic signal writing on a travelling blackened surface (Fig. 77). On the same surface the time is recorded by a writing-clock marking fifths of seconds.

The inner revolving screen by its revolution opens and shuts alternately for equal periods the circular holes in the fixed outer screen. The inner screen with its three tiers of windows is made in three pieces, each containing one tier of the windows. The piece containing the middle tier of openings is jointed in such a way that its openings can be set at any desired interval with the openings of the lowest tier. The highest tier is similarly jointed to the middle tier. In this way it can be arranged that the uppermost circular hole is open when the lower ones are closed, or is shut when the lower are closed, or is opened to any desired degree either before or after the lower; further, by removing the top gallery of the rotating screen it can be left permanently open. A similar relationship is also allowed between the middle holes and the lower.

By wearing weak prisms with their base-apex lines vertical, the images of the right-hand and left-hand holes can be brought to the same horizontal levels. The observer can then immediately fuse the four images to two by convergence. A horizontal fine thread halving each of the two middle holes, and similar but vertical threads halving the other two holes, serve to certify binocular vision to the observer. When the four holes are all allowed to act thus under appropriate convergent binocular gaze they are seen by the observer as two evenly lighted disks, one vertically above the other, and each cut into quadrants by a delicate black cross. By separately adjustable shutters any one, or any vertically edged fraction of one, of the disks can be separately screened out of vision.

The object of the above arrangement is to attain the following conditions. Images accurately similar are received by retinal areas fully visually conjugate. The areas are not only of the so-called 'geometrical identity', but are at the time of the observation in full binocular co-operation, owing to the concurrent convergence and accommodation. Extinction and illumination of the images occur

Sensual Fusion

pari passu in the two eyes, i.e. with like speed and in like direction. It can be synchronous or of any time-sequence desired. That the speed shall be similar for the two is insured by all the shutters being on the same spindle.

Each disk-shaped image will have on the retina a diameter of about 570μ. That is, when foveal vision is directed upon it, the image will occupy a practically rod-free area containing about 2800 cones. The direction of translation being the same for all the shutters the bright images on the two retinae are, if the shutters are set for simultaneous right and left images, commenced on 'identical' points of the two retinae, established progressively along 'identical' points, and finally extinguished in like manner progressively along 'identical' points. Or, conversely, if the shutters are set for accurately alternate right and left images the screening off begins in one eye at a spot and moment identical with those at which the turning on of the image commences in the other eye; so similarly it finishes. With the speeds of revolution used for the observations the time the shutter takes to expose or occlude completely each bright disk, varies between 0·011 and 0·002 sec. Error that might arise on this score is avoided by the consensual direction of movement of the right- and left-hand shutters.

That the 'retinal points' to which the images are thus applied synchronously or in desired sequence are truly 'identical' is certified, (1) by the paired physical images being seen single; (2) by the maximum disparation of the edges of the rotating shutters being about 7μ on the retina, whereas 350μ is about the vertical retinal disparation which limits binocular combination. Moreover, a contour travelling through a visual angle of 2° in $\frac{1}{90}$ sec., as in these observations, is not perceptible as a contour at all.

Difficulties due to change in pupil-width are excluded by artificial pupils. Equality of brightness of illumination of the four milk-glass-backed 8 mm. holes is obtained by making the straight-wire candle-shaped lamp of considerable, i.e. 12 cm. length, and fixing it accurately in the axis of the cylindrical screen. The rotating screen is blackened inside to minimize reflexion.

In this way two haploscopic images, one close above the other, are

Symmetrical Binocular Flicker

placed in the central field. The right and left components of each of these can be either synchronously or alternately compounded in each. The foveal gaze can be turned from one to the other of them when and as often as the observer desires, and in the fraction of a second by a slight, i.e. less than 3°, movement of the eyeballs. The comparison thus instituted is facile and sure.

A. SYMMETRICAL FLICKER

With the apparatus thus arranged various binocular combinations can be investigated and compared either one with another or with uniocular images.

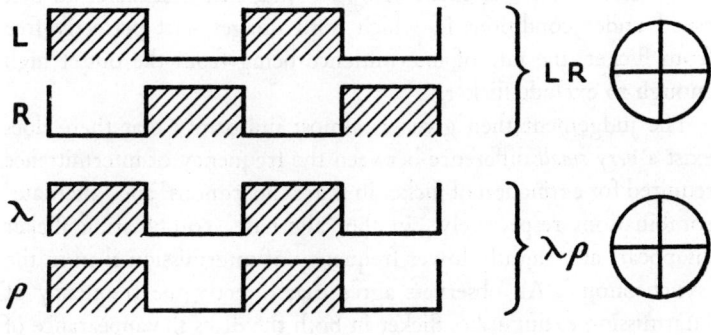

Fig. 78

As shown above, the apparatus allows of similar images being thrown on strictly and fully conjugate points of the two retinae, either synchronously right and left or alternately right and left, with a time accuracy not less than 0·0006 sec. for the slowest rates of intermission, and not less than 0·0001 sec. for the highest. The first comparison made (Exp. 1) may be to observe if there is any difference between the rates of intermittence for just perceptible flicker in two binocular images, one made with synchronous right and left illuminations, the other with alternate right and left illuminations. This arrangement is expressed graphically by the accompanying diagram (Fig. 78).

Sensual Fusion

The diagram makes the lower composite image the 'synchronous' one, but in the series of observations the 'synchronous' is sometimes the lower, sometimes the upper, and the observer is not informed which it may be. The observations may be made on the transition from flickering to unflickering sensation, or conversely on the transition from unflickering to flickering sensation; the observer in the latter has a more neutral approach to critical observation. Compared under rates of intermittence giving marked flicker in both images, observers find the flicker 'less' in the 'alternate' than in the 'synchronous' combination. This difference at the lower speeds inclines the observer to expect that complete extinction of the flicker will disappear the more readily in the image which at slow intermissions seems to flicker the less. Judgement is therefore best asked under conditions in which both images start perfectly free from flicker, the rate of intermittence being from the outset high enough to exclude flicker.

The judgement then given is almost uniformly that there does exist a *very small* difference between the frequency of intermittence required for extinction of flicker in the 'synchronous' and 'alternate' combinations respectively. In the 'alternate' combination flicker disappears at a slightly lower frequency of intermission than in the 'synchronous'. All observers agree that directly the frequency of intermission extinguishes flicker in both the disks the appearance of both is indistinguishably similar, and that there is then nothing to choose between the brightness of the two.

For almost all persons I have examined, a spot intermittently illuminated at a frequency of intermission just sufficient to extinguish flicker in it, when looked at with one eye only, still flickers slightly when looked at with both eyes. A like phenomenon is noticed by most observers when examined by the arrangement (Exp. 2) represented by Fig. 79.

The binocular arrangement, then, is said by them to require a slightly higher frequency for extinction of flicker than does the uniocular. Again, if under a frequency of intermission just securing extinction of flicker in either of the component uniocular images separately, one of these images, previously screened off, is readmitted,

Symmetrical Binocular Flicker

so that the pair act together with a synchronous arrangement of phase, a trace of flicker appears at once in the binocular image. It may be urged that this is due to the fresh retinal area being more sensitive to flicker, and it is true that the flicker so introduced tends soon to become less, but a residuum of the phenomenon seems to remain.

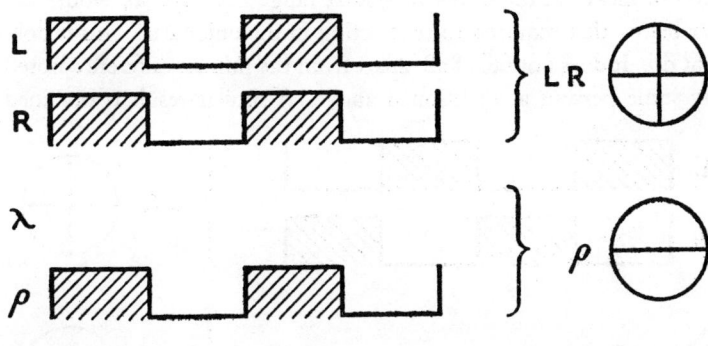

Fig. 79

Exp. 3. Conversely, under the arrangement indicated in Fig. 80, a number of the persons examined, but not all, decide that the binocular image requires for extinction of flicker a slightly lower frequency of intermittent illumination than does the uniocular. Also, a number of these persons, though not all, find that when the 'alternate right and left' combination is observed under a frequency of intermission of illumination just sufficient to extinguish its flicker, the screening out of one of the component uniocular images brings with it a slight appearance of flicker.

From these observations it appears that similar phases of flickering illumination if timed to fall coincidentally on conjugate retinal areas do *very slightly reinforce* each other in sensation, and if timed exactly alternately do very slightly *mutually reduce*. But the *broad outcome of the observations is that* so far from bright phases at one eye effacing dark phases at the corresponding spot of the other eye, *there is hardly a trace of any such interference*. To judge from its absence of influence on the flicker rate, the dark phase incident at retinal point A' does not, as regards sensual result, modify the bright phase synchronously incident at the conjugal retinal point A, and conversely. If the brightness of the bright phase or the darkness of the dark phase were lessened at A by A', the rate of frequency of stimulus for extinction of flicker must fall. But except in minute and perhaps equivocal degree it does not alter.

Sensual Fusion

As far as sensual effect goes, the light phases at the one eye practically do not, therefore, interfere or combine with the coincident dark phases at the other; and conversely. Nor do they, in the alternate left and right arrangement, add themselves as a series of additional stimuli to the like series of stimuli applied at the other eye. If they did the revolution rate of the cylindrical shutter required for extinction of flicker in the upper binocular range LR, Fig. 80, would fall far below that required for extinction in the uniocular. This it does not do. It does not fall at all, apart from the minute difference noted by some persons as mentioned above. A similar result is obtained

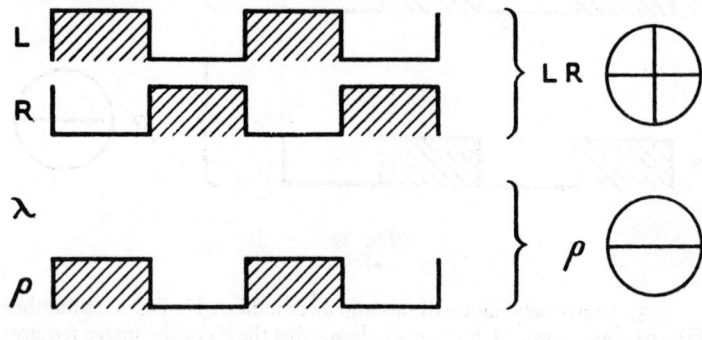

Fig. 80

under the, in some ways more decisive, conditions (Exp. 4) represented in Fig. 81.

With this arrangement no observer in my experiments has ever with certainty detected difference between the uniocular and binocular images in regard to either the apparent rate of the flicker when moderately coarse or the rate of intermission required for flicker extinction. This arrangement (Fig. 81) seems the most crucial for deciding the point. In the 'alternate right and left' arrangement (Fig. 78, LR, upper combination) the instants of change of phase falling together right or left, it might be that it did not matter as regards flicker sensation whether the direction of change was from light to dark or dark to light; the rates of intermission being the same right and left, and the instants of their incidence being synchronous, it might then be that as regards flicker the arrangement

Symmetrical Binocular Flicker

was only tantamount to the 'synchronous right and left' arrangement (Fig. 78, lower combination) or to the uniocular intermittence of the same rate. The arrangement (Fig. 81) avoids this dilemma. Moreover, it avoids both the minute reinforcement and the minute reduction of flicker inherent, according to the above experience, in the exactly 'synchronous' and 'alternate' arrangements. It may be termed for convenience of reference the 'intermediate' arrangement. The physiological stimulation it delivers to the conjugate retina is by any mode of count delivered at twice the rate of delivery for either retina considered apart from its fellow. *Yet the rate of revolution*

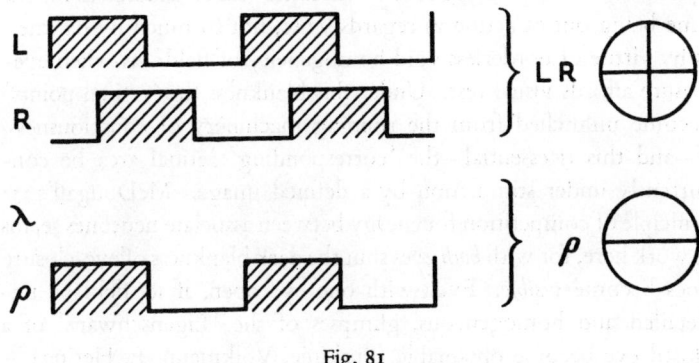

Fig. 81

of the cylindrical lantern required to extinguish flicker in this experiment remains for the binocular image the same as for the uniocular.

There arises the question whether we may regard the dark field covering the area correspondent with that to which in the other retina a bright image is presented, as non-existent visually. That assumption has been made above, and is indicated in the diagrams (Figs. 79, 80, 81). In them, where one image is represented as uniocular, the conjugate area of the other retina is left out of the diagram altogether, as though the latter retina were non-existent, or for the time being blind. This seems permissible, when care is taken to insure absence of all detail or contour from the dark field presented to the other retina, except for the one component of the compared binocular image. When that field is perfectly void of other

Sensual Fusion

contours, and unchanging and borderless, it is found to matter little what *depth* of darkness it has; it may be a shade of grey or even a fair white, without perceptibly influencing the sensual vibrations given by the flickering image before the other eye. The condition seems comparable with the familiar disability to see the dark field presented to one closed eye, when with the other eye the observer regards a detailed image.[166] For these reasons the visual image resulting from the presentation of the bright disk to one eye only, as in the arrangements shown by Figs. 79, 80, 81, was regarded as being a truly uniocular product, uncomplicated by any component from the other retina. The corresponding area of this latter was considered as for the time being out of action as regards sense, not so much by darkness as by virtue of borderless void homogeneity of field—as when eye-closure affords visual rest. Under this blankness the 'retinal points' become unhitched from the running machinery of consciousness, if—and this is essential—the 'corresponding' retinal area be concurrently under stimulation by a defined image. McDougall's[232] principle of competition for energy between associate neurones seems at work here, for with *both* eyes shut the dark blankness of eye-closure does become *visible*. Even with one eye open, if its field be undetailed and homogeneous, glimpses of the 'Eigenschwarz' of a closed eye become obtainable (Purkinje, Volkmann, E. Hering).

The accurately converse stimulation of the twin retinal areas might be expected to give some interference of the flicker sensations so generated. But the experimental evidence indicates absence (practically entire) of any interference between the flicker processes so initiated. The right and left 'corresponding retino-cerebral points' do not when tested by flicker reactions behave as though combined or conjugate to a single mechanism. Their sensual reactions retain individuality as regards time-relations even when completely confluent by reference to visual space.

B. ASYMMETRICAL FLICKER

In the foregoing experiments the flicker sensations of 'corresponding' areas of the two retinae appear (almost entirely) without influence one upon another. But in other experiments the flicker test reveals

Asymmetrical Binocular Flicker

very considerable mutual influence between reactions initiated at the corresponding area.

Suppose (Exp. 5) two binocular images LR and $\lambda\rho$ similarly combined from similar uniocular components, all individually equal in brightness and in intermission frequency. Suppose that of the components of one pair $(\lambda\rho)$ one (ρ) be replaced (Fig. 82) by an intermittent uniocular image (ρ'), of the same physical brightness as that giving the visual image ρ, but of considerably higher intermission frequency. In ρ' all flicker will disappear at slower speeds of revolution of the lantern than those required to extinguish flicker in L or R or λ. Fig. 82 represents the arrangement.

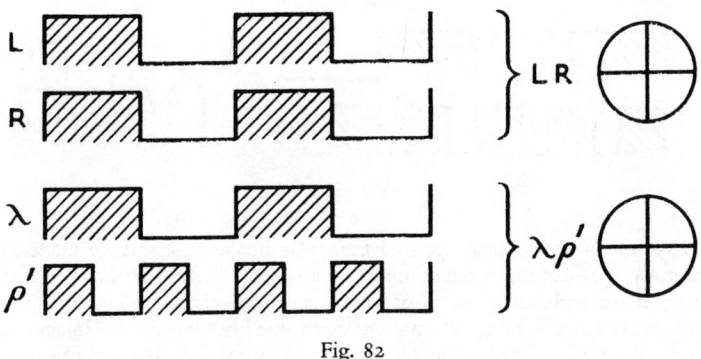

Fig. 82

The frequency of intermission required to extinguish flicker in $\lambda\rho$ is then found to be much lower than the frequency required for extinction of flicker in LR, or in L or R or λ separately. Thus the frequency for extinction of flicker in $\lambda\rho$ was found (observer H.H.) to average 52·2 phases per second as against 61·9 phases per second for LR, or for L, R, or λ separately.

Screening image ρ' out of the binocular combination $\lambda\rho'$, when the frequency of intermission was just high enough to free the $\lambda\rho'$ image from flicker, at once brought flicker into it; this disappeared immediately image ρ' was readmitted to the combination.

In this instance the intensity chosen for the steady illumination of the conjugate area was equal to that employed for the uniocular

Sensual Fusion

flickering image. The duration of the light phases and the dark per revolution of the lantern was equal, and the light and dark phases of the same intensity in both. But the phenomenon obtains also when the steady uniocular image is less bright (Exp. 6, Fig. 83) or more bright (Exp. 7, Fig. 84) than the flickering uniocular with which it is combined. The following example illustrates this (Exp. 6).

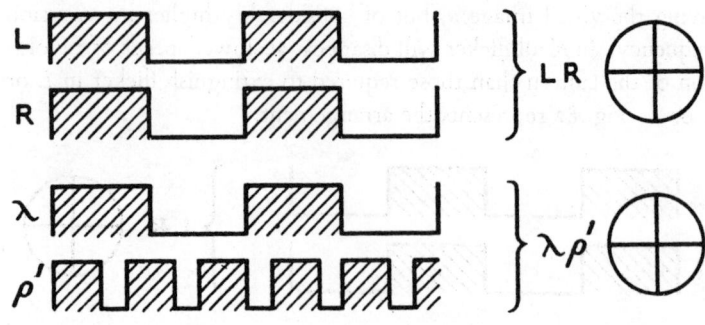

Fig. 83

Exp. 6. In the balanced pair of binocular images LR and $\lambda\rho$ made of carefully equalized intermittent uniocular images L, R, λ, and ρ the uniocular image ρ was replaced by one ρ' of five times greater rapidity of intermission and giving a steady image of only one-ninth the brightness of the images L, R, λ, and ρ when steady. The frequency of intermission required to extinguish flicker in the binocular image $\lambda\rho'$ (Fig. 83) was then found to be 72·1 phases per second, whereas in LR, and in λ, L and R separately, it was 75·5 phases per second as it had been in the previous. The steady sensation from image ρ' therefore damped the vibration of the flickering sensation from the conjugate spot under image λ by an amount represented by 3·4 phases per second.

Exp. 7 (Fig. 84) illustrates an observation in which for the image ρ in the binocular combination $\lambda\rho$ an image ρ' was substituted of three times higher frequency of intermission and giving a steady image of one-fifth greater brightness than the image L, R, and λ when steady. It was then found that the frequency of intermission required to extinguish flicker in the binocular image $\lambda\rho'$ (Fig. 84) was 57·8 alternate equal phases (of λ) per second. Whereas in LR, and in λ, L, and R, taken separately, the number of such phases required was 63·6 per second.

The image $\lambda\rho'$ was distinctly brighter visually than was LR, or any of the uniocular images λ, L, and R.

Asymmetrical Binocular Flicker

These observations show, as do the observations represented by Fig. 82, that it is not merely the reduction of brightness in the combined image $\lambda\rho$ in the arrangement shown by Fig. 83 that lessens the flicker in the latter. In fact, in the observations on the plan illustrated by Fig. 84 we have, for flicker photometry, the interesting case of a brighter intermittently illuminated surface flickering less than a duller one.

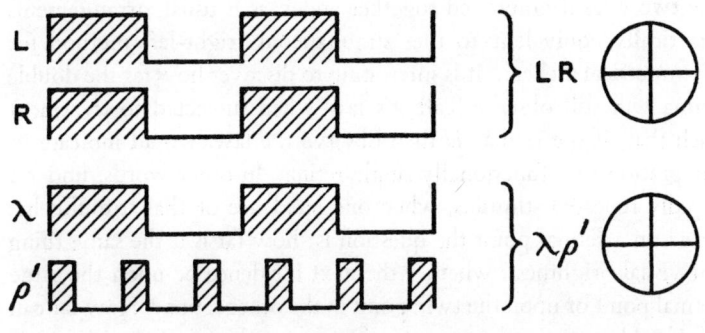

Fig. 84

Here the conditions of experiment suggest that the addition of the steady brightness at one eye to the dark phase of the intermittent at the 'corresponding spot' lightens the latter, and its addition to the phase of equal brightness with it leaves that practically unaltered.

That might be evidence of mutual interference between purely physiological processes initiated at the corresponding spots of the right and left retinae. But, on the other hand, the result at once suggests that the binocular product from a uniocular flickering and a uniocular unflickering image arises by a synthetic process akin to that which produces from a pair of individual uniocular brightnesses a binocular brightness near the arithmetic mean of the brightness of the two components. The rule of combination exemplified by these latter finds little solution by appeal to summation or interference of retinal and purely physiological processes.

Moreover, the supposition that the sensual reaction caused by a steady image acting at one of the pair of 'corresponding' areas, is interfering with or combining with the individual phases of reaction

Sensual Fusion

to the intermittent image at the fellow area, is exactly the supposition that the observations dealing with symmetrical flicker show to be untenable.

UNIOCULAR AND BINOCULAR COMPARISONS

With intermittent lights throughout a wide range of ordinary intensities Talbot's[14] law is unimpeachable for the single eye; and also for the two eyes if employed together under, as is usual, arrangements practically equivalent to the 'simultaneous' right-left method for 'symmetrical flicker'. It is interesting to discover how far the double retina will still observe Talbot's law when subjected to treatment such that, if the retina *did* then observe the law, would indicate its integration to a functionally single retina. In other words, under a rapidly repeated stimulus, when one incidence of that stimulus has acted on a retinal point the question is: how far is it the same thing for visual brightness, whether the next incidence be upon the same retinal point or upon the twin point in the other retina? How far can the double retina, when functioning for singleness of perception in binocular vision, be considered as functionally combined to a single retina, and how far does it then react as does a single retina, if examined for Talbot's law?

The 'alternate left-right arrangement' (Exp. 1, LR) supplies the required method of stimulation. With speeds of revolution of the lantern too high to allow flickering, the binocular image LR (Fig. 79) is seen to appear of brightness equal to $\lambda\rho$, and with the uniocular images λ or ρ taken singly. Therefore in the above sense, Talbot's law not only does *not* hold for the double retina considered as functionally single, but no *trace* of observance of the law is detectable. The two corresponding points are therefore in this respect *not* integrated to a single retinal surface.

It was often noted that with all four lantern images of equal luminosity, using intermission frequencies too rapid to allow flicker, the brightness of the binocular combination of any two did not distinctly exceed that of the uniocular. In certain instances the binocular combination did appear just distinctly the brighter. This was for instance the case when of the four lantern images the two on

Talbot's Law and Binocular Retina

the same horizontal level were combined by simple convergence. This excess of brightness is the well-known phenomenon examined by Jurin, Harris,[8] Fechner,[26] Aubert,[37] Valerius,[52] and others. But there occurred frequent instances in which no excess was observed in the brightness of binocular combinations over that of their carefully balanced uniocular components. In these observations the brightness of the physical images is however always much above the threshold of the light-adapted eye; and I have not made systematic observations with the eye dark-adapted. To obtain good conditions for comparison of the brightness of the binocular and uniocular images the following arrangement can be employed.

Exp. 8. Two images LR and $\lambda \rho \frac{1}{2}$ are placed in the visual field for mutual comparison. LR is composed of left-eye and right-eye equal and corresponding disk-shaped images as in previous experiments. $\lambda \rho \frac{1}{2}$ is composed of a left-eye image similar to L and R except that it lies just above or below them in the visual field. With λ's right half is combined the image of the right half of a lantern image similar again to the others, except that its left half is screened absolutely off into the blank undetailed darkness of the general field. When this is done the two opposite visual images LR and $\lambda \rho \frac{1}{2}$ regarded under perfectly steady ocular fixation are stable, and no difference of brightness is discernible between them. Moreover, no join is seen between the halves of $\lambda \rho \frac{1}{2}$ and no difference of brightness between the halves. After prolonged inspection of them rivalry becomes troublesome; but a judgement can be clearly arrived at before that happens.

In this experiment it might possibly be that equality of brightness between the halves of $\lambda \rho \frac{1}{2}$ is due to image $\rho \frac{1}{2}$ not really being in consciousness at all during the comparison. The image might possibly lapse under competition with the partly dissimilar correspondingly placed left-eye image λ. Experiments carried out by W. McDougall[223] give validity to such possible objection. The perceptibility of the horizontal bar in the right half of the image $\lambda \rho \frac{1}{2}$ is guarantee however that at least part of the uniocular image $\rho \frac{1}{2}$ is present. But to ascertain more surely whether image $\rho \frac{1}{2}$ is really during the visual equation co-operating in consciousness with λ the following further arrangement can be employed.

Exp. 9. (Fig. 85). With the revolving lantern so arranged that images L, R, λ, and $\rho \frac{1}{2}$ are all of equal brightness when steady and unflickering, $\rho \frac{1}{2}$ is given at a lesser frequency of intermission, so as to flicker while the others do

Sensual Fusion

not. A speed of revolution of lantern is then used at which just a trace of flicker is perceptible in $\rho\frac{1}{2}$ when binocularly combined with λ. The equation $LR = \lambda\rho\frac{1}{2}$ is then found to hold while flicker is still just traceable in the right half of $\lambda\rho\frac{1}{2}$. There is then no join seen between the halves of $\lambda\rho\frac{1}{2}$ nor any difference between the brightness of the halves. So long as ocular fixation is steady no rivalry disturbs the observation.

In this case there can, I think, be no question but that the one half of $\lambda\rho\frac{1}{2}$ is truly binocular, for the trace of flicker is perceptible during the actual performance of the comparison. Yet no difference of brightness is perceived between LR and $\lambda\rho\frac{1}{2}$, and the two lateral halves of $\lambda\rho\frac{1}{2}$ compared together seem of like brightness.

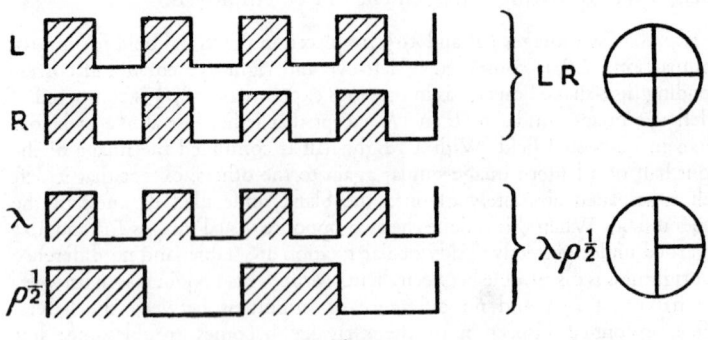

Fig. 85

Even when the binocular image does show the well-known slight excess of brightness over its uniocular components it, under some conditions (vide supra, 'alternate' arrangement), flickers no more or even less than they.

It is doubtful therefore to me whether the slight excess in brightness of the binocular image over its two equal uniocular components is really explicable as summation of the intensities of the reactions at the corresponding spots of the two retinae. Valerius[52] measured the increase to be one-fifteenth of the brightness of the uniocular image. Aubert's[37] diagram gives it as less than one-thirtieth. Aubert says it is not perceptible with brightness greater than that of white paper in diffuse daylight indoors.[65a]

In certain modes of experiment a uniocular image used as a standard for comparison might itself be suffering some reduction in

Uniocular and Binocular Brightness

brightness owing to slight combination with the dark field presented concurrently at the corresponding retinal area. But 'rivalry' should reveal such influence. A better definition and greater vividness of detail assured by better accommodation and convergence under binocular regard, might possibly give an appearance of greater brilliance and intensity. But these are only suggestions.

I conclude that, with ordinary intensities of illumination, although a binocular image does sometimes appear of slightly greater visual brightness than either of two similar uniocular images composing it, more often it has a visual brightness not perceptibly different from that of either of its two co-equal uniocular components. The case then falls within a general rule regarding binocular brightness attested by all observations I have on that subject. *A binocular brightness compared with its uniocular components is of value not greater than the greater of those, nor less than the lesser of them; when free from oscillations of rivalry its value is somewhat, but not far, above the arithmetic mean of the values of the two uniocular components as expressed by the measures of the physical stimuli yielding them.*

The various combinations cited in Experiments 2, 3, 4, 5, 6, 7, and 8 have all, when steady and unflickering, given brightnesses illustrating the above rule. Other illustrations are:

$\lambda = 1000,$ $\rho = 250,$ $\lambda\rho = 680,$
$\lambda = 1000,$ $\rho = 350,$ $\lambda\rho = 750,$
$\lambda = 1000,$ $\rho = 550,$ $\lambda\rho = 835,$
$\lambda = 1000,$ $\rho = 750,$ $\lambda\rho = 920,$
$\lambda = 1000,$ $\rho = 1000,$ $\lambda\rho = 1000.$

But I have not worked with combinations where the physical luminosity of one uniocular component has been less than one-thirteenth the physical luminosity of the other. It was near this limit that Aubert, and just beyond it that Fechner, noted decline of the darkening effect of the darker component. In my own few observations beyond that point the oscillations of rivalry have made judgement difficult. The more manageable examples are but demonstrations of 'Fechner's paradox', and fall under the above general rule. Hering[34] has suggested that rivalry is really occurring even

Sensual Fusion

with similar and right and left uniocular images; he says these react according to a law of 'complemental shares', and offers a theory, such as the name he gives implies, in explanation of the phenomenon. My Experiment 9 seems to offer difficulty to such a view.

Binocular combination of a less bright image with a more bright gives a visual image of less brightness than the latter (as stated in the rule above). But the application of the less bright physical image to the same uniocular area as the more bright gives a visual image of brightness greater than either.

As above described, a steady image presented on an area of one retina 'damps' the flicker of a flickering image concurrently presented at the corresponding area of the other. A steady image actually physically superposed on the same retinal area as a flickering one also reduces the latter's flicker: this latter is of course in accordance with Weber's law. The *modes* of interference seem incomparably different in the two cases; and experiment shows that the two interferences are quite often of different value.

Exp. 10 A. Binocular fusion of R and L gives flicker extinction at 65·5 phases per second.
Physical fusion of R and L gives flicker extinction at 59·4 phases per second. (Observer G.C.)
Binocular fusion of R and L gives flicker extinction at 106·6 phases per second.
Physical fusion of R and L gives flicker extinction at 100·3 phases per second.
R separately gives flicker extinction at 113·3 phases per second.
(Observer R.S.W.)

Finally, to touch on 'predominance of contours'. Its facts, established by so many workers, are among the most significant concerning the difference between binocular and uniocular fusion of visual reactions. I will merely give one illustration which seems specially instructive for the point before us.

Exp. 11. A steady unflickering disk-shaped image L is present to the left eye: across the disk is a narrow dark line. An image R of similar size and shape but without the dark line is presented to the corresponding area of the right eye. If the luminosity of L is progressively diminished, a value of luminosity is reached at which its cross-line, though visible when L alone is observed (e.g. right eye closed) is lost or uncertain in the binocular image RL. This reduction of the luminosity of L much exceeds the reduction at which

Uniocular and Binocular Contrast

its cross-line is lost when image R is concurrently thrown on the same area of the same retina, i.e. left retina. Thus, in one experiment the diminution of luminosity of L required for loss of the cross-line under the physical superposition of R and L on the same retina was 84 per cent, while the diminution of luminosity of L required for loss (or great uncertainty) of the line in the binocular image was 96 per cent.

Not only the ease, but the *mode* of disappearance of the cross-line, is significantly different in the two cases. In the 'physical superposition' the dark line became gradually thinner and fainter, and finally imperceptible, as the image L is lessened in luminosity. In the case of binocular fusion the dark line oscillates out of and back into sensation more and more, the disappearances predominating more and more as the darkening of L proceeds. At a reduction of 84 per cent of the luminosity of L the cross-line was steady, dark and sharp in the binocular image.

Our aim has been information as to the nature of the conjunction between the uniocular components in certain simple binocular sensations. The question concerns the nature of the tie between 'corresponding retinal points', meaning by 'retinal point' the retino-cerebral apparatus engaged in elaborating a sensation in response to excitation of a unit area of retinal surface.

That a sensation initiated from corresponding retinal points is commonly referred without ambiguity to a single *locus* in visual space has often been regarded (Newton,[5] Wollaston,[12a] Rohault,[3] Müller[20]) as evidence of community of the nerve apparatus belonging to the paired retinal points. Their visual image appears *single*. Wollaston supposed the twin points attached to one and the same nerve-fibre, which bifurcated at the chiasma. Rohault and Müller supposed the points to be served by twin fibres 'from one and the same ganglion-cell in the cerebral substance'. Later (cf. Aubert[37]), the visual singleness, spatial fusion of right and left impressions to a single perception, was taken to mean confluence of the nerve-processes, started in right and left retinae respectively, to 'a single common centre or point of the sensorium'. The discovery later still that the fibre-tracts from corresponding halves of the retinae

Sensual Fusion

both go to the occipital region of one and the same hemisphere has also been inferred to mean a spatially conjoint visual sensorium common to both retinae (e.g. Ramon-y-Cajal, Schäfer). But in such questions the inferences obtainable from mere anatomical features are equivocal and often remote in bearing. Were there to exist such a common mechanism situate as a unit at conjunction of the two convergent systems and were phases of excitement timed so as to arrive from one retina as exactly to fill pauses between excitations transmitted from the other, then there should be evidence of this in the time-relations of the phenomena induced. The state of excitement should tend to be maintained across periods that would otherwise checker it as pauses.

The retino-cerebral apparatus may be regarded as a structure of linked branching nerve-elements forming a system which expands as traced centrally from the retinal surface. It may be figured as a tree, with its stem at the retina and an arborization spreading into the brain, its ramifications there penetrating a vast cerebral field, interlacing with others in a cerebral forest composed of nervous arborizations. The simile fails, because in the nervous forest the arborizations make functional union one with another. Is the fusion of the perceptions adjunct to paired 'corresponding points' the outcome of a close concrescence of their neuronic or neuro-fibrillar arborizations, making of them practically a single upgrowth common to twin (right and left) stems rooted in the corresponding retinal units? If so, how low down, how close to their origin, are the twin systems grafted together, giving structural community to all the superstructure?

In the chain of nerve-elements attached to a sense-organ we infer in general that to the activities of the most peripheral links *per se* psychical events are not adjunct. Psychical processes, beginning with least complex and ascending toward development through many grades, attach to the chain in such a way that for the simplest only the more peripheral portions of the chain need be connected with the sense-organ, while for the more complex the central portions in addition become more extensively involved. But in the higher reactions of definite physical aspect, e.g. sense-perceptions, the lower

Binocular Fusion

apsychic and less definitely psychic activities are also implicate. Where from two sense-organs, e.g. two units of retinal surface, the two nerve-chain arborizations are mutually connected, so that the lower activities of the one affect by low-level side connexions the elements forming the other, there analysis must fail to distinguish in the full reaction what higher components may be separately referable to one only of the two individual chains. The processes apsychic, or so indefinitely psychic as to baffle introspection, at the root of those amenable to introspection, must by their coalescence defeat attempts to trace the final psychical product to either of its two possible sources, so long as both sources are open for its origination.

Were the nervous reactions initiated at twin points of the retinae *early* in its path along the retino-cerebral nerve-chain, to enter mechanisms common to both, there must, under 'alternate' or 'synchronous' right-left arrangement of stimuli (Fig. 78), be interference, algebraic summation, etc., a coalescence of events which, though apsychical in itself, would involve subsequent confusion of the sense-reactions of the two eyes. A state of things wholly different from this is revealed in the results of our experiments. And it would amount to the same thing whether two quickly successive flashes of a light fell both on one and the same member of a pair of 'corresponding points', or whether the first fell upon one member, the second upon the other. But the experiments show that the effect in the two cases is widely different. Talbot's law is not applicable to the double retina, that is, to the two retinae functioning together in binocular vision. The experimental results go to disprove the existence of any such fusion or interference between the apsychical or even the subperceptual events arising from corresponding retinal points. At most they indicate hardly discernible traces of such interference (Exp. 1). They indicate, on the contrary, that such simple forms of binocular perception as have been dealt with here are themselves fusions of elaborated uniocular *sensations*. Since left and right end-results emerge pure, 'hybridization' has not mixed the early stages in their evolution.

But the difference between the modes of stimulation left and right

Sensual Fusion

is a difference that, although it should be potent if the left and right *physiological* machinery were conjoined to unity, should constitute no difference when left stimulation is compared with right stimulation by the perceptual product which each yields. *The left eye and right eye flickering visual images, each viewed singly, do NOT* (apart from the faint cross-line for recognition) *differ to introspection.* If the sensations derived from the left eye and right eye respectively appear under introspection indistinguishably alike, what ground is there for mutual interference between them? It is much as though, of the left and right lantern images each were seen by one of two observers, with similar vision, and as though the minds of the two observers were combined to a single mind. It may be recalled that binocular unification of images, as we possess it, seems a comparatively late achievement of phylogenetic evolution.

When the visual product of the two retinae is thus regarded it is not surprising that Talbot's law fails for the binocular cyclopean retina. It fails because the binocular sensation is a fusion of uniocular sensation and from no two *similar* sensations can a resultant sensation be compounded different from its components. Were Talbot's law to hold in the above sense for the binocular retina there would, under the 'alternate left-right arrangement' (symmetrical flicker), at rates of intermission too high for flicker, result from an image L of brightness x, and an image R of similar brightness x, a combined image LR of brightness $x+x$, the value of the summed brightness being in accord with the Weber-Fechner rule of summation of sensual intensities. But, as shown, not only does this summation not occur, but nothing like it occurs. The binocular result most often does not perceptibly differ from either of its two co-equal components.

But the experiments with uniocular components dissimilarly flickering, and with flickering components concurrent with steady components, do evidence (unlike the other experiments) interference between the two eyes. This result might be interpreted as the outcome of community of the physiological mechanisms attaching to the paired 'corresponding retinal points'. But the other experiments negative the existence of this community. And the explanation just offered for the absence of interference in the other experiments will

Binocular Fusion

account for the presence of interference in these. From two components perceptibly differing between themselves in regard to some quality (e.g. flicker) a single combined sensual quality is obtained, intermediate between that of the two components taken singly. If the perceptible difference, e.g. in flicker, between the components is wide, the fusion is liable to phasic oscillations of predominance of one or other component. Where the difference in flicker is wide, such 'rivalry' between the right and left components is in fact not infrequently seen. One component may at the height of its phase be alone perceptible at the focus of attention, the other component being inhibited out of focal attention or even out of conscious vision altogether. The inference is that only *after the sensations initiated from right and left 'corresponding points' have been elaborated, and have reached a dignity and definiteness well amenable to introspection, does interference between the reactions of the two (left and right) eye-systems occur. The binocular sensation attained seems combined from right and left uniocular sensations elaborated independently.*

And in harmony with this view stands the evidence adduced for the rule formulated regarding the relation of binocular to uniocular brightness. Further, the difference between the sensual result of superposition of two similar images upon one and the same area of a single retina, and upon twin areas of the two retinae, could hardly be so great as it is, did apsychical or subsensual reactions underlying 'brightness' combine or interfere in the two retinal systems. The binocular combination must be a synthesis of a left-eye with a right-eye *sensation.* Similarly, the 'prevalence of contours' in binocular vision, and the phenomena of 'retinal rivalry', are explicable if each member of a pair of corresponding points yields a sensual entity which, when not widely dissimilar from that yielded by its twin point, fuses with that to a binocular sensation. In 'retinal rivalry' we have an involuntarily performed analysis of this sensual bicompound. The binocular perception in that case breaks down, leaving phasic periods of one or other of the simpler component sensations bare to inspection.

W. McDougall,[297] in applying to 'retinal rivalry' and 'prevalence of contours' his principle of competition of inter-related nerve-

Sensual Fusion

elements for energy, also argues a 'separateness of the visual cortical areas for the two eyes'. He brings forward striking experiments in evidence of this. In one of these[223] he shows that an after-image, left from excitation of one retina, is more strongly revived by subsequent weak diffuse excitation of that same retina than of its fellow. More recently, in experiments proving reinforcement of visual sensations by the activity of the ocular muscles, as evidenced by after-image observations, he[261a] shows that activity of the intrinsic muscles of an eye sends up to the brain an influence, reinforcing the activity of the cerebro-retinal tract of that eye, while it exerts no such effect upon the corresponding tract of the other eye, or exerts it in a minor degree only. With this separateness of the mechanisms, wherein are produced the sensations generated in the two retinae, our results by a different line of experimentation accord well.

The compounding together of right and left images really nonidentical but not widely dissimilar, is (Panum, Hering) the basis of visual 'relative depth-perception'. The compounding of visual images partly dissimilar—flickering with unflickering—seems a simpler case in the same category of synthetic actions. In our flicker experiments the visual components do not differ as to space-attributes, and their combination has therefore no resultant differential space-attribute. But the synthesis gives in each case a compromise between the components in regard to the attribute wherein they do differ; in the flicker experiments, that is in regard to the sensual steadiness of the brightness. This amounts to the same as the rule formulated above for binocular combination of brightness of different intensities, but steady.

Our experiments show, therefore, that during binocular regard of an objective image each uniocular mechanism develops independently a sensual image of considerable completeness. The singleness of the binocular perception results from union of these elaborated uniocular sensations. The singleness is therefore the product of a synthesis that works with already elaborated sensations contemporaneously proceeding.

The cerebral seats of right-eye and left-eye visual images are thus shown to be separate. Conductive paths no doubt interconnect them, but are shown to be unnecessary for visual unification of the two

Visual Fusion and Neural Union

images. The unification of a sensation of composite source is evidently associated with a neurone arrangement different from that which obtains in the synthesis of a reflex movement by the convergence of the reflexes of allied arcs upon its final common paths.

Here we seem to have therefore contemporaneity of itself sufficing for sensual synthesis, without necessarily any spatial fusion of the neural processes or mechanisms involved, i.e. without spatial confluence to a unit apparatus. As mentioned above, W. McDougall's experiments on after-images lead to a like conclusion. The foundation of new correspondences between retinal points in cases of squint (Tschermak) strengthen the same view. McDougall has recently well summarized the position. But it is one not generally admitted by physiologists or psychologists. Ziehen[242a] writes: 'Schon physiologisch ist die Verschmeltzung der beiden Netzhautbilder dadurch vorbereitet dass die Erregungen welche auf den linken Hälften beider Netzhäute auftreten, vermöge der eigenthümlichen partiellen Sehnerven-kreuzung *zusammen* in die rechte Grosshirnhemisphäre gelangen, und umgekehrt.' And this was the view of Joh. Müller and of Aubert, and is advanced on histological grounds by Ramon-y-Cajal.

The results bear also on the production of sensual reactions and states more complex than those of the examples taken. Hartmann, as quoted by McDougall, writes: 'Only because one part of my brain has a direct communication with the other is the consciousness of the two parts unified. Could we unite the brains of two human beings by a path of communication equivalent to cerebral fibres both would no longer have *two* but *one* consciousness'. There is no denying the extreme importance and the vast actual extent of the spatial conjunction of cerebral elements by conductive channels in sensual and perceptual reactions. Yet I cannot but think that its limitless postulation leads not so much to explanation of the high degree of unity of the individual mind as to an ultimate fallacy which Professor James has trenchantly termed that of 'the pontifical cell'. Pure conjunction in time without necessarily cerebral conjunction in space lies at the root of the solution of the problem of the unity of mind.

Sensual Fusion

Since convergence of the conductors from corresponding halves of the retinae to the same field of brain-cortex does not signify physiological conjunction of right and left sense-impressions, can we decipher at all what it does mean? To do so does not seem difficult, and displays strikingly the different value and directness of spatial union of conducting-paths for motor synthesis and for psychical respectively. In animals with overlapping visual fields the lateral movements of the eyeball have a mutual relation different from the ordinary relations of the movements of a unilaterally placed organ, e.g. a limb. Especially is this the case where the overlap of the visual fields is extensive, e.g. where the ocular axes are parallel. The horizontal movements of each eyeball are balanced about the primary line of vision of the globus in its habitual resting attitude, that is, in man, straight forward. That line sensually, as shown by introspective experiment, lies in the median sagittal plane of the head (Hering). Hence the term 'Cyclopean' has been applied to the biunial eye of human binocular vision. Finding the median vertical plane of sight of the resting eyeball to correspond with the median sagittal plane of the body, we may assume that the motor reflexes deal with the eyeball conformably with that; otherwise there would be discord between the reflexes and the sensations. Therefore we must in any general consideration of the taxis of the lateral movements of the two eyeballs transfer in thought each eyeball from its own actual sagittal plane to the median sagittal plane of the head; and this latter corresponds in the resting position with the sagittal median plane of the animal as a whole.

Each lateral muscle of the eyeball comes therefore to bear to the median plane of the body the same relation as does a limb on one side of the body. Thus, the external rectus muscle of the right eyeball bears the same lateral relation to the median sagittal plane of the body as does the right arm. And the internal rectus muscle of the left eyeball bears the same lateral relation to the median sagittal plane of the body as does the right arm. Now a general arrangement evident in the cerebral cortex is that the taxis of muscles lying to right of the median sagittal plane is entrusted to the left hemisphere, and *vice versa*. It is in accord with this that in animals with overlapping

Semidecussation of Optic Tracts

visual fields the horizontal movement of the eyes to one side should for *both* eyeballs be represented in *one and the same* hemisphere. And as a fact the conjugate movement is found represented for both eyeballs together in each hemisphere. If we regard, and it was shown above that we may do so, the median sagittal planes of both eyeballs as identical with the median sagittal plane of the head, they are identical with each other, and the scheme of cortical representation may be expressed thus: a point in the right retina and its twin point in the left demand each of them identical movement of the two eyeballs when, apart from convergence, those points excite their own replacement by the *fovea* (i.e. when initiating a gaze). It is obvious that the paths from the visual cortex of each side to the eyeball muscles—experiment shows such a path to exist—is connected therefore with both the right and left twin points. That is, it is a *common path*. The confluence of conductors from the two retinae to the same cortical field, though not uniting their retinal impressions, gives them access to a common efferent path which both must use.* At entrance to every common path lies, as shown before, a co-ordinating mechanism. A co-ordinative mechanism is thus obtained. This 'common path' with its bilateral twin origin impinges in its turn, directly or indirectly, on the motor neurones for the lateral eye-muscles, the *final common paths*. We have therefore to alter such a scheme as that furnished by Cajal by attaching his convergent paths to efferent paths, and by divesting their supposed nodal cortical point of its hypothetical powers as a sensual *Deus ex machina*. And we thus meet another instance of convergence of afferent paths leading to motor synthesis, but not, or only remotely, to sensual. Seen in this light the gulf between sensation and movement looms even wider than was allowed for in the tentative suppositions which prompted the above experiments on flicker.

We are thus warned against any hasty conclusion that the neural mechanisms which synthesize reflex movements illustrate in their arrangement also those concerned where sensual fusion is the

---

* Mott has likewise independently urged that the interpretation to be placed on this convergence of paths is motor rather than sensory. *Trans. Ophthalm. Soc.* (1905), vol. xxv, p. cii.

Sensual Fusion

phenomenon. But that does not invalidate a broad practical inference which study of the nervous system in regard to motor reaction allows. This inference is that toward the solution of the problems of motor taxis help is obtainable by appeal to characters evident in sensual reaction. This practical inference need not in the least involve any doctrinal attitude whatever toward the hypothesis of psycho-physical parallelism. It may proceed quite apart from that. It simply insists on the likeness of nervous reactions expressed by muscular and other effector-organs to reactions whose evidence is sensual. It insists on this likeness being close and fundamental enough to make each of the two classes of phenomena of use to the student of the other. A number of excellent investigators hold, on the opposite hand, that the study of the two should proceed apart even more rigidly than they do at present. Confusion has, it is true, been caused in both by the loose application of the terms of the one set of phenomena to the other. But to disregard the many significant similarities which exist between the two sets is, it seems to me, to throw away one of the best instruments for discovery in both. We saw how suggestive psychological data prove for classifying the various species of receptors considered as initiators of reflexes. The after-discharge of a nervous arc finds expression not only in reflex movement but in, for instance, a visual after-image. Centripetal impulses from eye-muscles reinforce visual (i.e. extero-ceptor) sensations (McDougall) just as centripetal impulses from the leg muscles reinforce reflex movement induced from the skin (extero-ceptor) of the foot. The 'immediate spinal induction' exemplified by reflexes has a counterpart in visual irradiation. Visual contrast, if translated into terms of reflex contraction, bears close resemblance to 'successive spinal induction'. The features of fatigue repeat themselves in both sets of phenomena. Receptors which initiate reflex movements adapted in regard to objects at a distance initiate as sense-organs sensations projected into circumambient sensual space. Receptors which initiate reflex movements advantageous in regard to some *locus* of the surface of the body itself, e.g. removal of irritation thence, initiate as sense-organs sensations referred to that same locus. Instances might be multiplied, but they have risen prominently in several of the fore-

Physiological and Psychical Signs of Neural Activity

going lectures, and are sufficiently before our minds now. A practical inference from them is that physiology and psychology, instead of prosecuting their studies, as some now recommend, more strictly apart one from another than at present, will find it serviceable for each to give to the results achieved by the other even closer heed than has been customary hitherto.

Besides this similarity of time-relation and other features between the physiological and the psychical signs of neural activity, another link connects the psychological and the physiological for the biologist. To the physiology of pure reflexes, that is, reflexes devoid of psychical accompaniment so far as introspection can discover, psychological interest nevertheless attaches, and on a very distinct ground. This ground of connexion is seen if inquiry is followed along the animal scale in the direction from higher forms to lower rather than by the usually more favourable reverse approach. This is partly because we directly observe psychical phenonema by introspection only, that is, only in ourselves; and the facts discovered by introspection are applicable to other beings the more readily the more those beings resemble ourselves, namely, are animals ranking near to man.

Pure reflexes are admirably adapted to certain ends. They are reactions which have long proved advantageous in the phylum, of which the existent individual is a representative embodiment. Perfected during the course of ages, they have during that course attained a stability, a certainty, and an ease of performance beside which the stability and facility of the most ingrained habit acquired during an individual life is presumably small. But theirs is of itself a machine-like fatality. Their character in this stands revealed when the neural arcs which execute them are separated, e.g. by transection of the spinal cord, from the higher centres of the nervous system. They can be checked, it is true, as we have seen, by collision with other reflexes as ancestral and as fatally operative as themselves (Lect. V and VI). To these ancient invariable reflexes, consciousness, in the ordinary meaning of the term, is not adjunct. The subject as active agent does not direct them and cannot introspect them.

Yet it is clear, in higher animals especially so, that reflexes are under

Sensual Fusion

control. Their intrinsic fatality lies under control by higher centres unless their nervous arcs are sundered from ties existing with those higher centres. In other words, the reactions of reflex-arcs are controllable by mechanisms to whose activity consciousness is adjunct. By these higher centres, this or that reflex can be checked, or released, or modified in its reaction with such variety and seeming independence of external stimuli that the existence of a spontaneous internal process expressed as 'will' is the naive inference drawn. Its spring of action is not now our question; its seat in the nervous system seems to correspond with that of processes of perceptual level. It is urgently necessary for physiology to know *how* this control—volitional control—is *operative* upon reflexes, that is, how it intrudes and makes its influence felt upon the running of the reflex machinery. How is the cough, or eye-closure, or the impulse to smile suppressed? How is the convergence of the eyeballs, innately associate to visual fixation of a near object, initiated voluntarily without recourse to fixation on an object? Or how is the innate respiratory rhythm voluntarily modified to meet the passing requirements of vocal utterance? No exposition of the integrative action of the nervous system is complete, even in outline, if this control is left without consideration. Reflexes ordinarily outside its pale can by training be brought within it. The actor, it is asserted, can shed tears at will or blush or blanch. Occasional instances are recorded of power to slow the rhythm of the heart at will; others, of power to suppress the reflex of swallowing when it has entered on its pharyngeal stage. Volitional movement can certainly become involuntary, and, conversely, involuntary movements can sometimes be brought under subjection to the will. From this subjection it is but a short step to acquisition of co-ordinations which express themselves as movements newly acquired by the individual. The controlling centres can pick out from an ancestrally given motor reaction some one part of it, so as to isolate that as a new separate movement, and by enhancement this can become a skilled adapted act added to the powers of the individual. In regard to the ring finger, the motor co-ordination ancestrally provided gives extension of that finger only in company with the fingers on each side of it. We can soon train ourselves to

Reflex and Volitional Action

lift the ring-finger alone without the others. The 'will' dissociates the ancestral co-ordination. Similarly we can acquire the power to move a part which neither reflexly nor otherwise would seem to come within the scope of our voluntary innervation, although of course there must be motor nerve and muscle upon which our innervation can operate. Thus, we can learn to retract the pinna of the ear; the movement is at first accompanied by other facial movement, but later with practice it becomes executable without other facial movement. A new reaction and co-ordination has been gained by the individual.

The transition from reflex action to volitional is not abrupt and sharp. Familiar instances of individual acquisition of motor co-ordination are furnished by the cases in which short, simple movements whether reflex or not, are by practice under volition combined into new sequences and become in time habitual in the sense that though able to be directed they no longer require concentration of attention upon them for their execution. As I write my mind is not preoccupied with how my fingers form the letters; my attention is fixed simply on the thought the words express. But there was a time when the formation of the letters, as each one was written, would have occupied my whole attention.

Volitional control of reflexes is a question of co-ordination not explicitly before us previously in these lectures. Its analysis has not indeed proceeded far. We may premise that some extension of the same processes outlined in Lect. V and VI, as operative in simultaneous combination and in successive combination of reflexes, must be operative in this control. There we saw reflexes modifying each other, and the more complex reactions being built up from simpler and more restricted ones. Some extension of the same process should, in view of our inferences regarding the nature of the dominance of the brain (Lect. IX), apply here also.

It is significant that, although the reflexes controlled are so often unconscious, consciousness is adjunct to the centres which exert the control. A biologist, Professor Lloyd Morgan, has urged that "the primary aim, object, and purpose of consciousness is control. Consciousness in a mere automaton is a useless and unnecessary

Sensual Fusion

epiphenomenon".* A somewhat similar thought rose incidentally to our lips in a previous lecture (Lect. IX). The pleasure-pain accompaniment of reflexes has often been interpreted as carrying that meaning. Certain it is that if we study the process by which in ourselves this control over reflex action is acquired by an individual, psychical factors loom large, and more is known of them than of the purely physiological *modus operandi* involved in the attainment of the control. Hence, psychological studies have been more numerous than physiological in this field. It is found that kinaesthetic sensations of the movement to be acquired or controlled, though helpful, are less important than the resident sensations from the part in its 'resting' state. These latter, with the power to focus attention upon them, appear, in a number of instances, to be a most necessary condition for the acquirement of the control. And in the monkey, voluntary control of a limb is largely lost when the limb has been rendered apæsthetic.157

A biological inference arises at this point. We have admitted that the organs to which psychosis is adjunct, namely, the brain, and especially in higher vertebrates the cerebral hemispheres, supply the surest touchstone to rank in the scale of animal creation. That is to admit, in other words, that development of these organs constitutes, on the whole, the best criterion to the success of an animal form in the competition which lies at the root of animal evolution. These organs, we have just seen, are the organs of nervous control; and that control is exercised mainly in the perfecting and readjusting of manœuvres of ancient heritage. The way in which we ourselves acquire a new skilled movement, the means by which we get more precision and speed in the use of a tool, the handling of an instrument, or marksmanship with a weapon, is by a process of learning in which nervous organs of control modify the activities of reflex centres, themselves already perfected for other though kindred actions. Our process of learning is accompanied by conscious effort. These nervous organs of control form, therefore, a special instrument of adaptation and of readjustment of reaction to suit better requirements which may be new. New adaptations whence the individual may reap benefit are thus attained. The more complex an organism, the

* *Introduction to Comparative Psychology* (London, 1894), p. 182.

Nervous Organs of Control

more points of contact it has with the environment, and the more frequently will it need readjustment amid an environment of shifting relationships. These nervous organs of control being organs of adjustment will be more prominent the further the animal scale is followed upward to its crowning species, man. And these organs which give adjustability to the running of the reflex machinery, as such, seem themselves—perhaps, by reason of their constant relative newness—to be among the most plastic in the body. In man and the species near him, these organs are most developed, and their mechanisms are cerebral. These cerebral mechanisms constitute the clearest criterion of evolutionary success. In these types it is cerebral function which best compasses that modification of old and that development of new reaction, which perfects the adaptation of the individual to the environment. The relatively high development in man of this organ for individual adjustment of reactions makes him the most successful animal on earth's surface at the present epoch. No doubt the greater part of all this adjustment of reaction will, in his case, as he stands now, come under intellectual activity. In him reason enables the individual profitably to forecast the future, and to act the more suitably to meet it, from memory of the past. Mere experience can, however, apart from reason, mould nervous reactions in so far as they are plastic. The *bahnung* of a reflex exhibits this faculty in germ. In the humble spheres of nervous activity, such as alone fall within the scope of these lectures, simple sensori-motor experience seems to count for more than reason in the actual process of acquiring new motor co-ordinations. Of course reason, directing effort, counts in the selection of the field of operation of motor experience. But the inefficacy, as a means to arrive at a new motor correlation, of instruction merely verbal, or of ideas constructed without motor experience, is common knowledge. To learn skating or racquets by simple cogitation or visual observation is, of course, impossible. Here mere sensori-motor experience is more valuable than any course of reasoning can be. Hence the training for a new skilled motor manœuvre must be simply *ad hoc*, and is of itself no training for another motor co-ordination—apart from the well-known mutual influence of training on symmetrical parts of the body. Yet, in high animal types, the connexion between skilled movements and the

Sensual Fusion

so-called 'motor' region of the cortex cerebri, and the defect in these which injury of that region entails, countenances the belief that the 'experience' involved in this training, though not rational, is cerebral. The compensation of co-ordinative defects which the cerebrum accomplishes after cerebellar or labyrinthine lesions, points to a similar conclusion. And we must remember that though the mere sensori-motor experience counts for so much in the mastering of a new movement, they are perceptual, and in man rational, processes which initiate, maintain, and guide effort toward acquirement of an act which is new.

We thus, from the biological standpoint, see the cerebrum, and especially the cerebral cortèx, as the latest and highest expression of a nervous mechanism which may be described as the *organ of, and for, the adaptation of nervous reactions*. The cerebrum, built upon the distance-receptors and entrusted with reactions which fall in an anticipatory interval so as to be *precurrent* (Lect. IX), comes, with its projicience of sensation and the psychical powers unfolded from that germ of advantage, to be the organ *par excellence* for the readjustment and the perfecting of the nervous reactions of the animal as a whole, so as to improve and extend their suitability to, and advantage over, the environment. These adjustments, though not transmitted to the offspring, yet in higher animals form the most potent internal condition for enabling the species to maintain and increase in sum its dominance over the environment in which it is immersed. A certain measure of such dominance is its ancestral heritage; on this is based its innate right to success in the competition for existence. But the factors and elements of that competition change in detail as the history of the earth proceeds. The creature has to be partially readjusted if it is to hold its own in the struggle· Only by continual modification of its ancestral powers to suit the present can it fulfil that which its destiny, if it is to succeed, requires from it as its life's purpose, namely, the extension of its dominance over its environment. For this conquest its cerebrum is its best weapon. It is then around the cerebrum, its physiological and psychological attributes, that the main interest of biology must ultimately turn.

BIBLIOGRAPHICAL REFERENCES

(1) DESCARTES, R. (1648). *Passions de l'âme.* Paris.
(2) DESCARTES, R. (1662). *De Homine* (ed. by Schuyl). Leyden.
(3) ROHAULT (1671). *Traité de physique,* Part I. Paris.
(4) DESCARTES, R. (1677). *De Homine* (ed. by de la Forge). Amsterdam.
(5) NEWTON, I. (1704). *Opticks.* Prop. 112.
(6) HALLER, A. VON (1752). *De partibus corporis humani sentientibus et nonsentientibus.* Göttingen.
(6a) SPALLANZANI (1768). *Sopra la reproduzione.* Modena.
(7) SMITH-KÄSTNER (1775). *Lehrbegriff d. Optik.*
(8) HARRIS (1775). *Opticks.* London.
(9) BICHAT (1805). *Rech. physiol. sur la vie et la mort,* III. Paris.
(10) BELL, C. (1811). *A New Idea of the Anatomy of the Brain.* London.
(11) MAGENDIE (1822). *J. physiol. exp.*
(12) BELL, C. (1823). *Philos. Trans.*
(12a) WOLLASTON (1824). *Philos. Trans.*
(12b) HERBART (1825). *Psychologie als Wissenschaft.* Königsberg.
(13) BELL, C. (1829). *Anatomy and Physiology of the Human Body,* by J. and C. Bell (7th ed., corrected by C. Bell). The passage referred to appears as a footnote, p. 110.
(14) TALBOT (1834). *Phil. Mag.* III (5), p. 327.
(15) PLATEAU, J. (1835). *Poggendorffs Ann.* XXXV, 457.
(16) GRAINGER (1837). *On the Structure of the Spinal Cord.* London.
(17) VOLKMANN (1838). *Müllers Arch.* p. 87.
(18) VOLKMANN (1842). *Müllers Arch.* p. 372.
(19) FLOURENS (1842). *Recherches expérimentale sur la fonction du système nerveux.* Paris.
(20) MÜLLER, J. (1843). *Elements of Physiology* (transl. by Baly). London.
(21) WEBER, E. H. & ED. (1846). *Omodei annali univers. di med.* CXVI, 225.
(22) TRAUBE, J. (1847). *Med. Zeitung Vereins Heilk.* V.
(23) MARSHALL HALL (1850). *Synopsis of the Diastaltic Nervous System.* London.
(24) PFLÜGER, ED. (1853). *Die sensor. Funkt. Rückenm.* Berlin.
(25) HARLESS (1858). *Abh. Baeyr. Akad. Phys.* XXXI.
(26) FECHNER (1860). *Abh. Akad. Wiss. Leipzig,* VII, 423.
(27) ROSENTHAL, J. (1861). *C.R. Acad. Sci. Paris,* I, 754.
(28) ROSENTHAL, J. (1861). *Untersuch. Naturl. Mensch. Tiere,* VIII, 312.
(29) BROCA, P. (1861). *Bull. Soc. anat.* Paris.
(30) ROSENTHAL, J. (1862). *Die Atembeweg. u. ihre Bezieh. z. nerve. Vagus.* Berlin.

Bibliographical References

(31) SETSCHENOW, J. (1863). *Physiol. Studien ü. d. Hemmungsmech. f. d. Reflexthät. d. Rückenm. u. Gehirn d. Frosch.* Berlin.
(32) SETSCHENOW, J. (1863). *Ann. Sci. Nat.* XIX, 109.
(33) SETSCHENOW, J. (1864). *Z. rat. Med.* XXIII, no. 6.
(34) HERING, E. (1864). *Beitr. Physiol.* Heft. V, 310. Leipzig.
(35) HUGHLINGS JACKSON (1864). *Lond. Hosp. Rep.* I, 459.
(36) CAYRADE (1864). *Les mouvements reflexes.* Paris.
(37) AUBERT (1865). *Physiol. Netzhaut*, p. 287. Breslau.
(38) SETSCHENOW, J. (1865). *Z. rat. Med.* XXVI, 292.
(39) V. CYON (1865). *Ber. Sächs. Ges. (Acad.) Wiss.* Leipzig.
(40) GOLTZ, F. (1865). *Centralbl. med. Wiss.* p. 705.
(41) V. CYON (1866). *Ludwigs Arbeiten.* Leipzig.
(42) VON BEZOLD & USPENSKY (1867). *Centralbl. med. Wiss.* p. 611.
(43) HERING, E. (1868). *Die Selbststeuerung d. Athmung durch d. Nervus Vagus. S.B. Akad. Wiss. Wien,* LVII, 2.
(44) BREUER, J. (1868). *S.B. Akad. Wiss. Wien,* LVIII, 2.
(45) GOLTZ, F. (1869). *Beiträge z. Lehre v. d. Funkt. d. Nervencentra d. Frosches.* Berlin.
(46) BASTIAN, C. (1869). *J. Ment. Sci.* London.
(47) FRITSCH & HITZIG, E. (1870). *Arch. physiol.* p. 300.
(48) NOTHNAGEL (1870). *Virchows Arch.* XLIX, 267.
(48a) HERING, E. (1872–4). *S.B. Akad. Wiss. Wien,* LXVI–LXX, Abt.iii.
(49) DUCHENNE, G. B. A. (1872). *L'électrisation localisée.* Paris.
(50) DARWIN, C. (1872). *Expressions of the Emotions.* London.
(51) FERRIER, D. (1873). *West Riding Lunatic Asylum Rep.* London.
(52) VALERIUS (1873). *Poggendorffs Ann.* CL, 17.
(53) HITZIG, E. (1874). *Untersuch. ü. d. Gehirn.* Berlin.
(54) GOLTZ & FREUSBERG (1874). *Pflüg. Arch. ges. Physiol.* VIII, 460.
(55) KRONECKER, H. (with W. STIRLING) (1874). *Festschr. z. Ludwig.* Leipzig.
(56) V. CYON (1874). *Pflüg. Arch. ges. Physiol.* VIII, 347.
(57) STIRLING, W. (1874). *Ludwigs Arbeiten*, p. 245. Leipzig.
(58) GOLTZ, F. (1874). *Pflüg. Arch. ges. Physiol.* IX, 552.
(59) EXNER, S. (1874). *Pflüg. Arch. ges. Physiol.* VIII.
(59a) FREUSBERG, A. (1874). *Pflüg. Arch. ges. Physiol.* IX, 358.
(60) FREUSBERG, A. (1875). *Pflüg. Arch. ges. Physiol.* X, 174.
(61) FREUSBERG, A. (1875). *Arch. exp. Path. Pharmak.* III, 17.
(62) DARWIN, C. (1875). *Insectivorous Plants.* London.
(63) ERB, W. (1875). *Berl. klin. Wschr.* no. 26.
(64) ERB, W. (1875). *Arch. Psychiat. Nervenkr.* V, 792.
(65) WESTPHAL, C. (1875). *Arch. Psychiat. Nervenkr.* V, 803.
(65a) AUBERT (1876). *Physiologische Optik*, p. 500. Leipzig.
(66) MOSSO, A. (1876). *Molesch. Untersuch.* II, 331.
(67) MAREY, E. J. (1876). *Trav. Laboratoire,* II. Paris.
(68) GERGENS (1876). *Pflüg. Arch. ges. Physiol.* XIII, 68.

Bibliographical References

(69) WUNDT, W. (1876). *Ueb. Reflex vorgang u. d. Wesen, central. Innervation.* Stuttgart.
(70) FERRIER, D. (1876). *Functions of the Brain.* London.
(70a) FLECHSIG, P. (1876). *Die Leitungsbahnen im Gehirn u. Rückenmark.* Leipzig.
(71) EXNER, S. (1877). *Arch. Anat. Physiol., Lpz.*, p. 567.
(72) ROMANES, J. (1877). *Philos. Trans.* CLVII.
(73) BABUCHIN (1877). *Arch. Anat. Physiol., Lpz.*, p. 66.
(74) LANGENDORFF, O. (1877). *Arch. Anat. Physiol., Lpz.*, p. 96.
(74a) LANGENDORFF, O. (1877). *Arch. Anat. Physiol., Lpz.*, p. 435.
(75) HUGHLINGS JACKSON (1877). *The Medical Examiner.* London.
(76) TSCHIRIEW, S. (1878). *Arch. Psychiat. Nervenkr.* VIII, 689.
(77) GRÜTZNER, P. (1878). *Pflüg. Arch. ges. Physiol.* XVII, 238.
(78) HUGHLINGS JACKSON (1878). *The Medical Examiner.* London.
(79) MARTIN, NEWELL & HARTWELL, E. M. (1879). *J. Physiol.* II.
(79a) WARD, J. (1879). *J. Physiol.* II.
(80) OTT, J. (1879). *J. Physiol.* II, 48.
(81) SPODE, O. (1879). *Arch. Anat. Physiol., Lpz.*, p. 115.
(82) JAMES, W. (1880). *Bost. Soc. Nat. Hist.*
(83) WUNDT, W. (1880). *Grundzüge der Physiol. Psychol.*
(84) SWINTON, A. H. (1880). *Insect Variety.* London.
(85) SPENCER, H. (1880). *Principles of Psychology.* London.
(86) SCHLÖSSER, E. (1880). *Arch. Anat. Physiol., Lpz.*
(87) GOLTZ, F. (1881). *Verricht. Grosshirns.* Strassburg.
(88) OTT, J. (1881). *J. Physiol.* III.
(89) KRONECKER, H. & MELTZER, S. J. (1881). *Arch. Anat. Physiol., Lpz.*, p. 465.
(90) KRONECKER, H. & MELTZER, S. J. (1881). *Mber. Berl. Akad. Wiss.* (24 Feb.).
(91) WALTON (1881). *J. Physiol.* III, 308.
(92) BUBNOFF, N. & HEIDENHAIN, R. (1881). *Pflüg. Arch. ges. Physiol.* XXVI, 137.
(93) MUNK, H. (1881). *Arch. Anat. Physiol., Lpz.*, p. 553.
(94) HEIDENHAIN, R. (1881). *Pflüg. Arch. ges. Physiol.* XXVI, 546.
(95) GAD, J. (1881). *Arch. Anat. Physiol., Lpz.*, p. 566.
(96) BERT, P. & MARCACCI (1881). *Lo sperimentali*, no. 10.
(97) FERRIER, D. & YEO, G. (1881). *Proc. Roy. Soc.* XXXII.
(98) RICHET, C. (1882). *Physiol. des Muscles et des Nerfs.* Paris.
(99) EXNER, S. (1882). *Pflüg. Arch. ges. Physiol.* XXVIII, 487.
(99a) GASKELL, W. H. (1882). *Philos. Trans.* p. 999.
(100) MELTZER, S. J. (1883). *Arch. Anat. Physiol., Lpz.* (Suppl. Bd.), p. 209.
(101) KRONECKER, H. & MELTZER, S. J. (1883). *Arch. Anat. Physiol., Lpz.* (Suppl. Bd.), p. 328.
(102) GAD, J. (1884). *66te Versamml. deutsch. Naturf. Aertze.*

Bibliographical References

(103) GASKELL, W. H. (1884). *Trans. 8th Internat. Med. Congress.* Copenhagen.
(104) SCHREIBER, J. (1884). *Deutsch. Arch. klin. Med.* XXXV, 254.
(105) JENDRÁSSIK, E. (1885). *Neurol. Centralbl.* p. 412.
(106) BEAUNIS, H. (1885). *C.R. Acad. Sci. Paris,* C, 918.
(106a) LANGE (1885). *Om Sindsbevägelser.* Copenhagen.
(107) MITCHELL & LEWIS (1886). *Medical News* (Feb. 13). Philadelphia.
(107a) BRUNTON, LAUDER T. (1887). *Text-book of Pharmacology* (3rd ed.), p. 168.
(108) GAD, J. (1887). *Arch. Physiol. Verhandl. phys. Ges.* (June), p. 468.
(109) BIEDERMANN, W. (1887). *S.B. Akad. Wiss. Wien,* XCIII (3), p. 8.
(110) EXNER, S. (1887). *Arch. Anat. Physiol., Lpz.,* p. 567.
(111) FRANCK, FR. (1887). *Leçons sur les fonct. cerveau.* Paris.
(111a) SCHÄFER, E. A. (1887). *Festschrift zu Karl Ludwig.* Leipzig.
(112) NANSEN, F. (1887). *Bergen's Museum.*
(112a) ALBERTONI (1887). *Arch. ital. Biol.* Part I.
(112b) TARCHANOW (1887). *Pflüg. Arch. ges. Physiol.* XL, 340.
(113) HERING, E. (1888). *Z.Theor. Vorgänge lebend. Substanz.* Prague.
(114) JAMES, W. (1888). *Scribner's Mag.* New York.
(115) GAD, J. (1888). *Eulenberg's Real-encycl.* XVI, 673.
(116) LOMBARD, W. P. (1888). *Amer. J. Psychol.* p. 8.
(117) BOWDITCH, H. P. (1888). *Boston Med. Surg. J.* no. 32.
(117a) SCHÄFER, E. A. & BROWN, SANGER (1888). *Philos. Trans.*
(118) HEAD, H. (1889). *J. Physiol.* X, 1.
(119) LOMBARD, W. P. (1889). *Arch. Anat. Physiol., Lpz.* (Suppl. Bd.), p. 292.
(119a) WERNICKE (1889). *Berliner Klin. Wschr.*
(120) BEAUNIS, H. (1889). *Arch. physiol norm. path.* p. 55.
(121) GAD, J. & JOSEPH, M. (1889). *Arch. Anat. Physiol., Lpz.,* p. 199.
(121a) MOTT, F. W. & SCHÄFER, E. A. (1890). *Brain,* XIII.
(122) BELMONDO & ODDI (1890). *Lab. di Fisiologia.* Florence.
(123) BOWDITCH, H. P. & WARREN, J. W. (1890). *J. Physiol.* XI, 25.
(124) JAMES, W. (1890). *Text-book of Psychology.* London.
(125) WALLER, A. D. (1890). *J. Physiol.* XI, 384.
(126) HAYCRAFT, J. (1890). *Brain,* XII, 516.
(127) BEEVOR, C. & HORSLEY, V. (1890). *Philos. Trans.* B, p. 128.
(128) MUNK, H. & OBREGIA (1890). *S.B. Akad. Wiss. Wien* (23 Jan.).
(128a) RAMON-Y-CAJAL (1890). *Gazett. med. Catalan.*
(129) BASTIAN, C. (1891). *Med.-chir. Trans.*
(130) STERNBERG, M. (1891). *S.B. Akad. Wiss. Wien,* C (3), 288.
(131) WALLER, A. D. (1891). *J. Physiol.* XII.
(131a) BOWLBY, A. (1891). *Med.-chir. Trans.*
(132) GOTCH, F. & HORSLEY, V. (1891). Croonian Lecture, Roy. Soc. Lond.
(133) POLIMANTI, O. (1892). *Arch. ital. Biol.* XXIII.
(133a) MUNK, H. (1892). *S.B. preus. Akad. Wiss.* XXXVI, 691.

Bibliographical References

(134) BEEVOR, C. (1892). *Brain*, Part 53, p. 51.
(135) GOLTZ, F. (1892). *Pflüg. Arch. ges. Physiol.* LI.
(136) SHERRINGTON, C. S. (1892). *J. Physiol.* XIII, 621.
(137) EWALD, J. R. (1892). *Endorgan d. Nervus Octavus.* Wiesbaden.
(138) SHERRINGTON, C. S. (1892). *J. Physiol.* XIII, Proc. (Feb.)
(139) SHERRINGTON, C. S. (1892). *Philos. Trans.* B, CLXXXIV.
(140) BRUNS (1893). *Neurol. Centralbl.*
(141) PIOTROWSKI, G. (1893). *J. Physiol.* XIV, 163.
(142) STERNBERG, M. (1893). *Die Sehnenreflexe.* Vienna.
(143) HEAD, H. (1893). *Brain*, Parts 61, 62.
(144) BAYLISS, W. M. (1893). *J. Physiol.* XIV, 303.
(144a) FERRIER, D. (1894). *Brain* (Spring Number).
(145) CYBULSKI & ZANIETOWSKI (1894). *Pflüg. Arch. ges. Physiol.* LVI.
(146) NAGEL, W. (1894). *Pflüg. Arch. ges. Physiol.* LVII, 495.
(147) LANGENDORFF & OLDAG (1895). *Pflüg. Arch. ges. Physiol.* LIX, 201.
(148) V. FREY (1894). *Ber. Sächs. Ges. (Akad.) Wiss.* Leipzig.
(149) EXNER, S. (1894). *Entwurf. z. einer physiol. Erklärung.*
(149a) LEE, F. S. (1894). *J. Physiol.* XVII, 192.
(150) LANGLEY, J. N. & ANDERSON, H. K. (1894). *J. Physiol.* XVI, 419.
(151) SHERRINGTON, C. S. (1894). *J. Physiol.* XVII, 27.
(152) SERGI (1894). *Dolore e Piacere.* Milan.
(153) SHERRINGTON, C. S. (1894). *J. Physiol.* XVII, 211.
(153a) MANN (1895). *Volkmanns Sammlung klin. Vorträge.*
(154) HERING, H. E. (1895). *Z. Heilk.* XVI.
(155) MÜNZER & WIENER (1895). *Prag. med. Wschr.* p. 481.
(156) FANO, G. (1895). *Arch. ital. Biol.* XXIV, 438.
(157) MOTT, F. W. & SHERRINGTON, C. S. (1895). *Proc. Roy. Soc.* LVII.
(157a) PORTER, T. W. (1895). *J. Physiol.* XVII, 455.
(158) BICKEL, A. (1896). *Pflüg. Arch. ges. Physiol.* LXV.
(159) HERING, H. E. (1896). *Prag. med. Wschr.* (July).
(160) STEINACH, E. (1896). *Pflüg. Arch. ges. Physiol.* LXIII, 495.
(161) GOTCH, F. (1896). *J. Physiol.* XX, 322.
(162) HERING, H. E. (1896). *Arch. exp. Path. Pharmak.* XXXVIII.
(163) WALLER, A. D. (1896). Croonian Lecture, *Philos. Trans.* B.
(164) GOTCH, F. & BURCH, G. (1896). *Philos. Trans.*
(165) LLOYD MORGAN, C. (1896). *Habit and Instinct.* London.
(166) HELMHOLTZ, H. V. (1896). *Physiol. Optik* (2nd ed.), p. 916. Hamburg.
(166a) GOLTZ, F. & EWALD, J. R. (1896). *Pflüg. Arch. ges. Physiol.* LXIII, 365.
(167) GOTCH, F. (1897). *J. Physiol.* XX.
(167a) ROSENTHAL, J. & MENDELSSOHN, M. (1897). *Neurol. Centralbl.* XXI.
(168) HERING, H. E. (1897). *Pflüg. Arch. ges. Physiol.* LXV.
(169) HERING, H. E. (1897). *Pflüg. Arch. ges. Physiol.* LXVIII.
(170) FOSTER, M. & SHERRINGTON, C. S. (1897). *Text-book of Physiology*, III. London.

Bibliographical References

(171) SHERRINGTON, C. S. (1897). *Proc. Roy. Soc.* LX, 365.
(172) V. FREY (1897). *Ber. Sächs. Ges. (Akad.) Wiss.* Leipzig.
(173) HERING, H. E. & SHERRINGTON, C. S. (1897). *Pflüg. Arch. ges. Physiol.* LXVIII.
(174) HERING, H. E. (1897). *Neurol. Centralbl.* no. 23.
(175) HOFBAUER, L. (1897). *Pflüg. Arch. ges. Physiol.* LXVIII.
(176) BICKEL, A. (1897). *Rev. méd. Suisse romande.*
(177) SERGI (1897). *Z. Psychol. Physiol.* p. 96.
(178) BETHE, A. (1897). *Arch. mikr.-Anat.* L, 629.
(178a) BETHE, A. (1897). *Pflüg. Arch. ges. Physiol.* LXVIII.
(179) HERING, H. E. (1898). *Pflüg. Arch. ges. Physiol.* LXX.
(180) CLIFFORD ALLBUTT (1898). *Syst. of Medicine*, III.
(181) VERWORN, M. (1898). *Beit. Physiol. Centralnervensystem.* Jena.
(182) SHERRINGTON, C. S. (1898). *J. Physiol.* XXII.
(183) SHERRINGTON, C. S. (1898). *Philos. Trans.* CXC.
(184) TOPOLANSKI, A. (1898). *Gräfes Arch.* XLVI, 452.
(185) BETHE, A. (1898). *Arch. mikr.-Anat.* LI.
(186) TSCHERMAK, A. (1898). *Arch. Anat. Physiol.* p. 291.
(187) GOLDSCHEIDER, A. (1898). *Die Bedeutung Reize Path. Therap. im Lichte Neuronlehre.*
(188) BAYLISS, W. M. & STARLING, E. H. (1899). *J. Physiol.* XXIV, 99.
(188a) BEER, TH., BETHE, A. & V. UEXKÜLL, J. (1899). *Biol. Centralbl.* XIX, no. 15.
(189) HUGHLINGS JACKSON (1899). *Brain*, XXII, 621.
(190) STEINACH, E. (1899). *Pflüg. Arch. ges. Physiol.* LXXVIII, 291.
(190a) HERING, H. E. (1899). *Zur Theorie Nerventhätigkeit.* Leipzig.
(191) DEMOOR, J. (1899). *Ann. Soc. Roy. Sci. Brux.* VIII.
(192) V. UEXKÜLL, J. (1899). *Z. Biol.* XXXVII, 381.
(193) MOORE, B. & REYNOLDS, H. W. (1899). *Physiol. Centralbl.* XII, 501.
(194) SHERRINGTON, C. S. (1899). Marshall Hall Address, *Med. Chir. Trans.* LXXXII.
(195) HERING, H. E. (1899). *Wien. Klin. Wschr.* no. 33.
(196) LOEB, J. (1899). *Vergleichende Gehirnphysiologie.* Leipzig.
(197) MELTZER, S. J. (1899). *New York Med. J.* (13, 20, and 27 May).
(198) ZWAARDEMAKER & LANS (1899). *Centralbl. Physiol.*
(199) BARKER, L. F. (1899). *The Nervous System.* New York.
(200) HUNT, REID (1899). *Amer. J. Physiol.* II, 396.
(201) HUBER, CARL G. (1899). *J. Morph.* XVI, 27.
(201a) SALOMONSON, J. K. A. W. (1900). *De Laar Neurones.* Amsterdam.
(202) HERING, H. E. (1900). *Prag. med. Wschr.* no. 25.
(203) BICKEL, A. (1900). *Arch. Anat. Physiol., Lpz.*
(204) BIEDERMANN, W. (1900). *Pflüg. Arch. ges. Physiol.* LXXX.
(205) SHERRINGTON, C. S. (1900). Schäfer's *Text-book of Physiology*, II.
(206) SCHÄFER, A. E. (1900). *Text-book of Physiology*, II.
(207) VERWORN, M. (1900). *Arch. Anat. Physiol., Lpz.* (Suppl. Bd.).

Bibliographical References

(208) VERWORN, M. (1900). Das Neuron, in *Anat. Physiol.* Jena.
(209) DONALDSON, H. (1900). *American Text-book of Physiology,* II.
(210) MERZBACHER, L. (1900). *Pflüg. Arch. ges. Physiol.* LXXXI.
(211) UEXKÜLL, V. J. (1900). *Z. Biol.* XXXIX.
(212) BAGLIONI, S. (1900). *Arch. Anat. Physiol., Lpz.* (Suppl. Bd., Physiol. Abt.), p. 193.
(213) LADD, G. T. (1900). *Descriptive Psychology,* p. 334.
(213a) SHERRINGTON, C. S. (1900). *Proc. Roy. Soc.* LXVI, 390.
(214) BONNIER, P. (1900). *L'Orientation.* Paris.
(215) MENDELSSOHN, M. (1900). 13th Cong. intern. de Med. Paris, Sect. of Physiology.
(216) LYON, E. P. (1900). *Amer. J. Physiol.* IV, 77.
(216a) LLOYD MORGAN, C. (1900). *Animal Behaviour.* London.
(217) LANGENDORFF, O. (1901). *Die physiologische Merkmale Nervenzelle.* Rostock.
(218) CHAUVEAU (1901). *Le pharynx.* Paris.
(219) LOEB, J. (1901). *Comparative Physiology of the Brain.* London.
(220) LANGLEY, J. N. (1901). *J. Physiol.* XXVII, 224.
(221) MISLAWSKI (1901). *Centralbl. Physiol.* XV, 481.
(222) FRÖHLICH, A. & SHERRINGTON, C. S. (1901). *J. Physiol.* XXVIII, 14.
(223) MCDOUGALL, W. (1901). *Mind,* X, no. 37.
(224) CLEGHORN, A. & STEWART, C. S. (1901). *Amer. J. Physiol.* V.
(225) GRÜNBAUM, A. & SHERRINGTON, C. S. (1901). *Proc. Roy. Soc.*
(226) WINKLER, C. & RYNBERGK, G. A. VAN (1901). *Proc. K. Akad. Wet.* Amsterdam.
(226a) MACWILLIAM, J. A. (1901). *Brit. Med. J.* (30 Nov.).
(227) V. UEXKÜLL, J. (1902). *Ergebnisse Physiol.* (First Series), II, 212.
(228) MERZBACHER, L. (1902). *Pflüg. Arch. ges. Physiol.* LXXXVIII.
(229) GRUNBAUM, A. & SHERRINGTON, C. S. (1902). *Proc. Roy. Soc.*
(230) TSCHERMAK, A. & KÖSTER, G. (1903). *Pflüg. Arch. ges. Physiol.* XCIII, 24.
(231) JONSTON, J. B. (1902). *J. Comp. Neurol.* XII, 87.
(232) MCDOUGALL, W. (1902). *Mind,* II, no. 43.
(233) HERING, H. E. (1902). *Ergebnisse Physiol.* (First Series), II, 503.
(234) MACDONALD, J. S. (1902). *Thompson-Yates Lab. Rep.* IV, 213.
(235) ZWAARDEMAKER & EYJKMAN (1902). *Onderz. physiol. Lab.* Utrecht. Hochsch. 5, III.
(236) DU BOIS REYMOND, R. (1902). *Arch. Anat. Physiol., Lpz.* (Suppl. Bd.), p. 27.
(237) MAGNUS, R. (1902). *Mitt. Stat. Zool. Neapel,* XV.
(238) YERKES, R. M. (1902). *Amer. J. Physiol.* VI, 440.
(239) V. BÄYER, H. (1902). *V. Z. allg. Physiol.*
(240) SEEMANN, J. (1902). *Pflüg. Arch. ges. Physiol.* XCI, 318.
(241) V. MONAKOW, C. (1902). *Ergebnisse Physiol.* (First Series), II, 563.
(242) BABÄK, E. (1902). *Pflüg. Arch. ges. Physiol.* XCIII, 134.

Bibliographical References

(242a) ZIEHEN, TH. (1902). *Leitfaden physiol. Psychol.* Berlin.
(243) MÜNZER & WIENER (1902). *Monats. Psychol. Neurol.* XII, 241.
(244) GOTCH, F. (1902). *J. Physiol.* XXVIII, 395.
(244a) LEWANDOWSKI, M. (1902). *J. Physiol. Neurol.* Bd. I, 72.
(245) BAGLIONI, S. (1903). *V. Z. allg. Physiol.* II, 556.
(245a) VERWORN, M. (1903). *Die Biogenhypothese.* Jena.
(246) BONDY, O. (1903). *V. Z. allg. Physiol.* II.
(247) FRÖHLICH, A. (1903). *V. Z. allg. Physiol.* II.
(248) BAGLIONI, S. (1903). *Centralbl. Physiol.* no. 23.
(249) BICKEL, A. (1903). *Mechanismus nervös. Bewegungsregul.* Stuttgart.
(250) HERRICK, C. J. (1903). *J. Comp. Neurol.* XII.
(251) SHERRINGTON, C. S. & LASLETT, E. E. (1903). *J. Physiol.* XXIX, 58.
(251a) WOODWORTH, R. S. (1903). *Le Mouvement.* Paris.
(252) SHERRINGTON, C. S. (1903). *J. Physiol.* XXX, 39.
(253) PARKER, G. H. (1903). *Amer. J. Physiol.* XVI, no. 1.
(254) LOEB, J. (1903). *Univ. of California Publication, Physiology.*
(255) YERKES, R. M. (with AYER, J. B.) (1903). *Amer. J. Physiol.* IX, 279.
(256) FANO, G. (1903). *Arch. ital. physiol.*
(256a) BRODMANN (1903). *J. Psychol. Neurol.* II, 79.
(257) YERKES, R. M. (1903). *Mark Anniv. Volume, Harvard Coll.* p. 359.
(258) YERKES, R. M. (1903). *Harvard Psychol. Studies,* I, 565.
(259) PHILIPPSON, M. (1903). *C.R. Acad. Sci. Paris.*
(260) FRÖHLICH, A. (1903). *Pflüg. Arch. ges. Physiol.* XCV.
(261) PHILIPPSON, M. (1903). *Bull. Acad. Roy. Belgique.*
(261a) MCDOUGALL, W. (1903). *Mind,* XIII, 473.
(262) MCDOUGALL, W. (1903). *Brain,* Part CII, p. 153.
(263) BETHE, A. (1903). *Allg. Anat. Physiol. Nervensyst.* Leipzig.
(264) INGBERT, C. (1903). *J. Comp. Neurol.* XIII, 53.
(265) INGBERT, C. (1903). *J. Comp. Neurol.* XIII, 209.
(266) BONNIER, P. (1903). *Un nouveau syndrome bulbaire.* Paris.
(267) STERNBERG, M. & LATZKO (1903). *Deutsch. Z. Nervenheilk.* XXIV, 209.
(267a) HITZIG, E. (1903). *Arch. Psychiat. Nervenkrank.* XXXVII.
(268) MAGNUS (1904). *Pflüg. Arch. ges. Physiol.* CII, 349.
(269) MUSKENS, J. L. (1904). *J. Physiol.* XXXI, 204.
(269a) CUSHING, H. (1904). *Johns Hopk. Hosp. Bull.* XV, 213.
(270) KIESOW, F. (1904). *Z. Psychol. Physiol.* XXXIII, 436; also earlier, *Philos. Stud.* XIV, 567.
(270a) LYON, E. P. (1904). *Amer. J. Physiol,* XII, 149.
(271) STOREY, T. A. (1904). *Amer. J. Physiol.* XII, 75.
(271a) FLECHSIG, P. (1904). *Ber. Sächs. Ges. (Akad.) Wiss.* Part I, p. 50, Part II, p. 177.
(272) ZWAARDEMAKER, H. (1904). *Arch. internat. physiol.* I, 1.
(272a) CAMPBELL, A. W. (1904). *Proc. Roy. Soc.* LXXII, 488.

Bibliographical References

(273) BIEDERMANN, W. (1904). *Pflüg. Arch. ges. Physiol.* CII.
(274) BONNIER, P. (1904). *Le sens des attitudes*. Paris.
(275) WOODWORTH, R. S. & SHERRINGTON, C. S. (1904). *J. Physiol.* XXXI, 234.
(276) YERKES, R. M. (1904). *Biol. Bull.* VI, 84.
(277) YERKES, R. M. (1904). *J. Comp. Neurol.* XIV, 124.
(278) HYDE, J. (1904). *Amer. J. Physiol.* X, 236.
(280) ROTHMANN (1904). *Arch. Psychiat.* XXXVIII, Heft 3.
(281) FRÖHLICH, A. (1904). *Pflüg. Arch. ges. Physiol.* CII.
(282) GROSSER, OTTO (1904). *Centralbl. Grenzgebiete Med. Chirurg.* VII, 25.
(283) HARRIS, W. (1904). *J. Anat. Physiol.* p. 399.
(284) RYNBERK, G. A. VAN (1904). *Petrus Camper*, III, 137.
(285) BAGLIONI, S. (1904). *V. Z. allg. Physiol.* IV, 113.
(286) FRÖHLICH, FR. (1904). *V. Z. allg. Physiol.* IV.
(287) SHERRINGTON, C. S. (1904). *J. Physiol.* XXXI, xvii. Proc.
(288) BAGLIONI, S. (1904). *Arch. Fisiol.* I, 575.
(289) RYNBERK, G. VAN (1904). *Arch. Farmacol. speri.* III, 7.
(290) SARGENT, P. E. (1904). *Bull. Com. Zoöl.*, Harv. Coll., XLV, iii, 131.
(291) CARLSON (1904). *Pflüg. Arch. ges. Physiol.* CI.
(292) HYDE, I. (1904). *Amer. J. Physiol.* X.
(293) BAGLIONI (1904). *Il policlinico*. Roma.
(294) PARI, G. A. (1904). *Arch. ital. Biol.* XLII.
(294a) BETHE, A. (1904). *Deutsch. Med. Wschr.* no. 33.
(295) PAWLOW, J. P. (1904). *Ergebn. Physiol.* (Third Series), I, 177.
(296) PHILIPPSON, M. (1904). *VI. Congr. intern. physiol.* Bruxelles.
(297) MCDOUGALL, W. (1904). *Brit. J. Psychol.* I, 114.
(298) WARRINGTON, W. B. & GRIFFITHS, F. (1904). *Brain*, XXVII, p. 297.
(298a) TSCHERMAK, A. (1904). *Institut impériale de Médecine experimentale*. St Petersburg.
(299) SHERRINGTON, C. S. (1904). *Brit. J. Psychol.* I.
(299a) EDINGER, L. (1904). *Vorlesungen nervösen Centralorg*. Leipzig, II.
(300) SHERRINGTON, C. S. (1904). *Brit. Assoc. Adv. Sci.· Rep., Camb.*, (Address to Sect. of Physiology).
(301) MCDOUGALL, W. (1904). *Proc. Psychol. Soc.; J. Psychol.*, no. 3.
(301a) LANGELAAN, J. W. (1904). *Proc. K. Akad. Wet.* Amsterdam.
(302) BEEVOR, C. E. (1904). Croonian Lectures, Roy. Coll. of Physicians, London.
(303) BIEDERMANN, W. (1905). *Pflüg. Arch. ges. Physiol.* CVII, 1.
(304) SHERRINGTON, C. S. (1905). *Proc. Roy. Soc.* LXXVI, 161, 269, and previous 'Notes' in Vols. LII, LIII, LX, LXI, LXIV and LXVI.
(305) YERKES, R. M. (1905). *Pflüg. Arch. ges. Physiol.* CVII, 207.
(306) MACDONALD, J. S. (1905). *Proc. Roy. Soc.* LXXVI.
(307) MACALLUM, A. B. (1905). *J. Physiol.* XXXII, 95.

Bibliographical References

(308) BOTTAZZI, F. (1905). *Gaz. internaz. Medicina*, VIII (April).
(309) PHILIPPSON, M. (1905). *Heger's Trav. Lab. physiol.* VII, no. 2.
(310) KALISCHER, O. (1905). *Abh. preus. Akad. Wiss.*
(311) EDKINS, J. S. (1905). *Proc. Roy. Soc.* LXXVI.
(312) LEWANDOWSKI, M. (1905). *Verh. physiol. Ges. Ber.*
(313) SOWTON, S. C. M. & SHERRINGTON, C. S. (1905). *Brit. Med. J.*, Report on Chloroform.
(314) MOTT, F. W. (1905). *Trans. Opt. Soc. Lond.*, XXV, ci.

BIBLIOGRAPHY OF WRITINGS

1884-1947

1884

On sections of the right half of the medulla oblongata and of the spinal cord of the dog which was exhibited by Prof. Goltz at the International Medical Congress of 1881 (with J. N. Langley [1]). *Proc. Physiol. Soc., J. Physiol.*, 1884 (Jan.), v, vi.

Secondary degeneration of nerve tracts following removal of the cortex of the cerebrum in the dog (with J. N. Langley [1]). *J. Physiol.* 1884 (June), v, 49-65, pl. 1-2.

1885

On secondary and tertiary degenerations in the spinal cord of the dog. *J. Physiol.* 1885 (Apr.), vi, 177-91, pl. 4-5.

1886

Preliminary report on the pathology of cholera Asiatica (as observed in Spain, 1885) (with C. S. Roy [1] and J. Graham Brown [2]). *Proc. roy. Soc.* 1886 (10 June), xli, 173-81.

Effect of ligature of the optic nerve in a rabbit. *Proc. Physiol. Soc., J. Physiol.*, 1886 (May), vii, xvi-xvii.

On a case of bilateral degeneration in the spinal cord, fifty-two days after hæmorrhage in one cerebral hemisphere (with W. B. Hadden [1]). *Brain*, 1886 (Jan.), viii, 502-11, pl. 1.

Note on two newly described tracts in the human spinal cord. *Brain*, 1886 (Oct.), ix, 342-51, pl. 1.

1887

Note on the anatomy of Asiatic cholera as exemplified in cases occurring in Italy in 1886. *Proc. roy. Soc.* 1887 (16 June), xlii, 474-7.

1888

The pathological anatomy of a case of locomotor ataxy, with special reference to ascending degenerations in the spinal cord and medulla oblongata (with W. B. Hadden [1]). *Brain*, 1888 (Oct.), xi, 325-35, pl. 1.

1889

On nerve-tracts degenerating secondarily to lesions of the cortex cerebri (Preliminary). *J. Physiol.* 1889, x, 429-32.

On formation of scar-tissue (with C. A. Ballance). *J. Physiol.* 1889 (Oct.), x, 550-76, pl. 31-3.

Bibliography of Writings

1890

Note on bilateral degeneration in the pyramidal tracts resulting from unilateral cortical lesion. *Brit. med. J.* 1890 (4 Jan.), I, 14.

On outlying nerve-cells in the mammalian spinal cord (Preliminary note). *Proc. roy. Soc.* 1890, XLVII, 144-6.

On the regulation of the blood-supply of the brain (with C. S. Roy [1]). *J. Physiol.* 1890, XI, 85-108, pl. 2-4.

Addendum to note on tracts degenerating secondarily to lesions of the cortex cerebri. *J. Physiol.* 1890, XI, 121-2.

Über die Entstehung des Narbengewebes, das Schicksal der Leucocyten und die Rolle der Bindegewebskörperchen (with C. A. Ballance). *Zbl. allg. Path. Anat.* 1890 (Oct.), I, 697-703.

A method to determine the quantity of blood in a living animal (with S. M. Copeman [1]). *Proc. Physiol. Soc., J. Physiol.*, 1890 (May), XI, viii-ix.

The effect of movements of the human body on the size of the spinal canal (with R. W. Reid [1]). *Brain*, 1890, XIII, 449-55.

Further note on degenerations following lesions of the cerebral cortex. *J. Physiol.* 1890, XI, 399-400.

Demonstration of ganglion cells in the mammalian spinal cord. *Proc. Physiol. Soc., J. Physiol.*, 1890 (Dec.), XII, xxxiv.

1891

On pilo-motor nerves (with J. N. Langley [1]). *J. Physiol.* 1891, XII, 278-91.

Note on Cheyne-Stokes breathing in the frog. *J. Physiol.* 1891, XII, 292-8, pl. 7.

Note on some functions of the cervical sympathetic in the monkey. *Brit. med. J.* 1891 (21 Mar.), I, 635.

Note on the nerve supply of the bladder and anus. *Brit. med. J.* 1891 (9 May), I, 1016.

Note on the knee-jerk. *St Thom. Hosp. Rep.* 1891, XXI, 145-7.

On outlying nerve-cells in the mammalian spinal cord. *Philos. Trans.* (1890), 1891, CLXXXIb, 33-48, pl. 3-4.

1892

The nuclei in the lumbar cord for the muscles of the pelvic limb. *Proc. Physiol. Soc., J. Physiol.*, 1892 (15 Feb.), XIII, viii-x.

Note toward the localisation of the knee-jerk. *Brit. med. J.* 1892, I, 545; Addendum to note on the knee-jerk. *Ibid.* (26 Mar.), 654.

Geminal nerve-fibres. Dichotomous branching of medullated fibres in the brain and spinal cord. *Proc. Physiol. Soc., J. Physiol.*, 1892, XIII, xxi-xxii.

Notes on the arrangement of some motor fibres in the lumbo-sacral plexus. *J. Physiol.* 1892, XIII, 621-772, pl. 20-3. (Preliminary note in *Proc. roy. Soc.* 1892 (14 Mar.), LI, 67-78.)

Bibliography of Writings

On varieties of leucocytes. *Zbl. Physiol.* 1892, VI, 399.
Sulla localizzazione del riflesso rotuleo. *G. Accad. Med. Torino*, 1892 (Dec.), XL, 951–9.
In memoriam W. B. Hadden, M.D. (Lond.), F.R.C.P. *St Thom. Hosp. Rep.* 1892, XXII, xix–xxi (unsigned).
Experiments in examination of the peripheral distribution of the fibres of the posterior roots of some spinal nerves (Preliminary note). *Proc. roy. Soc.* 1892 (2 Dec.), LII, 333–7 (full report 1894).
Experiments on animals (concerning the sensitiveness of the peritoneum; a polemic with Lawson Tait). *Lancet*, 1892 (Dec. 17), II, 1416–17; Experiments on living animals. *Ibid.* (31 Dec.), 1533; third letter *Ibid.* 1893 (28 Jan.), I, 221.

1893

Variations experimentally produced in the specific gravity of the blood. *J. Physiol.* 1893 (Jan.), XIV, 52–96, pl. 4 (with S. M. Copeman).
Note on the knee-jerk and the correlation of action of antagonistic muscles. *Proc. roy. Soc.* 1893 (Feb.), LII, 556–64.
Further experimental note on the correlation of action of antagonistic muscles. *Proc. roy. Soc.* 1893 (15 Apr.), LIII, 407–20. Abstr. bearing same title *Brit. med. J.* 1893 (10 June), I, 1218.
Experimental note on the knee-jerk. *Brit. med. J.* 1893 (23 Sept.), II, 685; also *St Thom. Hosp. Rep.* (1891), 1893, XXI, 145–7.
Note on the spinal portion of some ascending degenerations. *J. Physiol.* 1893 (Sept.), XIV, 255–302, pl. 13–18.
Remarks on L. A. Bidwell's paper 'Focal epilepsy; trephining and removal of small hæmorrhagic focus; no improvement; removal of part of leg centre after electrical stimulation; improvement.' *Brit. med. J.* 1893 (4 Nov.), II, 989.
Note on some changes in the blood of the general circulation consequent upon certain inflammations of an acute local character. *Proc. roy. Soc.* 1893 (11 Dec.), LIV, 487–8 (full report, 1894).
Experiments on the escape of bacteria with the secretions. *J. Path. Bact.* 1893 (Jan.), I, 258–78.
Sur une action inhibitrice de l'écorce cérébrale. *Rev. neurol.* 1893, I, 318–19.

1894

Note on experimental degeneration of the pyramidal tract. *Lancet*, 1894 (3 Feb.), I, 265. [Polemic reply by Horsley (10 Feb.), 370–1]; Second note by C. S. S. (17 Feb.), 439; Third note by C. S. S. (3 Mar.), 571.
Experimental note on two movements of the eye. *J. Physiol.* 1894 (19 July), XVII, 27–9.

Bibliography of Writings

On the anatomical constitution of the nerves of muscles. *Proc. Physiol. Soc.*, *J. Physiol.*, 1894 (23 June), XVII, xix–xx.

On the anatomical constitution of nerves of skeletal muscles; with remarks on recurrent fibres in the ventral spinal nerve-root. *J. Physiol.* 1894, XVII, 211–58, pl. 5–7.

Note on some changes in the blood of the general circulation consequent upon certain inflammations of an acute local character. *Proc. roy. Soc.* 1894, LV, 161–207.

Experiments in examination of the peripheral distribution of the fibres of the posterior roots of some spinal nerves. (I) *Philos. Trans.* (1893), 1894, CLXXXIV *b*, 641–763, pl. 42–52.

1895

Experiments upon the influence of sensory nerves upon movement and nutrition of the limbs (with F. W. Mott [1]). Preliminary communication. *Proc. roy. Soc.* 1895 (7 Mar.), LVII, 481–8.

Varieties of leucocytes. *Sci. Progr. Twent. Cent.* 1895 (Feb.), II, 415–30.

1896

A note on the physiology of the spinal cord. *St Thom. Hosp. Rep.* (1894), 1896, XXIII, 69–76.

Influence of simultaneous contrast on 'flicker' of visual sensation. *Proc. Physiol. Soc., J. Physiol.*, 1896 (14 Nov.), XX, xviii–xix.

Committee report on the life condition and infectivity of the oyster (with W. A. Herdman and others). *Brit. Ass. Rep.* 1896, 663; 1897, 363; 1898, 559–62.

1897

Cataleptoid reflexes in the monkey. *Proc. roy. Soc.* 1897 (21 Jan.), LX, 411–14; also *Lancet*, 1897 (6 Feb.), I, 373–4.

Experiments in examination of the peripheral distribution of the fibres of the posterior roots of some spinal nerves. (Preliminary abstract.) *Proc. roy. Soc.* 1897 (21 Jan.), LX, 408–11 (full report 1898).

On reciprocal innervation of antagonistic muscles. Third note. *Proc. roy. Soc.* 1897 (21 Jan.), LX, 414–17.

On reciprocal action in the retina as studied by means of some rotating discs. *J. Physiol.* 1897 (5 Feb.), XXI, 33–54.

Double (antidrome) conduction in the central nervous system. *Proc. roy. Soc.* 1897 (8 Apr.), LXI, 243–6.

Further note on the sensory nerves of muscles. *Proc. roy. Soc.* 1897 (8 Apr.), LXI, 247–9.

On the question whether any fibres of the mammalian dorsal (afferent) spinal root are of intraspinal origin. *J. Physiol.* 1897 (Mar.), XXI, 209–12.

Bibliography of Writings

The central nervous system, vol. 3 (with M. Foster [1]). Sir Michael Foster's *A Text Book of Physiology*, 7th ed., London, 1897. (In the 5th ed., 1890, 'Mr Langley' and 'Dr Sherrington' 'largely assisted' Foster in the preparation of the volume.)

The mammalian spinal cord as an organ of reflex action. Croonian Lecture. *Proc. roy. Soc.* 1897, LXI, 220–1. (Abstract. Published *in extenso* as Section IV of Experiments in examination, etc., *Philos. Trans.* 1898, CXC*b*, 45–186.)

Über Hemmung der Contraction willkürlicher Muskeln bei elektrischer Reizung der Grosshirnrinde (with H. E. Hering [1]). *Pflüg. Arch. ges. Physiol.* 1897, LXVIII, 221–8.

Antagonistic muscles and reciprocal innervation (with H. E. Hering). Fourth note. *Proc. roy. Soc.* 1897 (18 Nov.), LXII, 183–7.

The activity of the nervous centres which correlate antagonistic muscles in the limbs. *Rep. Brit. Ass.* 1897, 516–18.

Observations on visual contrast. *Rep. Brit. Ass.* 1897, 824–6.

Committee report on the physiological effects of peptone and its precursors when introduced into the circulation (with E. A. Schäfer and others). *Brit. Ass. Rep.* 1897, 531; 1898, 720; 1899, 605; 1900, 457; 1904, 342.

Committee report on the functional activity of nerve cells (with W. H. Gaskell and others). *Brit. Ass. Rep.* 1897, 512; 1898, 714–15.

1898

Experiments in examination of the peripheral distribution of the fibres of the posterior roots of some spinal nerves. (II) *Philos. Trans.* 1898, CXC*b*, 45–186, pl. 3–6 (rec. 12 Nov., 1896; read 21 Jan. 1897). Also *Thomp. Yates Lab. Rep.* 1898, I, 45–173.

Decerebrate rigidity, and reflex co-ordination of movements. *J. Physiol.* 1898 (17 Feb.), XXII, 319–32.

Cardiac physics. In Allbutt, *System of Medicine*, New York and London, 1898, V, 464–79 (2nd ed. revised by J. Mackenzie, 1909, VI, 3–25).

Further note on the sensory nerves of the eye-muscles. *Proc. roy. Soc.* 1898 (17 Nov.), LXIV, 120–1.

On the reciprocal innervation of antagonistic muscles. Fifth note. *Proc. roy. Soc.* 1898 (15 Dec.), LXIV, 179–81.

1899

The teaching of physiology and histology. *Brit. med. J.* 1899 (8 Apr.), I, 878.

On the spinal animal (Marshall Hall Lecture). *Med.-chir. Trans.* 1899 (23 May), LXXXII, 449–77, pl. 13–17. Abstract, *Brit. med. J.* 1899 (27 May), I, 1276; *Lancet*, 1899 (27 May), I, 1433; *Thomp. Yates Lab. Rep.* 1898, I, 27–44.

Tremor, 'tendon-phenomenon,' and spasm. In Allbutt, *System of Medicine*, 1899, VI, 511–24 (2nd ed., 1910, VII, 290–309).

Bibliography of Writings

On the relation between structure and function as examined in the arm. (Inaugural address.) *Trans. Lpool biol. Soc.* 1899, XIII, 1–20.
Inhibition of the contraction of voluntary muscles by electrical excitation of the cortex cerebri (with H. E. Hering [1]). *J. Physiol.* 1899, XXIII (Suppl. Rep. Internat. Congress), 31.
Inhibition of the tonus of a voluntary muscle by excitation of its antagonist. *J. Physiol.* 1899, XXIII (Suppl. Rep. Internat. Congress), 26.

1900

On the innervation of antagonistic muscles. Sixth note. *Proc. roy. Soc.* 1900 (18 Jan.), LXVI, 66–7. (*Thomp. Yates Lab. Rep.* 1899, I, 175–6.)
Experiments on the value of vascular and visceral factors for the genesis of emotion. *Proc. roy. Soc.* 1900 (10 May), LXVI, 390–403; Abstract, *Brit. med. J.* 1900 (14 July), II, 110.
The spinal cord. In *Text-book of Physiology*. Edited by E. A. Schäfer, Edinburgh and London, 1900, II, 783–883.
The parts of the brain below cerebral cortex, viz. medulla oblongata, pons, cerebellum, corpora quadrigemina, and region of thalamus. In *Text-book of Physiology*. Edited by E. A. Schäfer, Edinburgh and London, 1900, II, 884–919.
Cutaneous sensations. In *Text-book of Physiology*. Edited by E. A. Schäfer, Edinburgh and London, 1900, II, 920–1001.
The muscular sense. In *Text-book of Physiology*. Edited by E. A. Schäfer, Edinburgh and London, 1900, II, 1002–25.
Nature of tendon reflexes—a discussion of E. Jendrassik's paper before 13th Int. Congr. Med., *Lancet*, 1900 (18 Aug.), II, 530–1. Sur la nature des reflexes tendineux. *Res. Rap. Paris. Sect. Neurol.* 25–6; *C.R. XIII Int. Congr. Med.* 1900, Sect. Neurol. 149–55. Also *St Louis med. surg. J.* 1900, LXXIX, 197–8.
Lecture on *Physiology for Teachers* (29 Nov. 1900). Printed privately (1901) by The Childhood Society for the scientific study of the mental and physical conditions of children, 15 pp.

1901

The general anatomy and physiology of the nervous system. In Allchin, *Manual of Medicine*, 1901, III (*Diseases of the Nervous System*), 1–33.
The name of the red corpuscle: A suggestion. *Brit. med. J.* 1901 (23 Mar.), I, 742.
Über einige Hemmungserscheinungen im Zustande der sog. Enthirnungsstarre (decerebrate rigidity). *Wien. klin. Rsch.* 1901, XV, 774–5. (Nothnagel *Festschrift*) (with A. Fröhlich).
The spinal roots and dissociative anæsthesia in the monkey. *J. Physiol.* 1901 (23 Dec.), XXVII, 360–71, pl. 10.

Bibliography of Writings

Observations on the physiology of the cerebral cortex of some of the higher apes (with A. S. F. Grünbaum [1]). *Proc. roy. Soc.* 1901 (23 Nov.), LXIX, 206–9. Also *Thomp. Yates Lab. Rep.* 1902, IV, pt. 2.

An address on localization in the 'motor' cerebral cortex (with A. S. F. Grünbaum). *Brit. Med. J.* 1901 (28 Dec.), II, 1857–9. (Read before the Pathological Society, London, 17 Dec. 1901; also read before Vth Internat. Congress, Turin, abstract *Brit. med. J.* 1901 (12 Oct.), II, 1091–3.)

1902

Path of impulses for inhibition under decerebrate rigidity (with A. Fröhlich [1]). *J. Physiol.* 1902, XXVIII, 14–19.

Observations on 'flicker' in binocular vision. *Proc. roy. Soc.* 1902 (30 July), LXXI, 71–6.

A discussion on the motor cortex as exemplified in the anthropoid apes (with A. S. F. Grünbaum). *Brit. med. J.* 1902 (13 Sept.), II, 784, 785.

Committee report on the conditions of health essential to carrying on the work of instruction in schools (with E. W. Wallis and others). *Brit. Ass. Rep.* 1902, 483–96; 1903, 455; 1904, 348; 1906, 433; 1907, 421; 1908, 458.

Committee reports of special chloroform committee of the British Medical Association (with Dr Barr and others). *Brit. med. J.* 1902, II, 116–18; *ibid.* 1903, II, cxli–cxliii; 1904, II, 161–2; 1905, II, 180–1; 1906, II, 78–9.

Fatigue. A lecture to the Froebel Society, Owens College, Manchester. Abstract only, *Brit. med. J.* 1902 (25 Oct.), II, 1371.

Address to the Conference on the Hygiene of Social Life. *J. R. sanit. Inst.* 1902, XXIII, 311–17; abstract, *Brit. med. J.* 1902 (20 Sept.), II, 885–6, 991.

C. S. Roy, 1854–97. *Year Book of the Royal Society*, 1902, 231–5.

Note on the arterial supply of the brain in anthropoid apes (with A. S. F. Grünbaum [1]). *Brain*, 1902, XXV, 270–3.

Remarks at discussion on pathology of nerve degeneration. *Brit. med. J.* 1902 (27 Sept.), II, 928.

Note upon descending intrinsic spinal tracts in the mammalian cord (with E. E. Laslett). *Proc. roy. Soc.* 1902, LXXI, 115–21.

1903

The history of the discovery of trypanosomes in man. *Lancet*, 1903 (21 Feb.), I, 509–13 (with R. Boyce [1] and R. Ross [2]). Preliminary letter, *Lancet*, 1902 (22 Nov.), II, 1426; also *Brit. med. J.* 1902 (22 Nov.), II, 1680.

Observations on some spinal reflexes and the interconnexion of spinal segments (with E. E. Laslett). *J. Physiol.* 1903 (Feb.), XXIX, 58–96.

Remarks on the dorsal spino-cerebellar tract (with E. E. Laslett). *J. Physiol.* 1903 (Mar.), XXIX, 188–94.

Bibliography of Writings

Physiology and nervous diseases. An address delivered to 'Doctorate Graduates,' University of Chicago, October, 1903.

An address on science and medicine in the modern university (delivered at the opening of the new medical school, Toronto, 1903). *Brit. med. J.* 1903 (7 Nov.), II, 1193–6; also *Lancet*, 1903 (7 Nov.), II, 1273–6; *Science*, 1903 (27 Nov.), XVIII, 675–84.

Observations on the physiology of the cerebral cortex of the anthropoid apes (with A. S. F. Grünbaum [1]). *Proc. roy. Soc.* 1903 (11 June), LXXII, 152–5. (Also *Thomp. Yates Lab. Rep.* 1903, V, 55–8.)

Qualitative difference of spinal reflex corresponding with qualitative difference of cutaneous stimulus. *J. Physiol.* 1903 (Aug.), XXX, 39–46.

Address on medical science. *Canad. J. Med. Surg.* 1903, XIV, 321–32; *Dom. med. Mon.* 1903, XXI, 203–15.

On the dosage of the mammalian heart by chloroform (I) (with S. C. M. Sowton). *Brit. med. J.* 1903 (suppl.), cxlvii–clxi; *Thomp. Yates Lab. Rep.* 1903, V, 69–104.

Opening of discussion on applied hygiene for school teachers. *J. R. sanit. Inst.* 1903, XXIV, 27–31.

1904

On binocular flicker and the correlation of activity of 'corresponding' retinal points. *Brit. J. Psychol.* 1904 (Jan.), I, 26–60.

On certain spinal reflexes in the dog. *Proc. Physiol. Soc., J. Physiol.*, 1904 (19 Mar.), XXXI, xvii–xix.

A pseudaffective reflex and its spinal path (with R. S. Woodworth [1]). *J. Physiol.* 1904 (June), XXXI, 234–43.

On the dosage of the isolated mammalian heart by chloroform (II) (with S. C. M. Sowton). Appendix I to the Third Report of Special Chloroform Committee. *Brit. med. J.* 1904 (23 July), II, 162–8, 721; *Brit. Ass. Rep.* 1904, 761–2; and *Arch. Fisiol.* 1904 (Nov.), II, 140–1.

The correlation of reflexes and the principle of the common path. *Brit. Ass. Rep.* 1904 (18 Aug.), LXXIV, 728–41; also abstract *Brit. med. J.* 1904 (27 Aug.), II, 443; *Nature*, 1904, LXX, 460–6; *Pop. Sci. Mon.* 1904, LXV, 549–52.

Committee report on madreporaria of the Bermuda Islands (with S. J. Hickson and others). *Brit. Ass. Rep.* 1904, 299; 1905, 186; 1906, 325.

On the mode of functional conjunction of twin (corresponding) retinal points. *Arch. Fisiol.* 1904 (Nov.), II, 154–5.

1905

On reciprocal innervation of antagonistic muscles. Seventh note. *Proc. roy. Soc.* 1905 (6 Apr.), LXXVIb, 160–3.

On reciprocal innervation of antagonistic muscles. Eighth note. *Proc. roy. Soc.* 1905 (18 May), LXXVIb, 269–97.

Bibliography of Writings

Über das Zusammenwirken der Rückenmarksreflexe und das Prinzip der gemeinsamen Strecke. *Ergebn. Physiol.* 1905, IV, 797–850.

On the relative effects of chloroform upon the heart and upon other muscular organs. *Brit. med. J.* 1905 (22 July), II, 181–7. (Appendix I of Fourth Report of Special Chloroform Committee, see 1902.)

Physiology: its scope and method. From Oxford Lectures on *Methods of Science*, 1905, chap. 3, pp. 59–80.

The importance of longer hours of sleep at public schools. *Brit. med. J.* 1905 (2 Dec.), II, 1469–71 (unsigned).

Obituary. Sir John Burdon-Sanderson. *Brit. med. J.* 1905 (2 Dec.), II, 1491–2.

Training in hygiene for teachers. *J. R. sanit. Inst.* 1905, XXVI, 132–8.

1906

The Integrative Action of the Nervous System. New York, Charles Scribner's Sons, 1906, xvi+411 pp. [Cf. Curriculum vitae.]

On the innervation of antagonistic muscles. Ninth note. Successive spinal induction. *Proc. roy. Soc.* 1906 (15 Feb.), LXXVII b, 478–97.

On the proprioceptive system, especially in its reflex aspects. *Brain*, 1906, XXIX (Hughlings Jackson Number), 467–82.

Observations on the scratch-reflex in the spinal dog. *J. Physiol.* 1906, XXXIV, 1–50.

On the effect of chloroform in conjunction with carbonic dioxide on cardiac and other muscle (with S. C. M. Sowton [1]). Appendix III of Fifth Report of Special Chloroform Committee, see 1902, 1905. *Brit. med. J.* 1906 (14 July), II, 85–7.

Experiments in examination of the locked-jaw induced by tetanus-toxin (with H. E. Roaf [1]). *J. Physiol.* 1906 (Aug.), XXXIV, 315–31; abstract, *Lancet*, 1906 (22 Sept.), II, 810; *Brit. med. J.* 1906, II, 9.

The mechanism of 'locked jaw' produced by tetanus-toxin (with H. E. Roaf [1]). *Brit. med. J.* 1906, II, 1805.

1907

Appreciation of Sir Michael Foster. *Brit. med. J.* 1907, I, 351.

The Association and medical research. (Commenting on Mott's Review of *The Integrative Action of the Nervous System*), *Brit. med. J.* 1907 (16 Mar.), I, 657.

On reciprocal innervation of antagonistic muscles. Tenth note. *Proc. roy. Soc.* 1907 (18 Apr.), LXXIX b, 337–49.

Nerve as a master of muscle. *Not. Proc. roy. Instn*, 1907 (19 Apr.), XVIII, 609–18, and *Sci. Amer. Suppl.* 1908, LXV, 378.

Strychnine and reflex inhibition of skeletal muscle. *J. Physiol.* 1907 (Nov.), XXXVI, 195–204.

Bibliography of Writings

On reciprocal innervation of antagonistic muscles. Eleventh note. Further observations on successive induction. *Proc. roy. Soc.* 1907 (5 Dec.), LXXX b, 53–71; reprinted *Folia neuro-biol.* 1908 (Mar.), I, 365–83.
Spinal reflexes. *Brit. Ass. Rep.* 1907, 667.

1908

A discussion on the scientific education of the medical student. (Meeting of the British Medical Association.) *Brit. med. J.* 1908 (15 Aug.), II, 380; also *Lancet*, 1908 (15 Aug.), II, 480–1.
On reciprocal innervation of antagonistic muscles. Twelfth note. Proprioceptive reflexes. *Proc. roy. Soc.* 1908 (10 Dec.), LXXX b, 552–64; reprinted *Folia neuro-biol.* 1909, II, 578–88. Abstr. *Nature*, 1908, LXXVIII, 592.
On reciprocal innervation of antagonistic muscles. Thirteenth note. On the antagonism between reflex inhibition and reflex excitation. *Proc. roy. Soc.* 1908 (10 Dec.), LXXX b, 565–78; reprinted *Folia neuro-biol.* 1909, II, 589–602.
Committee report on body metabolism in cancer (with S. M. Copeman). *Brit. Ass. Rep.* 1908, 489–92; 1910, 297–300; 1911, 171.
Some comparisons between reflex inhibition and reflex excitation. *Quart. J. exp. Physiol.* 1908, I, 67–78.

1909

On plastic tonus and proprioceptive reflexes. *Quart. J. exp. Physiol.* 1909, II, 109–56.
Reciprocal innervation of antagonistic muscles. Fourteenth note. On double reciprocal innervation. *Proc. roy. Soc.* 1909, LXXXI b, 249–68; reprinted *Folia neuro-biol.* 1910, III, 477–96.
Discussion on the deep afferents; their function and distribution (Meeting of the British Medical Association). *Brit. med. J.* 1909 (11 Sept.), II, 679–90; also *Lancet*, 1909 (11 Sept.), II, 791–2.
A mammalian spinal preparation. *J. Physiol.* 1909, XXXVIII, 375–83.

1910

Obituary. W. Page May. *Brit. med. J.* 1910 (29 Jan.), I, 298.
Flexion-reflex of the limb, crossed extension-reflex, and reflex stepping and standing. *J. Physiol.* 1910 (Apr.), XL, 28–121.
Remarks on the reflex mechanism of the step. *Brain*, 1910 (June), XXXIII, 1–25.
Receptors and afferents of the third, fourth and sixth cranial nerves (with F. M. Tozer [1]). *Proc. roy. Soc.* 1910 (6 June), LXXXII b, 450–7; reprinted *Folia neuro-biol.* 1910, IV, 626–33.
Further remarks on the mammalian spinal preparation (with H. E. Roaf [1]). *Quart. J. exp. Physiol.* 1910 (Mar.), III, 209–11.

Bibliography of Writings

Notes on the scratch reflex of the cat. *Quart. J. exp. Physiol.* 1910 (Mar.), III, 213-20.

Brain, physiology of. In *Encyclopædia Britannica*, London and New York, 11th ed., 1910, IV, 403-13.

Note on certain reflex actions connected with the mouth. *Brit. dent. J.* 1910, XXXI, 785-90.

Committee report on mental and muscular fatigue (with W. MacDougall and others). *Brit. Ass. Rep.* 1910, 292; 1911, 174.

1911

On reflex rebound (with S. C. M. Sowton). *Proc. Physiol. Soc.*, printed but unpublished, 1911, 5 pp.

Reversal of the reflex effect of an afferent nerve by altering the character of the electrical stimulus applied (with S. C. M. Sowton). *Proc. roy. Soc.* 1911 (22 Mar.), LXXXIII b, 435-46; reprinted *Z. allg. Physiol.* 1911, XII, 485-98.

Motor localization in the brain of the gibbon, correlated with a histological examination (with F. W. Mott [1] and E. Schuster [2]). *Proc. roy. Soc.* 1911 (4 May), LXXXIV b, 67-74; reprinted *Folia neuro-biol.* 1911, V, 699-707.

Notes on the pilomotor system (with T. Graham Brown [1]). *Quart. J. exp. Physiol.* 1911 (June), IV, 193-205.

Muscle and nerve. In *Encyclopædia Britannica*, 11th ed. 1911, XIX, 44-50.

Spinal cord, physiology of. In *Encyclopædia Britannica*, 11th ed. 1911, XXV, 672-84.

Sympathetic system. In *Encyclopædia Britannica*, 11th ed. 1911, XXVI, 287-9.

On reflex inhibition of the knee flexor (with S. C. M. Sowton). *Proc. roy. Soc.* 1911 (29 June), LXXXIV b, 201-14.

The rôle of reflex inhibition. *Sci. Prog. Twent. Cent.* 1911 (No. 20), 584-610; trans. in *Scientia, Riv. Scienza*, 1911, IX, 226-46; abstract *Brit. med. J.* 1911 (25 Mar.), I, 690-1, and *Lancet*, 1911 (11 Mar.), I, 666.

Chloroform and reversal of reflex effect (with S. C. M. Sowton). *J. Physiol.* 1911 (July), XLII, 383-8.

Sir Rupert Boyce, 1863-1911. *Proc. roy. Soc.* 1911 (Sept.), LXXXIV b, 1-6.

Observations on the localization in the motor cortex of the baboon (*Papio anubis*) (with T. Graham Brown [1]). *J. Physiol.* 1911, XLIII, 209-18.

Observations on strychnine reversal (with A. G. W. Owen [1]). *J. Physiol.* 1911 (Nov.), XLIII, 232-41.

1912

Note on present problems of nervous function. In *Mélanges biologiques*, 1912, dédié à Charles Richet, pp. 371-9.

On the instability of a cortical point (with T. Graham Brown [1]). *Proc. roy. Soc.* 1912 (Mar.), LXXXV b, 250-77.

Bibliography of Writings

Bewegung und Leben. Address to the students at Utrecht, 1912 (May).
The rule of reflex response in the limb reflexes of the mammal and its exceptions (with T. Graham Brown [1]). *J. Physiol.* 1912 (May), XLIV, 125–30.
Some instances of uncertainty in reflex reactions. Delivered to British Medical Association, 26 July. Abstract, *Lancet*, 1912 (24 Aug.), II, 537.
Report of Departmental Committee on Sight Tests, Board of Trade, 1912 (10 May).

1913

Six chapters on physiology 'briefly explaining the principles which underlie the precepts and practice described in the other chapters of the book' (pp. 224–307). *A Manual of School Hygiene*, by E. W. Hope, E. A. Brown and C. S. S. (new edition, Cambridge University Press, 1913, xii + 311 pp.).
Reciprocal innervation and symmetrical muscles. *Proc. roy. Soc.* 1913 (13 Jan.), LXXXVI b, 219–32.
Nervous rhythm arising from rivalry of antagonistic reflexes: reflex stepping as outcome of double reciprocal innervation. *Proc. roy. Soc.* 1913 (20 Feb.), LXXXVI b, 233–61.
Note on the functions of the cortex cerebri (with T. Graham Brown [1]). *Proc. Physiol. Soc., J. Physiol.*, 1913, XLVI, xxii.
Reflex inhibition as a factor in the co-ordination of movements and postures. *Quart. J. exp. Physiol.* 1913 (June), VI, 251–310.
The sight tests of the Board of Trade (Polemic with F. W. Edridge-Green). *Lancet*, 1913 (14 June), I, 1691; (Edridge-Green's letters, *ibid.*, 1557, 1752–4, 1764).
Reciprocal innervation. Seventeenth Int. Congr. Med. *Brit. med. J.* 1913 (23 Aug.), II, 458–9.
An address on the provincial school of medicine and the provincial university. Delivered at the Prize distribution in the School of Medicine, University of Leeds. *Brit. med. J.* 1913 (4 Oct.), II, 844–6.
Rhythmic reflex produced by antagonizing reflex excitation by reflex inhibition. Ninth International Congress of Physiology. *Arch. int. Physiol.* 1913, XIV, 74.
Further observations on the production of reflex stepping by combination of reflex excitation with reflex inhibition. *J. Physiol.* 1913 (Nov.), XLVII, 196–214.
Reversal in cortical reactions (with T. Graham Brown [1]). *Arch. int. Physiol.* 1913, XIV, 72–3.

1914

Report on reciprocal innervation. *Trans. Int. Congr. Med.* 1913 (Sect. II, Physiol.), 1914, 85–93.
Acoustic reflexes in the decerebrate cat (with A. Forbes [1]). *Amer. J. Physiol.* 1914 (Nov.), XXXV, 367–76.

Bibliography of Writings

1915

Observations on reflex responses to single break-shocks (with S. C. M. Sowton). *J. Physiol.* 1915 (July), XLIX, 331-48.
Some observations on the bucco-pharyngeal stage of reflex deglutition in the cat (with F. R. Miller [1]). *Quart. J. exp. Physiol.* 1915 (Oct.), IX, 147-86.
Postural activity of muscle and nerve. *Brain*, 1915, XXXVIII, 191-234.
Simple apparatus for obtaining a decerebrate preparation of the cat. *Proc. Physiol. Soc., J. Physiol.*, 1915 (3 July), XLIX, lii-liv.
Committee report on the structure and function of the mammalian heart (with S. Kent). *Brit. Ass. Rep.* 1915, 226-9; 1916, 304; 1917, 122.

1916

A simple apparatus for illustrating the Listing-Donders law. *Proc. Physiol. Soc., J. Physiol.*, 1916 (15 July), L, xlvi-xlix.

1917

Observations on the excitable cortex of the chimpanzee, orang-utan and gorilla (with A. S. F. Leyton [1]). *Quart. J. exp. Physiol.* 1917, XI, 135-222.
Reflexes elicitable in the cat from pinna vibrissæ and jaws. *J. Physiol.* 1917 (Dec.), LI, 404-31.
Observations with antitetanus serum in the monkey. *Lancet*, 1917 (29 Dec.), II, 964-6.
Recent physiology and the war. *Not. Proc. roy. Instn*, 1917, XXII, 1-3, and *Science*, 1917, XLVI, 502-4.

1918

Stimulation of the motor cortex in a monkey subject to epileptiform seizures. *Brain*, 1918 (Mar.), XLI, 48-9.
Brevity, frequency of rhythm and amount of reflex nervous discharge, as indicated by reflex contraction (with N. B. Dreyer [1]). *Proc. roy. Soc.* 1918 (Oct.), XCb, 270-82.
Observations on the sensual rôle of the proprioceptive nerve-supply of the extrinsic ocular muscles. *Brain*, 1918 (Dec.), XLI, 332-43.

1919

Mammalian Physiology. A Course of Practical Exercises. Oxford, Clarendon Press, 1919, xii + 156 pp.
Note on the history of the word 'tonus' as a physiological term. Contribution to *Medical and Biological Research Dedicated to Sir William Osler*, New York, 1919, I, 261-8.

Bibliography of Writings

1920

Sir William Osler. Obituary. *Brit. med. J.* 1920 (10 Jan.), 1, 65.

Postural activity of muscle. Cavendish Lecture, West London Medico-chirurgical Society. *Brit. med. J.* 1920 (21 Aug.), II, 288. (Apparently never printed *in extenso*.)

Gateways of sense. Huxley Lecture, Birmingham University, 26 November 1919. *Brit. med. J.* 1920 (4 Dec.), II, 875. (Apparently never printed *in extenso*.)

1921

On the myogram of the flexor-reflex evoked by a single break-shock (with K. Sassa [1]). *Proc. roy. Soc.* 1921 (May), xcii*b*, 108–17.

Break-shock reflexes and 'supramaximal' contraction-response of mammalian nerve-muscle to single shock stimuli. *Proc. roy. Soc.* 1921 (May), xcii*b*, 245–58.

Albert Sidney Leyton. Obituary. *Brit. med. J.* 1921 (8 Oct.), II, 579.

Anniversary address delivered before the Royal Society of London, 30 November 1921. *Proc. roy. Soc.* 1922 (Jan.), c*a*, 353–66; *ibid.* xciii*b*, 1–14, extract bearing title: The maintenance of scientific research. *Nature*, 1921 (8 Dec.), cviii, 470–1.

Sur la production d'influx nerveux dans l'arc nerveux réflexe. *Arch. int. Physiol.* 1921 (Dec.), xviii, 620–7. (Volume dedicated to Léon Fredericq.)

1922

Note on the after-discharge of reflex centres. In *Libro en honor de Santiago Ramon y Cajal*, Madrid, 1922, pp. 97–101.

Some points regarding present-day views of reflex action. Address to Royal Society, Edinburgh, 20 March 1922. Abstract, *Nature*, 1922 (8 Apr.), cix, 463.

Some aspects of animal mechanism. Presidential Address, British Association for the Advancement of Science, Hull. *Brit. Ass. Rep.* 1922 (Sept.), 1–15; *Brit. med. J.* 1922 (9 Sept.), II, 485–6. Also *Nature*, 1922, cx, 346–52; *Vet. Rec.* 1922, II, 762–6; *J. Ment. Hygiene*, 1923, xvii, 1–19.

Inaugural address delivered at the opening of the Biological Building, McGill University, Montreal, 5 October 1922. Printed privately, Murray Printing Co., Ltd., Toronto, 1922, 8 pp.

Anniversary address delivered before the Royal Society of London, 30 November 1922. *Proc. roy. Soc.* 1923, cii*a*, 373–88, and xciv*b*, i–xvi. Extract under title: The use of a pancreatic extract in diabetes. *Nature*, 1922 (9 Dec.), cx, 774; also *Brit. med. J.* 1922 (9 Dec.), II, 1139–40.

1923

The position of psychology. Address to National Institute of Industrial Psychology, 20 March 1923. Abstract, *Nature*, 1923 (31 March), cxi, 439. (Apparently never printed *in extenso*.)

Bibliography of Writings

Stimulus rhythm in reflex contraction (with E. G. T. Liddell [1]). *Proc. roy. Soc.* 1923 (May), xcv*b*, 142–56. Appendix on separation key by C.S.S.

A comparison between certain features of the spinal flexor reflex and of the decerebrate extensor reflex respectively (with E. G. T. Liddell [1]). *Proc. roy. Soc.* 1923 (July), xcv*b*, 299–339.

Recruitment type of reflexes (with E. G. T. Liddell [1]). *Proc. roy. Soc.* 1923 (Oct.), xcv*b*, 407–12.

Anniversary address delivered before the Royal Society of London, 30 November 1923. *Proc. roy. Soc.* 1924 (Jan.), cv*a*, 1–16; *ibid.* xcv*b*, 485–99; *Nature*, 1923 (8 Dec.), cxii, 845–8; *Brit. med. J.* 1923 (8 Dec.), ii, 1113–14.

1924

Reflexes in response to stretch (myotatic reflexes) (with E. G. T. Liddell [1]). *Proc. roy. Soc.* 1924 (Mar.), xcvi*b*, 212–42.

Problems of muscular receptivity. *Nature*, 1924 (21 and 28 June), cxiii, 732, 892–4, 929–32.

Notes on temperature after spinal transection, with some observations on shivering. *J. Physiol.* 1924 (May), lviii, 405–24.

Anniversary address delivered before the Royal Society of London, 1 December 1924. *Proc. roy. Soc.* 1925 (Jan.), cvii*a*, 1–14; *ibid.* xcvii*b*, 254–67; *Nature*, 1924 (6 Dec.), cxiii, 840–1.

1925

Recruitment and some other features of reflex inhibition (with E. G. T. Liddell [1]). *Proc. roy. Soc.* 1925 (Feb.), xcvii*b*, 488–518.

Remarks on some aspects of reflex inhibition. *Proc. roy. Soc.* 1925 (Feb.), xcvii*b*, 519–45.

The late Sir Clifford Allbutt. Obituary. *Brit. med. J.* 1925 (7 Mar.), i, 495.

Further observations on myotatic reflexes (with E. G. T. Liddell [1]). *Proc. roy. Soc.* 1925 (Oct.), xcvii*b*, 267–83.

An address on avenues in medicine. Delivered at the opening of the winter session of the London (Royal Free Hospital) School of Medicine. *Mag. Lond. (Roy. Free Hosp.) School Med. for Women*, 1925, xx, 133–41; *Lancet*, 1925 (10 Oct.), ii, 741–3. Abstract under title: Medicine as a career for women. *Brit. med. J.* 1925 (19 Oct.), ii, 667–8.

Address at the unveiling of the Wheatstone Memorial at Gloucester, 19 October 1925. *Nature*, 1925 (31 Oct.), cxvi, 659.

J. N. Langley. Obituary. *Brit. med. J.* 1925 (14 Nov.), ii, 925.

Anniversary address delivered before the Royal Society of London, 30 November 1925. *Proc. roy. Soc.* 1926, cx*a*, 1–15; *ibid.* 1926, xcix*b*, 107–21; *Nature*, 1925 (5 Dec.), cxvi, 833–5.

The Assaying of Brabantius and Other Verse. Oxford University Press, 67 pp.

Bibliography of Writings

1926

Addition latente and recruitment in reflex contraction and inhibition. *Livre à Charles Richet*. Paris, 1926, 3 pp.

Observations on concurrent contraction of flexor muscles in the flexion reflex (with R. S. Creed [1]). *Proc. roy. Soc.* 1926 (June), c*b*, 258–67. Appendix on double mirror myograph by C.S.S.

Reflex fractionation of a muscle (with S. Cooper [1] and D. E. Denny-Brown [2]). *Proc. roy. Soc.* 1926 (Nov.), c*b*, 448–62.

1927

Interaction between ipsilateral spinal reflexes acting on the flexor muscles of the hind-limb (with S. Cooper [1] and D. E. Denny-Brown [2]). *Proc. roy. Soc.* 1927 (Feb.), cI*b*, 262–303.

Whither?—A footnote. *Nature*, 1927 (5 Feb.), CXIX, 205.

Lister and physiology. *Nature*, 1927 (23 Apr.), CXIX, 606–8; *Brit. med. J.* 1927 (9 Apr.), I, 653–4; *Lancet*, 1927 (9 Apr.), I, 743–4.

Ernest Henry Starling. Obituary. *Brit. med. J.* 1927 (14 May), II, 905.

Second Listerian Oration. *Canad. med. Ass. J.* 1927 (18 June), 17, II, 1255–63.

Dunham Lectures, 1927 (Harvard Medical School); 10 October, Observations on stretch reflexes; 13 October, Modes of interaction between reflexes; 17 October, Some factors of co-ordination in muscular acts. Abstract: *Bost. med. surg. J.* 1927, CXCVII, 812 (not published *in extenso*).

Keith Lucas (1879–1916). *Dictionary of National Biography*, 1912–21. [Supplement III], Oxford University Press, 1927.

Committee report on colour vision, with particular reference to classification of colour blindness (with H. E. Roaf and others). *Brit. Ass. Rep.* 1927, 307–8.

1928

Foreword [p. v] to L. J. J. Muskens, *Epilepsy, Comparative Pathogenesis, Symptoms, Treatment*. London, Baillière, Tindall and Cox, 1928, xiv + 435 pp.

Sir Dawson Williams. Obituary. *Brit. med. J.* 1928 (10 Mar.), I, 418.

Eulogy of Harvey. The Harvey Tercentenary Celebrations, Royal College of Physicians, 14 May 1928. *Brit. med. J.* 1928 (19 May), I, 866–8; *Lancet*, 1928 (19 May), I, 1034–5.

Some physiological data toward functional analysis of a simple reflex centre. *Arch. Sci. biol.* 1928 (June), XII, 1–7. Bottazzi Birthday Volume.

Introduction [pp. xi–xiii] to F. Mason, *Creation by Evolution. A Consensus of Present-day Knowledge as set forth by Leading Authorities in Non-technical Language that all may understand*. New York, Macmillan, 1928, xxii + 392 pp.

A mammalian myograph. *Proc. Physiol. Soc., J. Physiol.*, 1928, LXVI, iii–v.

The instability of a single vortex-row. *Nature*, 1928 (1 Sept.), CXXII, 314.

Bibliography of Writings

Subliminal fringe in spinal flexion (with D. E. Denny-Brown [1]). *J. Physiol.* 1928, LXVI, 175-80.
Sir David Ferrier. *Proc. roy. Soc.* 1928 (Nov.), CIII b, viii-xvi.

1929

Life in upper Canada in 1827. By B. Aldren. Remarks on foregoing letter by C. S. S., *Canad. med. Ass. J.* 1929 (Jan.), XX, 65-7.
Some functional problems attaching to convergence. Ferrier Lecture. *Proc. roy. Soc.* 1929 (Sept.), CV b, 332-62; and *Brit. med. J.* 1929, I, 1136-7.
Mammalian Physiology. A Course of Practical Exercises (with E. G. T. Liddell [1]). 2nd ed. Oxford, Clarendon Press, 1929, xii + 162 pp.
Improved bearing for the torsion myograph (with J. C. Eccles [1]). *Proc. Physiol. Soc., J. Physiol.*, 1929 (Dec.), LXIX, i.
Brain, physiology of. *Encyclopædia Britannica*, London and New York, 1929, 14th ed., IV, 1-9. Rewritten; see also 1910.
The spinal cord—physiology. *Encyclopædia Britannica*, London and New York, 1929, 14th ed., XXI, 220-8. Rewritten; see also 1911.
The sympathetic system. *Encyclopædia Britannica*, London and New York, 1929, 14th ed., XXI, 702-4. Rewritten; see also 1911.

1930

Reflex summation in the ipsilateral spinal flexion reflex (with J. C. Eccles [1]). *J. Physiol.* 1920 (Mar.), LXIX, 1-28.
Numbers and contraction-values of individual motor-units examined in some muscles of the limb (with J. C. Eccles [1]). *Proc. roy. Soc.* 1930 (June), CVI b, 326-57.
Flexor reflex responses to successive afferent volleys (with J. C. Eccles [1]). *Proc. Physiol Soc., J. Physiol.*, 1930 (July), LXX, xxv-xxvii.
Notes on the knee extensory and the mirror myograph. *J. Physiol.* 1930 (Aug.), LXX, 101-7.
Nervous integrations in man. In Cowdry, *Human Biology and Racial Welfare* (with J. F. Fulton [1]), New York: Paul B. Hoeber, 1930 (pp. 246-65).

1931

Studies on the flexor reflex:
  I. Latent period (with J. C. Eccles [1]). *Proc. roy. Soc.* 1931 (Mar.), CVII b, 511-34.
  II. The reflex response evoked by two centripetal volleys (with J. C. Eccles [1]). *Ibid.* 535-56.
  III. The central effects produced by an antidromic volley (by J. C. Eccles alone). *Ibid.* 557-85.
  IV. After-discharge (with J. C. Eccles [1]). *Ibid.* 586-96.

Bibliography of Writings

V. General conclusions (with J. C. Eccles [1]). *Proc. roy. Soc.* 1931 (Mar.), cviib, 597–605.
VI. Inhibition (with J. C. Eccles [1]). *Ibid.* 1931, cixb, 91–113.
Quantitative management of contraction in lowest level co-ordination. Hughlings Jackson Lecture. *Brain*, 1931 (Apr.), liv, 1–28. Also abstr. *Brit. med. J.* 1931, I, 207–11.

1932

State of the flexor reflex in paraplegic dog and monkey respectively (with J. F. Fulton [1]). *J. Physiol.* 1932 (May), lxxv, 17–22.
Concluding remarks to discussion on tonus of skeletal muscle. Internat. Neurol. Congress, Berne, 1931. *Arch. Neurol. Psychiat., Chicago,* 1932 (Sept.), xxviii, 676–8.
Chromatolysis of motor-horn cells. *Proc. Physiol. Soc., J. Physiol.* 1932 (May), xii, 11–12P.
Reflex Activity of the Spinal Cord (with R. S. Creed, D. Denny-Brown, J. C. Eccles, E. G. T. Liddell [1]). Oxford, Clarendon Press, 1932, viii + 184 pp.
Degeneration of peripheral nerves after spinal transection in the monkey (with S. Cooper [1]). *Proc. Physiol. Soc., J. Physiol.,* 1932 (Nov.), lxxvii, 18P.
Inhibition as a co-ordinative factor. Nobel Lecture delivered at Stockholm, 12 December 1932. Stockholm, P. A. Norstedt, 1933, 12 pp.

1933

The Brain and its Mechanism. The Rede Lecture delivered before the University of Cambridge, 5 December 1933. Cambridge University Press, 1933, 36 pp. 2nd issue, November 1937.

1934

Reflex inhibition as a factor in co-ordination of muscular acts. *Rev. Soc. argent. Biol.* 1934 (Nov.), x, 510–13.
Review of Hallowes, K. D. *The Poetry of Geology.* In *Sci. Progr.* 1934 (July), xxix, 165.
Periodicals and reference. [Review of *World List.*] *Nature,* 1934 (22 Sept.), cxxxiv, 435–7.
Language distribution of scientific periodicals. [Analysis of *World List.*] *Nature,* 1934 (9 Oct.), cxxxiv, 871–2.

1935

Sir Edward Sharpey-Schafer and his contributions to neurology (Sharpey-Schafer Memorial Lecture). *Edinb. med. J.* 1935 (Aug.), xlii, 393–406.
Functional problems of convergence of nerves. *Orv. Hetil.* 1935 (Sept.), lxxix, 1050–1.
Santiago Ramón y Cajal, For. Mem. R.S. Obituary. *Obit. Notes Roy. Soc.* 1935 (Dec.), No. 4, 425–41.

Bibliography of Writings

1936

The chastening. *Cornhill Magazine*, 1936 (Aug.), CLIV, 140.

1937

The wise Ulysses. *Cornhill Magazine*, 1937 (Jan.), CLV, 38.
Community. *Cornhill Magazine*, 1937 (May), CLV, 701.
Sir Squire Sprigge. *Lancet*, 1937 (26 June), I, 1554.
Review of Horton and Aldredge, *Johannes de Mirfeld of St Bartholomew's Smithfield: His Life and Works*. In *Medium Ævum*, 1936, III, 236–40.
Scientific endeavour and inferiority complex. Review of Ramón y Cajal, *Recollections of My Life*. In *Nature*, 1937 (9 Oct.), CXL, 617–19.
Preface to *Le tonus des muscles striés* by G. Marinesco, N. Jonesco-Sisesti, O. Sager and A. Kreindler. Académie Roumaine, *Études et Recherches*, Bucharest, 1937 [pp. vii–viii].
Langley, John Newport. In *Dictionary of National Biography*, 1922–30 [Supplement IV], Oxford University Press, 1937, 479–81.
Ferrier, Sir David. In *Dictionary of National Biography*, 1922–30 [Supplement IV], Oxford University Press, 1937, 302–4.
Paget, Stephen. In *Dictionary of National Biography*, 1922–30 [Supplement IV], Oxford University Press, 1937, 649–51.

1938

The Society's Library. *Notes Rec.* [Roy. Soc., Lond.], 1938, I, 21–7.

1940

Gower's tract and spinal border-cells (with Sybil Cooper). *Brain*, 1940, LXIII, 123–34.
The Assaying of Brabantius, and Other Verse. Sm. 8vo. 2nd ed., enlarged, 1940, Oxford University Press.
Man on his Nature. The Gifford Lectures, Edinburgh, 1937–8. 8vo. illustrated. Cambridge University Press, 1940, v+413 pp. Reprinted 1942, 1946; in U.S.A. 1942.

1942

Goethe on Nature and on Science. 8vo. The Deneke Lecture, 1942; Lady Margaret Hall, Oxford. Cambridge University Press. 41 pp.

1946

The Endeavour of Jean Fernel. 8vo. illustrated. Cambridge University Press, 1946, x+223 pp.

Bibliography of Writings

1947

Spanish translation of *The Endeavour of Jean Fernel*, 1947. (In the Press.)
'*Marginalia.*' Contribution to volume in honour of Charles Singer. Edited by Dr Ashworth Underwood.
The re-Christening of Physiology. Article contributed to volume in honour of Prof. Van Rynberk. Amsterdam, 1947.
The Integrative Action of the Nervous System. A new edition, with an Introduction. Edited by Samson Wright. Cambridge University Press, 1947.

INDEX

[*Figures in heavy type refer to numbered items in the Bibliography.*]

Actinian, 131, 313
Action-current of nerve, 70
Adaptation, 324
    the cerebrum and, 386
Adapted reactions, reflexes as, 236–69, 351
Adequate stimulus, 11, 91, 245, 344
Affective tone, 231, 256, 265, 266, 319, 326, 330–3
Afferent arc, 7, 53, 109
After-discharge, 13, 27–35, 50, 75, 101, 105, 289, 384
    analogous to positive after-image, 33
    clonic, in flexion-reflex, 29; in scratch-reflex, 30
    cut short by inhibition, 33, 105
    duration of stimulus and, 29
    in crossed extensor-reflex, 31
    intensity of stimulus and, 27
    prolonged in cooled frog, 31
After-image, 33, 384
Aiptasis saxicola, 131, 313
Albertoni, 272 **112a**
Allbutt, Clifford, 73 **180**
Allied reflexes, 120, 121–36, 145, 170, 290, 347, 354
All-or-nothing principle, 70, 73
Alternating reflexes, 146, 201–3
Ameiurus, 131, 313
Anaesthetics, 14, 80, 82
Anderson, H. K., Langley, J. N., &c., 38 **150**
Anelective receptors, 228, 316, 318
Anger, 260, 262
Anodon, 85
Antagonistic muscles, 84, 201–3, 280–6
    reflexes, 137–45, 186–91, 204, 230, 289, 322, 354
Anthropoid apes, motor cortex of, 273–9, 288, 290
Anthropomorphic interpretation, 237
Anticipatory reactions, 326–33
Aorta, 100
Apathy, 17, 233
Arachne, 240

Arthropoda, 41, 85, 240, 315
Ascidia, 334, 337
Asphyxia, 80
Associative recall, 331, 351
Astacus, 85, 107, 239, 251, 295, 329
Asterias, 240
Atrophy of muscles, 248
Atropin, 305
Attention, 234
Attitude, 301–4, 336–43, 350; *and see* Postural reflexes
Aubert, 371, 372, 373, 375 381 **37, 65a**
Auerbach's plexus, 64
Aurelia aurita, 170
Autonomic system (Langley), 318
Axis-cylinder, fluidity of, 16
Axones, 41
Ayer, J. B., **255**

Babäk, E., **242**
Babuchin, 38 **73**
v. Baeyer, 14, 80 **239**
Baglioni, S., 67, 69, 71, 80, 109, 118, 135, 206 **212, 245, 248, 285, 288 293**
'Bahnung', 13, 178, 185, 207
Ballance, C., 272
Barblets, 321
Barker, L. F., **199**
Barometric pressure and sensation, 338
Bastian, C., 248, 271 **46, 129**
Bayliss, W. M., 114 **144**
    & Starling, E. H., 3, 237, 312, **188**
Beagle, 330
Beaunis, H., **106, 120**
Bee, 251
Beer, Th., **188a**
Beevor, C., 272, 284 **134, 302**
    & Horsley, V., 272, 273, 277, 279, 290 **127**
Behaviour of animals, 238
Bell, C., 38, 271, 287 **10, 13**
Bell-Magendie law, 38, 80
Belmondo, 144 **122**
Bergmann, 80

421

Index

Bernard, C., 109
Bert, P. & Marcacci, 96
Bethe, A., 14, 17, 39, 41, 42, 64, 81, 119 **178, 178a,** 185, **188a,** 263, **294a**
Bezold, A., **42**
Bichat, 257 **9**
Bickel, A., **158,** 176, 203, 249
Biedermann, W., 9, 31, 70, 80, 85, 107, 183 **109,** 204, 273, 303
Bile-duct, 11
Binocular brightness compared with uniocular, 369, 373
Binocular contrast compared with uniocular, 375
Binocular flicker, 357–81; symmetrical, 361; asymmetrical, 366
Binocular fusion, 356–84
Biogen-hypothese, 197
du Bois-Reymond, R., 16, 38 **236**
Bonnier, P., 340, 341 **214, 266, 274**
Bottazzi, F., **308**
Bowditch, H. P., **117**
& Warren, J. W., 178 **123**
Bowlby, A., 248 **131a**
Brachioplegia, 278
Brachiopod, 334
Brain, dominance of the, 308–52
integration by the, 351
organ for adaptation of reactions, 385
relation to 'distance-receptors', 348
Breuer, J., 100 **44**
Broca, 271 **29**
Broca's centre, 290
Brodmann, 280 **256a**
Brondgeest, 304
Bruns, L., 248 **140**
Brunton, Lauder T., 195 **107a**
Bubnoff, N. & Heidenhain, R., 178, 280, 282 **92**
Burch, G., Gotch, F., &, 67 **164**

Cajal, Ramon y, 14, 23, 86, 143, 147, 233, 280, 376, 381, 383 **128a**
Campbell, A. W., 279, 280 **272a**
Carcinus, 14, 81, 240
Carlson, 291
Carmarina, 119, 120
Cayrade, 36
Central sulcus, genua of, 277

Centrality, significance of, in the nervous system, 115, 312
Centres, rank of, 313
Cercopithecus callithrix, 296
Cerebellum, ganglion of proprio-ceptive system, 346
Cerebral cortex, 178, 270–307, 351, 355, 380–7
employs reciprocal innervation, 280–99
extirpation, 278
genesis of, 348
inhibitory influence of, 280
interrelation of the two hemispheres, 289, 382
modifying reflexes, 305
motor reactions of, compared with spinal, 290, 305
reinforcing influence of, 178
'silent' fields of, 279
unequal motor representation in, 291
Cerebral sulci, variability of, not functional boundaries, 276
Chauveau, A., 183 **218**
Chelae, 329
Chemo-receptors, 313, 317, 318, 325, 326
Chick, 331
Child, 255, 258, 332
Chimpanzee, motor cortex of, 273
Chloroform, 80, 82, 114, 255, 280
Chorda tympani, 85
Chordata, 319
Chromatolysis, 248
Cleghorn, A., **224**
Clonic action, 65
from cortex, 289
in flexion-reflex, 26–31, 289
in scratch-reflex, 31, 201, 289
Clover-fly, 251
Coelenterate, 119
Cohnheim, O., 42
Combination of reflexes, 134, 135
simultaneous, 150–80
successive, 182–235
Cometula, 240
Common path, 53, 224, 310, 312, 320, 346, 350
principle of final, 117–51, 233, 354, **383**
Common paths, profusion of, 147

Index

Comparative psychology, 307
Compensatory reflexes, 146, 201, 204–6, 214, 337, 340
'Complication', 8, 346, 352
reflex, 131, 313
Conation, 330–3
Conative feeling, 330–3
Condensation of receptor distribution, 346
Conduction, 5, 8
in nerve-cell, 2, 15
in nerve-trunks, 13–18, 80–3
in reflex-arc, 13–18, 33, 80–3
intracellular and intercellular, 5, 15, 16, 17
reversible and irreversible, 13, 16, 38–42
speed of, 18–25
synaptic, 16, 17, 18, 81
Conductor, 6, 309
Conjunctival reflex, 239
Consummatory reactions, 329–33
Contracture, hemiplegic, 250, 303, 304
Contrast, visual, 208, 384
Co-ordination, contribution to, by receptor, 13
Co-ordination in the compound reflex, 116–235
in the reflex sequence, 182–235
in the simple reflex, 8, 36–115
in the simultaneous compound reflex (reflex 'pattern'), 152–81
Corneal reflex, 239
Cortex, cerebral, *see* Cerebral cortex
Crayfish, 85, 107, 239, 251, 295, 329
Croak-reflex, 9
Crossed extension-reflex of leg, 31, 73, 76, 79, 84, 98, 100–5, 108, 123, 129, 137, 142, 146, 150, 164, 167, 191, 206–10, 223, 225, 249
Crossed stepping-reflex, 189, 190, 225
Curare, 114
Cushing, H., 277 **269a**
Cushny, A., 112
Cybulski & Zanietowski, 70 **145**
'Cyclopean' eye, 382
v. Cyon, 100, 114, 195 **39, 41, 56**

Darkness in visual field, 365

Darwin, C., 10, 236, 258, **261**, 305 **50, 62**
Darwin and reflex purpose, 1, 10, 236, 305
Decerebrate rigidity, 89, 252, 299–305, 337
Defecation, 305
Degeneration, Wallerian, 17
method of successive, 51–5
Deglutition, 69, 100, 183, 322, 326, 329, 332
Deiter's nucleus, 342
Déjerine, 279
Delay, reflex, 18–25
Demoor, J., 23 **191**
Dendrites, 41
Depressor nerve, 100, 114
Descartes, R., 257, 286, 288 **1, 2, 4**
Diaphragm, 67, 68, 206
Diaschizis, 245
Differentiation and integration correlated, 343
Diffuse nervous system, 39–42, 311–14
Disgust, 261–3
Distance-receptors, 306, 324–9, 332–5
the cerebrum the ganglion of, 348–52
Disynaptic arc, 53
Donaldson, H., 116, 148 **209**
Double-joint muscles, 109, 112, 284
Double-sign reflexes, 83, 137, 200
Drosera, 251
Duchenne, G. B. A., 162 **49**
Duval, 23

Earthworm, 183
Echinus, 113, 313
Eckhard, C., 9
Edinger, L., **299a**
Edkins, J. S., 3 **311**
Effective threshold, 309
Effector, 6, 309
Ehrlich, P., 143, 233, 237
'Eigenschwarz', 366
Elasmobranch, 349
Emotions, bodily resonance of, 256–69
disgust, 262
exteriorization of, 252–6, 257–8; Darwin's description, 257, 261; Spencer's description, 258; in Goltz's decorticate dog, 263, 266, 267

423

Index

Emotions, James-Lange theory of, 259
  Lloyd Morgan's views, 265, 268
  psycho-physical relationship, 259; experimentally tested, 260
  visceral changes not necessary, but secondary to emotion, 265
End-effect, 5
  rhythm of, 13, 42–66
  intensity of, 13, 70–80
End-plate, 55
Erb, W., **63, 64**
Ewald, J. R., 206, 248, 303 **137, 166a**
Excitability, selective, 12
Exner, S., 14, 21, 87, 126, 135, 178, 182, 280, 299 **59, 71, 99, 110, 149**
Extensor-thrust, 67–9, 75, 88, 90, 91, 93, 109, 150, 176, 239, 249
Extero-ceptive field, 131–4, 316–22, 324, 340, 345
Extero-reflexes, 129–36, 316–23
Eyeball movements, 274–5, 277, 280–1, 285–6, 289, 337, 382
Eyelid-reflex, 45
Eyjkman, Zwaardemaker &, **235**

Fano, G., **156, 256**
Fatigue, 13, 215–24
  in sense organs, 224
  reflex, analysis of, 217; changes in, 215; earlier in scratch than flexion reflex, 215; fresh reflex overcomes fatigued reflex, 223; form of negative induction 223; inhibition compared with, 222
Fechner, 371, 373 **26**
Fechner's paradox, 373
Ferrier, D., 271, 272, 281, 295 **51, 70, 97, 144a**
Fick, A., 70
Figure, reflex, 166–70
Final common path, *see* Common path relatively indefatigable, 224
Flechsig, P., 278, 279, 280 **70a, 271a**
Flexion-reflex, 18, 19–25, 71, 72, 79, 83, 86, 88–100, 103, 108–11, 125, 133, 134, 137, 140–3, 146, 150, 152–4, 158–63, 166–70, 181, 188–90, 205, 206, 208, 214, 215–16, 225, 234, 240, 244, 249, 288, 354

Flicker-sensation, alternate, 362–6, 370, 377
  asymmetrical, 366–70
  binocular, 356–83
  symmetrical, 362–6
  synchronous, 361–6
  uniocular, 363–7
Flourens, 271 **19**
Fly, 239, 251
Focus of effect of a reflex, 152, 240
Foster, M., **170**
Franck, Fr., 19, 87 **111**
Franz, 307
Fredericq, L., 240
Freusberg, A., **54, 59a, 60, 61**
v. Frey, 12, 227 **148, 172**
Fritsch & Hitzig, E., 271, 273 **47**
Frog, 9, 130, 182, 239, 252, 322, 327, 339, 341, 342, 349, 351
Fröhlich, A., 101, 255 **222, 247, 260, 281, 286**

Gad, J., 38 **95, 102, 108, 115**
  & Joseph, M., 14 **121**
Gall-bladder, 10–11
Ganglia, antennary of *Carcinus*, 14
  spinal, 14, 320
  sympathetic, 15, 320
Gaskell, W. H., 196, 197, 207, 325 **99a, 103**
van Gehuchten, 14, 86, 143
Gergens, 9 **68**
Gerlach, 156
Geryonid, 119
Goldscheider, A., 16, 157 **187**
Golgi, C., 143, 156, 233
Goltz, F., 3, 9, 149, 225, 241, 242, 256, 263, 265, 266, 267 **40, 45, 54, 58, 87, 135, 166a**
Gorilla, motor cortex of, 273–80
Gotch, F., 77, 87 **132, 161, 167, 244**
  & Burch, G., 67 **164**
Grainger, 239 **16**
Grasshopper, 239, 252
Gravity, as a stimulus, 316, 336
Grey-matter, delay of conduction in, 18–25
Griffiths, F., **298**
Grosser, O., **282**
Grünbaum, A. F., 273, 290 **225, 229**

Index

Grützner, P., 92 77
Gustatory organs, 326

Hairs, 46, 164, 341
Hall, Marshall, 9, 241 23
v. Haller, A., 10 6
Harless, 25
Harris, 371 8
Harris, W., 283
Hartmann, 381
Hartwell, E. M., Newell Martin &, 173 79
Harvey, W., 233
Haycraft, J. B., 126
Head, H., 118, 143
  diaphragmatic slip, 67, 68
Head, physiological conception of the, 335–7
Heidenhain, R., 304 94
  Bubnoff, N., &, 178, 280, 282 92
v. Helmholtz, H., 18 166
Hemiplegic contracture, see Contracture
Herbart, 313, 352 12b
Hering, E., 100, 208, 366, 373, 380, 382 34, 43, 48a, 113
Hering, H. E., 109, 252, 281, 284 154, 159, 162, 168, 169, 173, 174, 179, 190a, 195, 202, 233
Herrick, C. J., 131, 313
'Higher' and 'lower' in regard to organisms, 236
Hitzig, E., 273 53, 267a
  Fritsch &, 271, 272 47
Hofbauer, L., 175
Homarus, 329
Horsley, V., 132
  Beevor, C., &, 273, 277, 279, 290 127
Huber, C., 201
Hughlings Jackson, *see* Jackson, Hughlings
Hunt, Reid, 200
Hunter, J., 147, 312
Hyde, Ida, 278, 292
Hydra, 310

Immediate (or direct) spinal induction, 78, 120–35, 185, 207, 384
Incremental reflex, 22–5
Indifference between reflexes, 148–9
Induction, spinal, immediate (or direct), 78, 120–35, 185, 384
  successive (or indirect), 207–14, 384

Ingbert, 333 264, 265
Inhibition, 13, 65, 83–106, 133–51, 159, 192, 241, 327
  action of strychnine and tetanus toxin on, 107–13, 292–9
  central, 101
  compared with fatigue, 222
  from cortex, 280–99
  J. S. Macdonald on, 197–200
  nature of, 192–200
  'neutral' in character, 195
  not 'neutral' in character, 196
  of knee-jerk, 88–90
  peripheral, 84, 85
  rebound after, 207
  reciprocal, 83–107, see Reciprocal inhibition
  vagus on heart, 196, 197
Initial reflex, 24
Injury-current of nerve, 16
Innuus rhesus, 273
Insecta, 334
Integration, by nervous agency, 2, 308–53
Intensity of reflex, 26, 70–9, 93, 152–6, 232
  crossed and direct reflexes compared, 225
  grading of, 70; abolished by strychnine, 71; in crossed extensor-reflex, 73, 79; in extensor thrust, 75; in flexion-reflex, 71; in reflex sequence, 224–7; in scratch-reflex, 71
Intensity of stimulus, 13, 26, 27, 51, 150, 155
  effect on refractory phase, 49
  effect on fatigue, 220
  effect on prepotence of reflex, 224–7
Interaction of reflexes, 116–51
  partial, 145
Intercellular conduction, *see* Conduction, intercellular
Intercostal movement, 173
Interference between reflexes, 137–43, 145, 149–51, 190–4, 200, 310, 386
  reversible, 142
Internal capsule, stimulation of, 281, 284
Internuncial paths, 118, 147, 328, 342, 348
Intero-ceptive field, 317, 320, 321, 344
Intestinal peristalsis, 312

Index.

Intracellular conduction, *see* Conduction, intracellular
Irradiation of reflexes, 77, 79, 152–6, 160–6, 168–9, 176–81
   accessibility of motor neurones, 160–3
   effect of intensity of stimulation, 152
   in certain directions and not in all, 156
   in long spinal reflexes, 163
   in spinal shock, 153
   neurone threshold and, 156–8
   Pflüger's law of spread, 165
   role of segmental proximity of afferent and efferent roots, 160
   rules of spread in spinal reflexes, 160–6
   short and long reflexes compared, 158–9
Irreversible conduction, 13, 16, 38–42

Jackson, Hughlings, 271, 289, 303, 304, 314 **35, 75, 78, 189**
James, W., 259 *et seq.*, 381 **114, 124**
   'law of forward conduction', 38 **82**
Jamin, 249
Jaw, innervation of movements of, 290, 291, 295–8
Jendrássik, E., 178 **105**
'Jerk' phenomena, 86, 88, 134, 213, 248, 279, 302, 337
Johnston, J. B., 231
Joseph, M., Gad, J., &, **121**
Jurin, 371

Kalischer, O., 159 **310**
Ketten-reflexe (Loeb), 182, 335
Kicking in reflex defecation, 305
Kiesow, F., 227 **270**
Knee-jerk, 86, 88, 134, 213, 248, 279, 337
'Knock-out' blow, 342
Köster, G., Tschermak, A., &, 100, 114 **230**
Krause, 277, 333
Kronecker, H.
   & Meltzer, S. J., 100, 183, 298 **89, 90, 101**
   & Stirling, W., 44 **55**
Kuhne, W., 38

Labyrinth, relation to cerebellum, 136, 206, 248, 334, 347
   role of, 336–44

Ladd, G. T., 213
Lange, 259, 265 **106a**
Langelaan, J. W., **301a**
Langendorff, O., 92, 345 **74, 74a, 147, 217**
Langley, J. N., 14, 318 **220**
   & Anderson, H. K., 38 **150**
Lans, Zwaardemaker, &, 45 **198**
Laryngeal nerve, superior, 101
Laslett, E. E., 251
Latent period, 13, 18–25, 92
Latzko & Sternberg, M., 255 **267**
Lauder Brunton, *see* Brunton
Law of Bell and Magendie, 38, 80
Law of forward direction of conduction (James), 38
Law of Talbot, 370, 377, 378
Laws of reflex-action, of Pflüger, 163–6
Lee, F. S., 206 **149a**
v. Lenhóssek, 86, 143
Lewandowsky, M., 250, 303 **244a, 312**
Lewis, Mitchell, &, 178 **107**
'Lichthof', 208
Lloyd Morgan, *see* Morgan
Localization in motor cortex, 270–307
'Local sign' in reflexes, 124–9, 248–51
Lockjaw, 295–9
Locomotion, 344, 350
   and receptive range, 334
   in dog, 68, 213
   in *Medusa*, 64
Loeb, J., 182, 206, 335 **196, 219, 254**
Lombard, W., 178, 222 **116, 119**
Lotze, 236
'Lower' and 'higher' as applied to organisms, 236
Luciani, L., 272, 303, 340
Ludwig, C., 161
Lugaro, 23
Lyon, E. P., 206 **216, 270a**

Macallum, A. B., 200 **307**
Macdonald, J. S., 16, 68, 197, 198, 200 **234, 306**
McDougall, W., 202–4, 224, 366, 371, 379, 381, 384 **223, 232, 261a, 262, 297, 301**
MacWilliam, J., **226a**
Magendie, 38, 271 **11**
Magnus, R., 64 **237, 268**

Index

Malapterurus, 38, 67, 77
Man, motor cortex of, 277
Mann, G., 272, 303 **153a**
Marcacci, Bert, P., &, 96
March of spinal and cortical reaction, 289
Marey, E., 44, 45 **67**
Mark time reflex, 211–13
Martin, Newell, & Hartwell, E. M., 173 **79**
Material me', 324
Median line, reflexes of, 322
Median sagittal plane, relation of cortical reactions to, 289, 384
Medusa, 17, 39, 44, 49, 57, 64, 69, 78, 170, 250, 312
Meltzer, S. J., 100, **197**
& Kronecker, H., 100, 298 **89, 90, 101**
Membrane at cell-junctions, 16
Membrane, synaptic, 42
Memory, 229, 331
Mendelssohn, M., **167a, 215**
Merzbacher, L., 71 **210, 228**
Mesencephalo-spinal path, 330
Metamerism, 314, 320, 343, 345
Milieu interne, 4
Mimetic movement, 254–67
Minimum visibile, 186
Mislawski, 206 **221**
Mitchell & Lewis, 178 **107**
v. Monakow, 53, 140, 245, 276, 279 **241**
Monti, 23
Moore, B. & Reynolds, H. W., 14 **193**
Morgan, Lloyd, 238, 265, 268, 331, 387 **165, 216a**
Mosso, A., 182 **66**
Motor area of cerebral cortex, 270–307, 382, 386
Motor neurone, 52, 143, 309
Mott, F. W., 272, 279, 280, 329, 383 **157, 314**
& Schäfer, E. A., 281, 290 **121a**
Müller, J., 375, 381 **20**
Munk, H., 272 **93, 133a**
& Obregia, 281 **128**
Münzer & Wiener, **155, 243**
Muskens, J. T., 206 **269**

Nagel, W., 17, 131, 206, 313 **146**

Nansen, F., 86 **112**
Nerve-net, 39–42, 57, 314
Neuroglia, 14
Neuromuscular cells, 309
Neurone, motor, 52, 143, 309
threshold, 156
Neutrality of reflexes, 148, 290, 305
Newton, I., 375 **5**
Nicotine, 14
Nissl's chromatolysis, 248
Noci-ceptive path, in lateral spinal columns, 255
reflexes, 91, 227–32, 249, 252–5, 322, 330–2
Noci-ceptors; 227–32, 318, 330, 344
Nothnagel, 65, 66, 255 **48**

Obregia, Munk, H., &, 281 **128**
Oddi, 144 **122**
Oesophageal reflex, 183
Oestral period in spinal animal, 265
Oldag, Langendorff &, 92 **147**
Olfacto-phrenic arc, 350
Opening of mouth, 253, 295–8
Ophioglypha, 113
Ophiurus, 240
Optic chiasma, 375, 383
Optic nerve, 70, 333
Orang-utan, motor cortex of, 273
Otocyst, 170, 334, 336, 342
Ott, J., **80, 88**
Oxygen and reflexes, 13, 80

Pain-endings, 227–30, 318
Pain nerves, 227–30, 253
path in spinal cord, 253–5
visceral, 10
Pallio-spinal path, 330
Paneth, 272
Panum, 380
Parallelism of ocular axes, 382
Paralysis, after cortical lesion, 278
Pari, G., 71 **294**
Parker, G. H., 130 **253**
Path, private, 117, 346
'Pattern', reflex, 166–73
Pawlow, J., 295
Perceptual image, 355
Perikarya, 14, 21, 81
Permeability of synaptic membrane, 42

Index

Perspective figures, 172
Pflüger, E., 78, 163-6, 236 **24**
Pflüger's laws, 78, 163-6
Philippson, M., 68, 213, 239 **259, 261, 296, 309**
Photo-receptors, 323, 333, 336, 346
Phrenic neurones, 245
Phrenic reflex, 206
Pigeon, destruction of labyrinth in, 342
Pinna-reflex, 10, 91
Piotrowsky, G., 85, 107 **141**
Plateau, J., **15**
Pluricellular conductor, 39
Plurireceptive summation, 125-9, 309
Plurisegmental discharge, 159
Plurisegmental integration, 314, 343, 345
Polarized conduction, 39
Polimanti, O., **133**
Porter, T. W., **157a**
Post-central convolution, not motor, 273, 277, 280
  thalamic path to, 329
Postural reflexes, 205, 230, 232, 336-44
Postures, segmental and total, 326, 340-3, 344
Poteriodendron, 6, 309, 310
Pouting, indicating displeasure, 255
Pre-central convolution, 271-82
Precurrent reactions, 326, 329-30
'Predominance' of contours, 374
Prepotent reflexes, 225, 228-31, 319
Prevalence of contours, 379
Principle of competition for energy (McDougall), 200-4, 366
Private path, 117, 346
Proprio-ceptive field, 132, 133, 206, 316, 320, 335-44
Proprio-ceptive reflexes, 132-5, 205-6, 304
Proprio-ceptive system, and the head, 335-43
  cerebellum is head ganglion of, 346-8
  includes labyrinth, 336-43
Proprio-ceptors, 130
Proprio-spinal nerve-tracts, 52-6
Pseudaffective reflexes, 252-6
  chloroform and ether cry, 255
  decorticate infant's cry, 255
  detailed description of, 253
  prepotent generally, 229-32
  role of thalamus, 255
  used to determine central pain pathway, 252
Psycho-physical parallelism, 384
Pulmono-phrenic arc, 350
Purkinje, 366
Purpose in reflexes, 236-40, 304
Purring, not elicited in decerebrate animal, 256, 278
Pyramidal tract, 330

Ramon y Cajal, *see* Cajal
Rebound, reflex, 206, 207-13
  due to superactivity following inhibition, 212
  flexion following extensor thrust (as in locomotion), 213
  in alternating reflexes, 213
  not due to repose of centre, 212
Reception, 5, 309-28
Receptive fields, 45, 90, 121-31, 159, 162, 176, 316-19, 322-8
  eliciting bulbo-spinal reflexes, 166
  extero-ceptive, *see* Extero-ceptive field
  intero-ceptive, *see* Intero-ceptive field
Receptive fields, proprio-ceptive, *see* proprio-ceptive field
  of extensor-thrust, 67 *q.v.*
  of flexion-reflex, 90 *q.v.*
  of scratch-reflex, 45 *q.v.*
  not identical with spinal root fields, 176
Receptive range, 333-5
Receptor, 12, 227-32
  a factor in co-ordination, 13
Receptors, classification of, 317
  distance, 324-9, 330, 333-5
  symmetrical, 149, 322
Reciprocal inhibition of reflexes, 83-113
  action of strychnine on, 107-13, *see* Strychnine
  diagram of neural plan, 108
  in deglutition, 100
  in vascular reflexes, 100; reversed by drugs, 114
  McDougall's views on, 202-4
  of after-discharge, 105
  of clonic spasm, 101, 106
  of crossed extensor-reflex, 100, 102, 104, 105

428

Index

Reciprocal inhibition of decerebrate rigidity, 89, 100
of extensor thrust, 90, 105
of flexor-reflex, 99
of ipsilateral vasto-crureus by internal saphenous and hamstring nerve (always), 110; action reversed by strychnine, 111, 204; action reversed by tetanus toxin, 111
of knee-jerk, 86
of respiration (vagus), 100
of tonic (postural) reflexes, 232
specific inhibitory central afferent terminals, 107
Reciprocal innervation, *see* Reciprocal inhibition
and cerebral cortex, 280–99
Reflex, an artificial abstraction, 116
Reflex action, defined, 5
subjection to 'volition', 385–7
Reflex-arc, 7, 46, 51–7, 157, 319
characteristics of conduction in, 13
conduction in reflex and nerve trunk compared, 13
disynaptic, 53
of scratch-reflex, 51–3
role of cell body (perikaryon), 14
role of dendrites, 14
role of neuroglia, 14
role of surfaces of separation, 15–17
role of synapse, 17, *q.v.*
Schaltzellen in, 53
the primitive, 308–11
Reflex attitude, *see* 'Posture'
Reflexes, abdominal, 164
action of anaesthetics on, 80; oxygen-lack on, 80; strychnine on, 71. 81, *q.v.*
adapted reactions, 236–69
adequate stimuli for, 9–13
after-discharge, *q.v.*
alliance of proprio-ceptive and extero-ceptive, 133–5, 206
allied, 121–30; allied inhibitory, 136–7
alternating, 201, 213; rebound in, 213
antagonistic, 137–45
'bahnung' (facilitation), 37, 134, 135
central interaction not algebraical summation, 119
chain, 182
cleansing (*wisch*), 252

common path, 149–51, 234–5; final, 53, 117
common paths, number of, 147–8
compared with neuromuscular transmission, 16
compensatory, 204; of proprioceptor origin, 206
'complication', 8, 131
compound, 152–235
convergence on common path, 149–51
co-ordination in, 8–18
cortical control of, 386; reaction combined with, 305
crawling of earthworm, 183
croak, 9
dart of frog's tongue, 182
deglutition, 183, *q.v.*
delay, 18–25
direct spinal induction, 78, 120–35, 185, 207, 384
double sign, simultaneous and successive, 84
elicited from receptive surface and nerve trunk, 9
enable organism to dominate its environment better, 237
extensor thrust, 9, 67, *q.v.*
facilitation ('bahnung'), 37
fatigue, *q.v.*
final common path, 53, 117; *see* Final common path
focal area of receptive field more effective, 130
incremental, 22–5
indifference, mutual, between reflexes, 148–9, 200–6
induce opposed reflex, 214
induction, *see* Reflexes, Spinal Induction
inertia and momentum in, 34
inhibition, central, 101; *see* Reflexes, Reciprocal Inhibition; peripheral, 84, 85; *see* Inhibition
initial, 24
intensity of, *q.v.*
interaction between, 116–51
interference between, 137–43, 145, 149–51
interference, partial, 145
irradiation, *q.v.*

Index

Reflexes, irreversible conduction, 38
law, of bilateral symmetry of reflex action (Pflüger), 164; of forward conduction, 38; of homonymous conduction of unilateral reflexes (Pflüger), 164; of irradiation (Pflüger), of headward spread, (denied), 165; of unequal intensity of bilateral reflexes (Pflüger), 164 less resistant than nerve trunks, 80
local sign in, 248-52, *q.v.*; in various species of animals, 251
long, 159, 343
mark time, 211-13; followed by rebound, 211; inhibited from tailskin, 211
median line, 232
motor root does not represent reflex figure, 173-6; fibres not functionally co-operative collection, 175
nerve cells, function of, 81
noci-ceptive, 253, *q.v.*
nodal points in reflex arcs, 143-5
nodal points in reflex arc mechanisms of co-ordination, 147
pattern, 8
Pflüger's laws, 163; see Reflexes, law
pinna, 10
prepotence in combined afferent stimulation, 119
prepotent, 183; affective reflexes generally, 229-32; noci-ceptive reflexes generally, 229-31
private path, 118
proprio-ceptive, *q.v.*
pseudaffective, 252-6, *q.v.*
purpose in, 236-41, 304; in pseudaffective reflexes, 252; in various type reflexes, 238; shown by local sign, 250
rebound, *q.v.*
reciprocal inhibition, *q.v.*
reciprocal innervation, 83-113, 235, see Reciprocal inhibition
reflex figure, 8, 166-73; areas (10 predominant) eliciting bulbo-spinal reflexes, 164; motor root does not represent, 173-6
reinforcement, 176-81; form of summation, 178

reversible interaction between reflexes, 142
rhythmic, unaffected by deafferenting operative limb (scratch-, *wisch*reflex), 252
scratch, *q.v.*
sequence, factors determining, 207; fatigue, 207; functional species of reflex, 207; intensity of competing stimuli, 207; spinal induction, 207
sexual clasp of frog, 231
sexual, in spinal dog, 265
shake, 165
shock, spinal, see Spinal shock
short, 159, 343
simple, 7-115
simultaneous combination, 152-80
simultaneous double sign, 84
species of, in reflex sequence, 227-34
spinal induction, 207; immediate, only between allied reflexes, 207; successive, 207; see Reflexes, successive indirect induction
spinal shock, 241-50, *q.v.*
stepping, 201, 214
stimulus rhythm and response, 42-7; compared in reflex and nerve muscle preparation, 42; stimulus rhythm different from response rhythm, 43, see Refractory phase, Stimulus
strychnine and tetanus toxin, 107-13, *q.v.*
successive combination, 182-235
successive double sign, 84
successive indirect induction, 207-14, 384; crossed extensor augmented by precurrent flexion-reflex, 209, 210; form of rebound, 207; from central stimulation of knee extensor nerve, 210; in reflex sequence, 207-14; rebound exaltation following inhibition, 211; reflex induces opposed reflex, 214; resembles visual contrast, 208
summation, 36-8, 91, 93, 119, 121; 'bahnung', facilitation, 37, 185; of subliminal stimuli, 36, 185; pluricellular, 310, 311; relation to reinforcement, 178; temporal, 13
swallowing, *q.v.*

Index

Reflexes, tail, *q.v.*
  threshold lowered by preceding excitation, 185
  tonic (postural), *q.v.*; easily inhibited, 232
  torticollis, 164
  transition from one reflex to another, 188, 191, 192
  type reflex, 129
  variability of response, 233
  vasomotor, 10; in spinal animal, 243, 264
  visceral (from bile duct), 10
  wag of tail, 164
  wider combination of, 135
  wisch (cleansing), 252
Refractory phase in reflexes, 13, 44–65, 137
  affected by internal conditions, 69
  akin to inhibition, 65
  duration varies with reflex, 69
  in crossed stepping reflex, 65
  in extensor thrust, 68
  in *Medusa*, 57–65
  in reflex swallowing, 69
  in scratch reflex, 45, 53, 63
  locus of, 53
  not overcome by increasing stimulus-intensity, 49
Reinforcement, reflex, 176–81
Reissner fibre, 328
Renaut, 23
Resistance, spinal, 156–8
  relation to action of strychnine, 111
Respiratory regulation, 206
Restriction of distribution a factor in integration, 345–6
Retrogradation, 268
Reymond, du Bois, *see* du Bois-Reymond
Reynolds, H. W. & Moore, B., 14 193
Rhizostoma, 39, 41, 57
Rhythmic reflexes, 34, 35, 45–67
Rhythmic response from cortex, 295
Richet, C., 33, 36, 85, 107 **98**
Rigor mortis, onset delayed by deafferentation, 338
  speedy onset when preceding tonus high, 337
Rohault, 375 3

Romanes, J., 17, 41, 44, 170, 171 **72**
Röntgen rays, no receptors for, 316
Rosenthal, J., 195 **27, 28, 30, 167a**
Rotating lantern, 356–61
Rothmann, 280
van Rynberk, **226, 284, 289**

Salomonson, J., **201a**
Sargent, P., **290**
Schäfer, E. A., **43**, 272, 276, 281, 376
  111a, 117a, 121a, 206
Mott, F. W., &, 290
Schaltzelle (v. Monakow), 53, 140, 245
Schlösser, E., **86**
Schopenhauer, 256
Schreiber, J., **104**
Scratch-reflex, 10, 20, 31, 34, 35, 45–65, 71, 74, 79, 91, 103, 120–30, 133, 137–43, 146, 147, 150, 154, 165, 180, 184, 186–94, 201, 214, 215–23, 239, 240, 245–7, 249, 288
Seemann, J., **240**
Segment, nervous integration of the, 319–22
Segmental arrangement of nervous system, 314–15
  of motor cortex, 278
Segmental postures, 341–6
Segmental reflexes, 230, 336–44
  leading, 322–3
Segments, neural integration of series of, 314–15, 343, 345
Selachian, 330
Selective excitability, 13, 227, 316, 317
Self-regulation of respiratory arcs, 100
Semicircular canals, 336
Sensation, projicience of, 324
Sensitivity of viscera, 10, 12
Sensual fusion, 353–85
Sensual 'objects', 356
Sensual percept, 356
Sergi, 260 **152, 177.**
Setschenow, 36, 65 **31, 32, 33, 38**
Sexual reflexes, 231, 265, 325
Shake-reflex, 165, 239
Sherrington, C. S., **136, 138, 139, 151, 153, 157, 170, 171, 173, 182, 183, 194, 205, 213a, 222, 225, 229, 251, 252, 275, 287, 299, 300, 304, 313**
Shock, spinal, *see* Spinal shock

431

Index

Siluroid fishes, 131
Simia satyrus, motor cortex of, 273
Simultaneous combination of reflexes, 150–80
Skeletal muscles, tonus of, see Tonus
Smith-Kästner, 7
Sowton, S. C. M., 80 **313**
Spallanzani, **6a**
Species of reflex, effect on prepotence, 228–32
Spencer, Herbert, 258, 344, 348 **85**
Spinal induction, immediate (or direct), 78, 120–35, 185, 207, 384
successive (or indirect), 207–14, 384
Spinal nerve-root, afferent, 85, 171, 176, 177, 301, 319
co-ordination and the, 173-6
efferent, 173–6, 320
Spinal shock, 241–50, 351
aboral only, 241
blood-pressure fall, not due to, 244
descending paths, role of, 247
diaschizis between *Schaltzellen*, 245
difference on two sides, 250
different reflexes affected differently, 249
fatigue, resemblance to, 245
Goltz's view ('collection of inhibitory phenomena'), 241, 245
in man, 248
isolation dystrophy after, 248
more severe in fore-limbs than in hind-limbs, 242
recovery from, order of, 249
reflex changes in, 241–50
scratch-reflex in, 246, 247
secondary transection, not after, 243
species difference in, 247, 249
synaptic transmission, defective in, 245
trauma, not due to, 242, 244
Spode, O., 81
'Spontaneous' reflex, 109, 208
Stannius, 109
Starling, E. H., Bayliss, W. M., &, 3, 237, 312 **188**
Stefani, 303
Steinach, E., 9, 14 **160, 190**
Stepping-reflex, 66, 211, 212
Sternberg, M., 134, 178 **130, 142**
Latzko, &, 255 **267**

Stewart, C., **224**
Stimulus, adequate, 12, 91, **227**
efficacy of electrical, 12
intensity of, see Intensity
mass as a, 316
nocuous, see Noci-ceptive
'object' as a, 346
prolongation of, 29
threshold value of, 12
Stirling, W., 36, 37 **57**
(with H. Kronecker), **55**
Storey, T. A., **271**
Strychnine, 71, 107–14, 135, 156, 161, 174, 292–9, 302
central action of, 107–13
central inhibition reversed by, 111, 113; attributed to augmenting central excitation (rejected), 112; converting central inhibition into excitation, 112. See Tetanus toxin, Inhibition, Reciprocal inhibition
Sulcus centralis, genua of, 277
Summation, 13, 36–8, 91, 93, 119, 121, 178, 310
Swallowing, see Deglutition
Swinton, A. H., 84
Sympathetic system, 318
Synapse, 15–17, 21, 42, 144–5, 321
setting of the, 22, 25
different resistances at, 157
Synaptic conduction, 13, 143, 157
Synaptic membrane, see Synapse
Synaptic nervous system, 311–14

Tail, 201, 211, 212, 225, 322
Talbot, **14**
Talbot's law, 370, 377, 378
Tamburini, 272
Tango-receptors, 319, 341
Tarchanow, **112b**
Teleology and physiology, 1, 235
Tetanus toxin, 111–14, 292–9, 302
Thorndyke, 307
Threshold, effective, 309
of neurone, 156
selective, 227, 228, 318
variability of, 13, 37
Threshold-stimulus, 12, 309, 310
Tiaropsis indicans, 119, 251

432

Index

Tonic reflexes, 232, 299–304, 337–43, 347–8
   as basis of attitude, 339–43
Tonus-labyrinth, 136, 248, 336–43
Tonus, reflex, of skeletal muscles, 86, 87, 299–304, 337–43
Topolanski, A., 285 **184**
Torpedo, 77
Tortoise, 239, 324
Touch-spots, 316
Traube, J., **22**
Trauma, as a stimulus, 242
Tremor in fatigue, 215
Troglodytes niger, motor cortex of, 274, 275
Tschermak, A., 200, 237, 280, 329, 381 **186, 298a**
   & Köster, G., 100, 114, **230**
Tschiriew, S., **76**
Tunicate, 63

v. Uexküll, J., 113, 204, 237, 307, 313 **188a, 192, 211, 227**
Unity of a motor centre, 78
Uspensky, 144 **42**

Vagi, 196, 197, 264, 288
Valerius, 371, 372 **52**
Vasomotor reflexes, 11, 242–4, 259, 264, 321
Vertebrate, 69, 315
Verworn, M., 2, 13, 80, 101, 144, 197, 309 **181, 207, 208, 245a**
Vibrissae in reflex responses, 164, 253
Viscera, sensitivity of, 10, 12
   reflexes from, 69, 321
Visceral (intero-ceptive) field, 317, 351
Vocalization, reflex, 253, 255
Vogt, 279

Volkmann, 288, 366 **17, 18**
Vorticella, 6, 308, 310

Waller, A. D., 70, 80, 87 **125, 131, 163**
Wallerian degeneration, 17
Walton, 71 **91**
Ward, J., **79a**
Warren, J. W., Bowditch, H. P., &, 178 **123**
Warrington, W. B., 317 **298**
Wasp-larvae, 331
Weber, E. H., 288 **21**
Weber-Fechner rule, 378
Weber's law, 374
Wernicke, 303 **119a**
Westphal, 87 **65**
White rami of sympathetic system, few afferent fibres in, 317
Whytt, R., 241
Wiener, Münzer &, **155, 243**
'Willed' movements, 285, 305, 385–90
   Descartes' views, 286
Winkler, C., **226**
Winslow, 162
Winterstein, 13
Wollaston, 375 **12a**
Woodworth, R. S., 252, 295 **251a, 275**
Wundt, W., 14, 31, 70, 195, 200, 304 **69, 83**

Yeo, G., Ferrier, &, **97**
Yerkes, R. M., 307 **238, 255, 257, 258, 276, 277, 305**

Zanietowski & Cybulski, **145**
Ziehen, Th., 381 **242a**
Zwaardemaker, H., 69, 125, 183 **272**
   & Eyjkman, **235**
   & Lans, 45 **198**

CLASSICS IN PSYCHOLOGY
An Arno Press Collection

Angell, James Rowland. **Psychology: On Introductory Study of the Structure and Function of Human Consciousness.** 4th edition. 1908

Bain, Alexander. **Mental Science.** 1868

Baldwin, James Mark. **Social and Ethical Interpretations in Mental Development.** 2nd edition. 1899

Bechterev, Vladimir Michailovitch. **General Principles of Human Reflexology.** [1932]

Binet, Alfred and Th[éodore] Simon. **The Development of Intelligence in Children.** 1916

Bogardus, Emory S. **Fundamentals of Social Psychology.** 1924

Buytendijk, F. J. J. **The Mind of the Dog.** 1936

Ebbinghaus, Hermann. **Psychology: An Elementary Text-Book.** 1908

Goddard, Henry Herbert. **The Kallikak Family.** 1931

Hobhouse, L[eonard] T. **Mind in Evolution.** 1915

Holt, Edwin B. **The Concept of Consciousness.** 1914

Külpe, Oswald. **Outlines of Psychology.** 1895

Ladd-Franklin, Christine. **Colour and Colour Theories.** 1929

Lectures Delivered at the 20th Anniversary Celebration of Clark University. (Reprinted from *The American Journal of Psychology*, Vol. 21, Nos. 2 and 3). 1910

Lipps, Theodor. **Psychological Studies.** 2nd edition. 1926

Loeb, Jacques. **Comparative Physiology of the Brain and Comparative Psychology.** 1900

Lotze, Hermann. **Outlines of Psychology.** [1885]

McDougall, William. **The Group Mind.** 2nd edition. 1920

Meier, Norman C., editor. **Studies in the Psychology of Art: Volume III.** 1939

Morgan, C. Lloyd. **Habit and Instinct.** 1896

Münsterberg, Hugo. **Psychology and Industrial Efficiency.** 1913

Murchison, Carl, editor. **Psychologies of 1930.** 1930

Piéron, Henri. **Thought and the Brain.** 1927

Pillsbury, W[alter] B[owers]. **Attention.** 1908

[Poffenberger, A. T., editor]. **James McKeen Cattell: Man of Science.** 1947

Preyer, W[illiam] **The Mind of the Child: Parts I and II.** 1890/1889

The Psychology of Skill: Three Studies. 1973

Reymert, Martin L., editor. **Feelings and Emotions: The Wittenberg Symposium.** 1928

Ribot, Th[éodule Armand]. **Essay on the Creative Imagination.** 1906

Roback, A[braham] A[aron]. **The Psychology of Character.** 1927

I. M. Sechenov: Biographical Sketch and Essays. (Reprinted from *Selected Works* by I. Sechenov). 1935

Sherrington, Charles. **The Integrative Action of the Nervous System.** 2nd edition. 1947

Spearman, C[harles]. **The Nature of 'Intelligence' and the Principles of Cognition.** 1923

Thorndike, Edward L. **Education: A First Book.** 1912

Thorndike, Edward L., E. O. Bregman, M. V. Cobb, et al. **The Measurement of Intelligence.** [1927]

Titchener, Edward Bradford. **Lectures on the Elementary Psychology of Feeling and Attention.** 1908

Titchener, Edward Bradford. **Lectures on the Experimental Psychology of the Thought-Processes.** 1909

Washburn, Margaret Floy. **Movement and Mental Imagery.** 1916

Whipple, Guy Montrose. **Manual of Mental and Physical Tests: Parts I and II.** 2nd edition. 1914/1915

Woodworth, Robert Sessions. **Dynamic Psychology.** 1918

Wundt, Wilhelm. **An Introduction to Psychology.** 1912

Yerkes, Robert M. **The Dancing Mouse** and **The Mind of a Gorilla.** 1907/1926